THE BRITISH HOMOEOPATHIC ASSOCIATION

# Family Encyclopedia of Homoeopathic Remedies

Dr Peter Webb, a graduate of Peterhouse, Cambridge, and St Mary's Hospital Medical School, London, was a GP for sixteen years during which time he trained to be a homeopath. He is a member of the Royal College of Physicians and has diplomas in Child Health, Obstetrics and Gynaecology.

D1494003

**Note**

This book is intended as a reference volume only, not a manual for self-treatment.

Every effort has been made to ensure the contents of this book are accurate and current. Medical and pharmaceutical knowledge is constantly changing and the application of it to particular circumstances depends on many factors. Therefore readers are urged always to consult a qualified medical specialist for individual advice. The writer, researchers and publishers of this book cannot be held liable for any errors or omissions, or action that may be taken as a consequence of using it.

THE BRITISH
HOMOEOPATHIC
ASSOCIATION

# Family Encyclopedia of Homoeopathic Remedies

Dr Peter Webb

MA, MB, MRCP, MFHom.

ROBINSON
London

Robinson Publishing Ltd
7 Kensington Church Court
London w8 4SP

First published in the UK by
Robinson Publishing Ltd 1997

A copy of the British Library Cataloguing in
Publication Data is available from the British Library.

ISBN 1-85487-469-1

Printed and bound in the EC

10 9 8 7 6 5 4 3 2

# *Contents*

## Part I: Common Illnesses and Their Remedies

## Disorders of the Muscles and Skeleton 295

*Ankle problems: sprained ankle, fractured ankle, other ankle problems.
Ankylosing spondylitis. Backache: arthritis of the spine, lumbago,
prolapsed intervertebral discs. Bone pain. Cervical spondylitis. Cramps.
Writer's cramp. Dupuytren's contracture. Elbow disorders. Fibrositis.
Fractures. Ganglion. Gout. Hip disorders. Infective arthritis. Knee
problems. Osteoarthritis. Poliomyelitis.* Polymyalgia rheumatica.
*Psoriatic arthritis. Reiter's syndrome. Repetitive strain injury (RSI).
Restless limbs. Rheumatoid arthritis. Shoulder disorders and frozen
shoulder. Tenosynovitis. Tubercular arthritis.*

## Problems of the Nervous System 339

Physical problems: *Bell's palsy, chorea (including Huntington's
chorea), epilepsy, migraine, motor neurone disease, multiple sclerosis,
Parkinson's disease, trigeminal neuralgia.* Mental problems:
*alcoholism, anger, anxiety and phobias, depression, grief,
homesickness, jealousy, mania, manic depression, mischievous
behaviour, quarrelsome behaviour, schizophrenia.*

# Part II: Problems of Newborn Babies, Infants, Children and Adolescents

## Newborn Babies 391

*Birthmarks. Circumcision. Colic. Difficult delivery. Feeding
difficulties. Fever. Gastroenteritis. Nappy rash. Jaundice. Night
crying. Seborrhoeic eczema. Septic spots. Sticky eyes. Umbilical
hernia. Urinary tract infections.*

## Infants 404

*Balanitis. Bedwetting. Bronchiolitis. Constipation. Coughs. Croup.
Dental problems. Dyslexia. Ear infections. Encopresis. Feeding
difficulties. Febrile convulsions. Gastroenteritis. Head banging.
Infectious diseases: chicken pox, diphtheria, measles, meningitis,
mumps, rheumatic fever,* roseola infantum, *rubella, scarlet fever
and scarletina, tetanus, whooping cough. Sleep problems. Still's
disease. Teething. Temper tantrums.*

# Part III: Special Disorders of Adults

Text in SMALL CAPITALS indicates that there is an entry for this condition. If no page number is given, look in the index to find it.

# Acknowledgements

I acknowledge the considerable help and support that my wife, Frances, has given me while I have been writing this book. Without her encouragement in coping with the unknown territory of computers, I would have found the task that much more difficult. I therefore wish to dedicate this book to her.

I would also like to acknowledge and thank:

- Dr Christopher Caldwell-Nichols, a friend who daily helped me find my way out of many mazes to locate missing files.
- Mr Lawrence Jones, for introducing me to the necessary computer soft- and hardware.
- Mrs Enid Segall, General Secretary of the British Homoeopathic Association, who has kept me fully briefed about the writings of Dr Margaret Tyler that were not included in her *Pointers* booklets.
- And finally Mark, Victoria and Tristan, who have all helped me out on many occasions with the intricacies of the computer.

# Preface

Some years ago, Dr Margaret Tyler published a series of booklets entitled *Pointers to the Common Remedies of Certain Common Illnesses*, based on articles she had written for the British Homeopathic Association. This book uses Dr Tyler's work as a backbone, but certain sections have been expanded in order to cover a wider range of illnesses. In recent years, a number of new ailments have become more prominent – for example, myalgic encephalomyelitis (ME); repetitive strain injury (RSI); anorexia nervosa, bulimia, Crohn's disease and multiple sclerosis (MS). These have been included in this book to show how homeopathy can be used as a method of therapy in these cases.

This book is intended to be user-friendly so that readers can treat certain illnesses with homeopathic remedies, and to that end, dosage and potency schedules have been included. **However, it is important to realize that a precise medical diagnosis should be established before using homeopathic remedies and this means getting medical advice as required.** Nevertheless, homeopathy can be used as a truly complementary therapy, working alongside conventional medicine. Indeed, the two therapies used together can have an effect that is greater than when one is used alone. There are, however, always occasions when conventional medical therapy is the preferred choice. Never forget: when in doubt about a diagnosis, consult a medical practitioner.

# What is Homeopathy?

Homeopathy was demonstrated as a method of therapy in 1806 by a German physician called Samuel Hahnemann. He found that, when he took liquefied Peruvian bark (*Cinchona officinalis* [China]), he developed symptoms similar to those of people suffering from an illness then called "marsh fever" and now known as malaria. In a series of experiments, he gave this bark to people with malaria and found that they recovered.

This "like cures like" principle led Hahnemann to coin the word "homeopathy" to describe this form of therapy – *homoeos* being the Greek for "similar" and *pathos* the Greek for "suffering". The "like cures like" principle – also known as the "similar" principle – is the basis of homeopathy. The closer the match between clinical (physical) symptoms and the drug picture (the symptoms that the drug produces in healthy individuals), the better the therapeutic effect.

## How are homeopathic remedies made?

Homeopathic remedies are primarily based on natural substances – common plants and seeds, common metals and their salts, insects and snake venoms, for example. Some – called *nosodes* – are made from diseased tissue. An example is a glandular fever nosode, which is made from tissue from an infected lymph gland. However, as will be shown, none of the tissue actually ends up in the homeopathic remedy, and so there is no danger of catching a disease from it. (*See* p. 95 for more information on Hahnemann's miasm theory, from which nosodes were developed.)

All homeopathic remedies are dissolved – if necessary, after being ground down to a powder – into an alcoholic solution called a "mother tincture". By diluting these tinctures, Samuel Hahnemann was able to get rid of any toxic side-effects. And by experimenting on himself, his friends and his family, he found that, paradoxically, the weaker the solution became, the stronger the homeopathic/therapeutic effect. Hahnemann diluted his remedies until there was only one drop of the active ingredient in every 100 parts of the remedy. He also showed that it was by vigorous shaking, known as *succussion*, that the homeopathic/therapeutic effect was conferred.

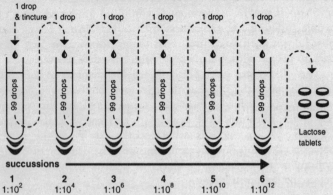

## Preparation of the 6c Potency

1 drop & tincture — 1 drop — 1 drop — 1 drop — 1 drop — 1 drop

99 drops

Lactose tablets

succussions →

| 1 | 2 | 3 | 4 | 5 | 6 |
|---|---|---|---|---|---|
| $1:10^2$ | $1:10^4$ | $1:10^6$ | $1:10^8$ | $1:10^{10}$ | $1:10^{12}$ |

The potency strength recommended in this book is the 6c and 30c range (although occasionally the 200c potency is used, as is the neat mother tincture). This means that the original mother tincture has been diluted by a factor of one part in 100, and this process of dilution is then repeated 6, 30 or 200 separate times (see the above illustration for the preparation of the 6c potency).

The resulting solutions are called *potentized*.

These diluted solutions are sprayed on to lactose or sucrose tablets. (If a person has an intolerance of dairy products, the lactose-based tablets should be avoided and sucrose-based tablets used instead.) The remedies can also be given as a liquid – 2 drops is one dose for older children and adults, and babies and very young children (up to the age of one) take 1 drop. The remedy can also be prepared as a powder (or the tablets themselves can be crushed into powder form) or it can come in granular form (one dose = approximately 10 granules). There is no therapeutic difference between any of these preparations. The preference for the remedy type is purely personal for adults and older children. Practical considerations obviously apply when administering remedies to babies, when the liquid form is the easiest to use.

## How are the remedies taken?

It is important to remember that remedies should be sucked in the mouth and not swallowed. It doesn't matter whether the remedy is placed under or on the tongue. If tablets are taken, they can be nibbled and not just passively sucked. It is ideal but not essential that the remedy is not touched by hand, to avoid contamination with chemicals from soaps and creams. Instead it should be placed in a clean receptacle and then conveyed to the mouth.

It is also preferable that caffeine (found in tea, coffee, chocolate and cola drinks), peppermint and substances containing codeine (sometimes found in pain-killing tablets) are avoided while using homeopathic remedies. This is because these substances interact with the action of the remedies and diminish their therapeutic action. Herbal teas (but not peppermint) and plain water are ideal drinks. Paracetamol and ibuprofen (Nurafen) are suitable pain-killing tablets. A suitable alternative to chocolate is the sweet made from carob beans.

Prednisolone – a common steroid drug used for a wide range of conditions, including arthritis, skin diseases, allergies and eye inflammation – has a major effect in diminishing the therapeutic action of homeopathic remedies, but this should never be discontinued when considering using such therapy. As I have said before, homeopathy can be used in a complementary way with conventional medicine. If you have been prescribed prednisolone by your doctor, the dosage schedule of the homeopathic remedy has to be readjusted. This will mean using the 30c potency instead of the 6c potency and taking this twice a day for a longer period of time. If the recommended potency is 30c, the dosage and the duration of treatment will have to be doubled.

One of the advantages of using homeopathy as a form of treatment for very young children, and particularly babies, is that they don't have to be woken in order for the remedy to be given. The single or double drop can simply be put on to the lips or the exposed tongue.

Before taking a remedy, nothing should be eaten or drunk for a few minutes, and the same applies after the remedy has been taken. It used to be advised that 30 minutes should elapse either side of taking a remedy, but work with animals using homeopathic remedies has shown that there is still a therapeutic effect even if this rule is not strictly followed.

In the lists of remedies given in the following pages, the source of each one has been put in brackets after the name.

It is important to realize that, although some of the plant sources are poisonous – for example, belladonna is obtained from deadly nightshade – the homeopathic method of preparation by extreme dilution means that, theoretically, there are no molecules of the original substance in the final preparation. The remedy, however, still has a therapeutic effect and, of course, is totally safe to take.

## What is a remedy picture?

Each remedy has certain specific effects on various parts of the body. These were initially discovered by Hahnemann by giving mother tincture to himself, his family and his friends, all of whom were healthy at the time. They noted any symptoms that they developed as a result, and a profile was built up for each substance. This is called its *remedy picture*.

## What is an aggravation?

Occasionally a homeopathic remedy may "overstimulate" the body, causing a temporary worsening of symptoms. This is known as an *aggravation*. Although uncommon, it does cause concern. In fact, from a homeopathic point of view, it indicates that the correct remedy has been selected. By immediately stopping the remedy, the aggravation will slowly subside. The aggravation can be stopped more quickly by drinking several cups of strong coffee, which will serve as an antidote to the remedy.

## What is the constitutional remedy?

We are all very different types of people with personal likes and dislikes and differing emotional responses. Homeopathy is the only method of therapy that recognises these differences. Such variations provide "symptoms" from which a specialist homeopath is able to determine a specific remedy, which is known as the *constitutional remedy*.

# PART I

# *Common Illnesses and Their Remedies*

# Upper Respiratory Tract Illnesses

This section includes all problems of the respiratory tract above the voice box (larynx) and includes the common cold, influenza, post viral fatigue syndrome (PVFS), myalgic encephalomyelitis (ME), influenza, sore throats, glandular fever and coughs. For the treatment of CROUP, see the section devoted to problems of young children (p. 407).

## The common cold

The symptoms of the cold – bunged-up nose, runny nose, cough, sore throat, headache – are caused by certain viruses for which there are, as yet, no known conventional treatments. Although a cold is unpleasant, if no treatment is given it will probably resolve on its own after one to two weeks. However, a cold can lead on to other problems such as BRONCHITIS or ASTHMA (if the person has a predisposition to one of these illnesses), as well as a general feeling of heaviness and malaise. The initial treatment advice for a person suffering from a cold is to rest and drink plenty of fluids and take paracetamol to give symptom relief.

However, not only does homeopathy give symptom relief, it also has a curative effect. To treat the common cold from a homeopathic point of view, it is important to determine whether there are any predisposing factors that may have been instrumental in "causing" the common cold. While the general measures of treatment – rest and drinking plenty of fluids – will still apply, when using the homeopathic approach it is generally found that symptoms resolve more quickly than by doing nothing. Should the person need pain relief, paracetamol can be given. It will not interfere with the action of the homeopathic remedy.

Homeopathically, it is possible to identify certain *predisposing factors* that have influenced the development of a common cold and from which a specific remedy can be selected. Examples of suitable specific remedies are described with their remedy pictures below. When choosing a remedy, the clinical (physical) symptoms should be matched with the symptoms shown in the remedy picture, remembering the principle of "like cures like". The selection process applies equally to babies, children and adults.

> It is difficult if not impossible to give tablets to babies and very young children. However, a liquid remedy will do just as well. One drop is a single dose for babies, and two drops is the dose for older children. Follow the dosage schedule given for the 'A, B, C' rule below.

If the predisposing factors for a cold are not clear, the simple "A, B, C rule" applies:

**A** stands for *Aconitum napellus* (monk's-hood). Using the 30c potency, give one dose immediately the symptoms start. This usually stops the cold from progressing. If the symptoms do continue, the remedy can be taken every hour using the 6c potency, for a maximum of six doses. If there is no improvement, go on to:

**B**, which stands for *Belladonna* (deadly nightshade). Using the 30c potency, give one dose immediately, and then continue with the 6c potency, to be given four times a day.
If after two days there is no improvement, go on to:

**C**, which stands for *Calcarea carbonica* (calcium carbonate). Using the 30c potency, give one dose twice a day. Then continue with the 6c potency three times a day until the symptoms begin to resolve. At that stage, discontinue the treatment.

# Predisposing factors for colds, and their remedies

If the possible "cause" – or predisposing factor – of the cold is more certain, the following lists of remedies will help. For each indication, the remedies are listed in the probable order of preference, but check the remedy pictures at the end of this section to accurately match the physical symptoms of the cold with the precise remedy. Using the 30c potency, carry out the following dose schedule:

- Give one dose twice a day for two days.
- Reduce to one dose daily for a maximum of five days.

If there is no sign of improvement after 36 hours of using the first remedy, begin to consider a new remedy by consulting the remedy pictures at the end of this section. Follow the same dosage schedule as for the first remedy.

If the cold has been brought on by cold and dry weather:

- *Aconitum napellus* (monk's-hood)
- *Bryonia* (wild hops)
- *Hepar sulphuris* (Hahnemann's calcium sulphide)
- *Nux vomica* (poison-nut)

If the cold has been brought on by cold and wet weather:

- *Calcarea carbonica* (calcium carbonate)
- *Dulcamara* (bittersweet)
- *Rhus toxicodendron* (poison ivy)

If the cold has been brought on by sitting in a draught:

- *Arsenicum album* (arsenic trioxide)
- *Belladonna* (deadly nightshade)

- *Hepar sulphuris* (Hahnemann's calcium sulphide)
- *Natrum carbonicum* (sodium carbonate)
- *Nux vomica* (poison-nut)
- *Sulphur*
- *Dulcamara* (bittersweet)
- *Mercurius solubis* (ammonium nitrate salt of mercury)

If the nasal discharge is causing redness around the nose:

- *Allium cepa* (red onion)
- *Arsenicum album* (arsenic trioxide)
- *Gelsemium* (yellow jasmine)
- *Kali iodatum* (potassium iodide)
- *Mercurius solubis* (ammonium nitrate salt of mercury)
- *Nux vomica* (poison-nut)
- *Sulphur*

If the nasal discharge is associated with tears causing redness around the eye margin:

- *Euphrasia* (eyebright)

If the nasal discharge is blood-stained:

- *Allium cepa* (red onion)
- *Arsenicum album* (arsenic trioxide)
- *Belladonna* (deadly nightshade)
- *Hepar sulphuris* (Hahnemann's calcium sulphide)
- *Phosphorus*
- *Pulsatilla* (wind flower)

If the nasal discharge contains crusts of gummed-up catarrh:

- *Calcarea carbonica* (calcium carbonate)
- *Kali bichromium* (potassium bichromium)
- *Phosphorus*
- *Tuberculinum* (nucleo-protein from tubercular abscess)

If the nasal discharge is greenish in colour:

- *Kali bichromium* (potassium bichromium)
- *Kali iodatum* (potassium iodide)
- *Mercurius solubis* (ammonium nitrate salt of mercury)
- *Pulsatilla* (wind flower)

If the nasal discharge is smelly:

- *Hepar sulphuris* (Hahnemann's calcium sulphide)
- *Mercurius solubis* (ammonium nitrate salt of mercury)
- *Calcarea carbonica* (calcium carbonate)
- *Kali bichromium* (potassium bichromium)
- *Natrum carbonicum* (sodium carbonate)
- *Pulsatilla* (wind flower)

If the nasal discharge is yellowish in colour:

- *Calcarea carbonica* (calcium carbonate)
- *Hepar sulphuris* (Hahnemann's calcium sulphide)
- *Kali bichromium* (potassium bichromium)
- *Kali iodatum* (potassium iodide)
- *Mercurius solubis* (ammonium nitrate salt of mercury)
- *Phosphorus*
- *Pulsatilla* (wind flower)
- *Tuberculinum* (nucleo-protein from tubercular abscess)

If the nasal discharge is associated with vomiting:

- *Ipecacuanha* (ipecac root)

If the nasal discharge is associated with a lack of thirst:

- *Pulsatilla* (wind flower)
- *Gelsemium* (yellow jasmine)

If the symptoms from the nasal discharge are worse while in a warm room:

- *Pulsatilla* (wind flower)

- *Tuberculinum* (nucleo-protein from tubercular abscess)
- *Allium cepa* (red onion)
- *Mercurius solubis* (ammonium nitrate salt of mercury)
- *Nux vomica* (poison-nut)

If the symptoms of the nasal discharge are made markedly worse on entering a warm room:

- *Bryonia* (wild hops)

If the symptoms are associated with a sore throat:

- *Mercurius solubis* (ammonium nitrate salt of mercury)
- *Nux vomica* (poison-nut)
- *Phosphorus*

# Remedy pictures for the common cold

The remedies listed above now have their "pictures" described in more detail. Physical symptoms can then be more closely linked with the remedy picture, remembering to use the basic homeopathic principle of "like cures like". The dosage schedule is the same as the one at the beginning of the section (and applies to both adults and children).

### *Aconitum napellus* (monk's-hood)

Very sudden onset of symptoms from exposure to cold – in particular, cold, dry winds. The throat is sore, it is red in colour and there is an associated high fever. The voice box (larynx) is sensitive to the touch and very sensitive to inhaled air. Any cough is hoarse, dry, loud and spasmodic. The person is restless, anxious and frightened. The symptoms tend to be worse at night.

### *Allium cepa* (red onion)

The cold is associated with streaming eyes and nose, with or without a headache. The nasal discharge makes the nose and eyes sore. The tears are profuse and colourless. The person is hot and thirsty and worse in the evening. He or she feels worse in a warm room and better in the open air. The voice box is very tender to the touch, and there seems to be a permanent tickle in it. The cough seems to split and tear the voice box, and this symptom is worse when cold air is inhaled.

### *Arsenicum album* (arsenic trioxide)

The nasal discharge is thin and watery, resulting in a sore lip. The nose is continually stuffed up. The sneezing is profuse. Sufferers are excessively cold and cannot get near enough to a fire in order to get warm or wrap up with enough clothes. They are very neat and tidy, and very restless and anxious. They feel better by having their heads elevated and by having plenty of warm drinks. There is a deterioration of symptoms towards the middle of the night.

### *Belladonna* (deadly nightshade)

Sufferers are red, hot but not perspiring. They feel bunged up and have a throbbing headache, and possibly an earache. The throat is sore, very red and shiny. The voice is hoarse, and the voice box is painfully dry. It is as if the voice box is inflamed and swollen with breathing like snoring and a danger of suffocation. The cough is dry, and tears and scrapes at the throat.

### *Bryonia* (wild hops)

Starts as a cold with sneezing, nasal discharge, and tears giving pain in the eyes and the head. All this leads to hoarseness and catarrh going down the back of the throat to the voice box, possibly resulting in a chest infection. The cough is dry and spasmodic and is generally worse at night, after eating or drinking, on entering a warm room or after taking a deep breath. There is little production of sputum. The person is irritable and thirsty for long drinks and wants to lie still and be left alone.

### *Dulcamara* (bittersweet)

This is indicated when the cold results from getting wet or chilled when overheated, or when the weather is cold and wet; this includes the possibility of snow. The symptoms are worse when moving from a hot environment to a cold one, and in the open air. The cold is associated with a stiff neck and sore throat, and the back and limbs feel painful. There is a profuse watery discharge from the nose and eyes.

### *Euphrasia* (eyebright)

The cold is characterised by a colourless nasal discharge and a marked tearful state. The nasal discharge and tears cause much soreness. The nasal catarrh runs backwards down to the voice box, giving a cough that is worse during the day and better at night when lying down. Paradoxically, the nasal symptoms are worse at night when lying down.

### *Gelsemium* (yellow jasmine)

The nasal catarrh is associated with warm, moist and relaxing weather (that is, the reverse of the remedy pictures for *Hepar sulphuris* and *Dulcamara*). The nasal discharge makes the nostrils very sore and painful, as if hot water is being poured through them, and the symptoms are better when the person is near a heat source. The body is heavy and tired, giving a frontal headache. The person is not at all thirsty.

### *Hepar sulphuris* (Hahnemann's calcium sulphide)

The nasal discharge is associated with much sneezing. It is initially watery and then becomes thick, yellow and smelly. Sufferers are hypersensitive to touch, pain, draughts and/or cold, and they feel better in mild, wet weather. Should the symptoms go on to the chest, stop the remedy and switch to *Phosphorus*.

### *Ipecacuanha* (ipecac root)

The cold is associated with nausea and/or vomiting.

### *Kali bichromium* (potassium bichromium)

The nasal catarrh is thick, yellow or greenish, ropey, stringy or jelly-like. The nose becomes red and swollen from the acrid watery nasal discharge, which is offensive and can be drawn out of the nostrils in long strings. There is a pressure pain in the root of the nose.

### *Kali iodatum* (potassium iodide)

The cold results from exposure to damp weather. The nose is red, and swollen from the acrid nasal discharge. The eyes smart and easily develop tears. The person develops a frontal headache from the catarrhal inflammation of the frontal sinuses. The inflammation can also extend to the eyes, throat and chest. The tongue is white and there is a profuse thirst. The person alternates between feeling hot and dry and being drenched with sweat. The heat is associated with shivering.

### *Mercurius solubis* (ammonium nitrate salt of mercury)

The nasal discharge is offensive and makes the nose sore. The throat is particularly sore. The tongue is furred, with teeth marks around the edges. There is periodic sweating, and when this occurs, the symptoms deteriorate. The breath smells offensive.

### *Natrum carbonicum* (sodium carbonate)

There is a constantly runny nose that is provoked by the slightest draught. Symptoms deteriorate every other day, and they are entirely relieved by sweating (the reverse remedy picture of *Mercurius solubis*).

### *Natrum muriaticum* (sodium chloride)

The overall characteristics of this remedy are that sufferers have a craving for salt, and hate any form of fuss. They tend to bear grudges easily and can be difficult to live with. There is an associated cough with a bursting headache. Urine can spurt out involuntarily during a bout of coughing, particularly in older people.

### *Nux vomica* (poison-nut)

The overall characteristics of this remedy are that sufferers are irritable (compare this with *Aconite* where they are anxious). At the start of the cold, the nose is stuffed up and dry, the throat is rough (as if scraped) and there is a lot of sneezing. The whole body feels cold, and sufferers don't warm up in front of a fire or by putting on any amount of clothing. They feel even colder when moving in bed. The person shivers after drinking and when in contact with the open air.

## Remedies for the final stages of a cold

The selected remedy – here given with its remedy picture – should be given as one 30c dose daily until the symptoms have finally cleared up.

### *Calcarea carbonica* (calcium carbonate)

The person who matches this remedy has much sweating of the scalp, and feels very cold.

### *Sulphur*

Sufferers get overheated and sweat easily. They feel comfortable at night with their feet sticking out of the bed to cool them down. They tend to be untidy and argumentative. They have a preference for fatty food, and get particularly hungry at 11.00 am.

*Tuberculinum* (nucleo-protein from tubercular abscess)

Particularly suited for persons with a family history of tuberculosis. They are always catching colds and always feel tired. They feel worse in a warm room and have a fear of dogs.

## Prevention of the common cold

There is no known treatment for preventing the common cold, but some people have found that by taking a high dose (at least 1 gram) of vitamin C a day, plus one daily garlic capsule, and by avoiding undue stress, getting enough sleep and eating a proper diet, they manage to avoid catching colds.

# *Influenza*

True influenza is characterized by a high fever, muscle ache – particularly eye ache – and prostration, caused by specific viruses.

The conventional treatment is bed rest, having plenty of fluids to drink and fever reduction by taking paracetamol or similar.

There are eight homeopathic remedies that can be used in a complementary way with the above advice. Pick the one whose "picture" suits the physical symptoms the closest, and treat with one dose of 30c potency twice a day for three days. Then reduce the potency strength to 6c and take the remedy every six hours for a maximum of twenty doses.

The following remedies are listed in the probable order of importance.

*Aconitum napellus* (monk's-hood)

Characterized by sudden onset of fever, with chilliness, the body throbbing with the pulse, and great restlessness from anxiety. A remedy that is associated with the onset of symptoms during cold, dry weather with a bitterly cold wind (the reverse of the picture for *Gelsemium*).

### Gelsemium (yellow jasmine)

Characterized by generalized heaviness. The head, eyelids and limbs feel heavy. Occurs in mild weather (the reverse of *Aconitum*). There is a bursting headache, starting from the neck and extending over the scalp to the forehead and eyes; this headache is relieved by urinating. The person does not feel at all thirsty.

### Eupatorium perfoliatum (thoroughwort)

The main characteristic of this remedy is intense pain in the limb bones and back as if the bones are broken, as a result of which, the person dares not move for fear of pain (the reverse of *Pyrogen*). There is a bursting headache, as well as shivering associated with chills in the back (like *Gelsemium* and *Pyrogen*). The eyeballs feel sore (like *Bryonia* and *Gelsemium*). There may be vomiting of bile. Like "break-bone fever".

### Pyrogen (artificial sepsin)

This is indicated for a fever associated with violent pulsations of the heart and blood vessels and intense restlessness. The pulse can become very rapid: the ratio between the pulse and the temperature is distorted, so that when the temperature is high, the pulse is low, and vice versa. Sufferers feel very cold so that no fire can warm them up (like *Nux vomica* and *Gelsemium*). They feel a creeping chilliness in the back, with a thumping heart. They also have a bursting headache and experience intense restlessness. They find that the bed feels hard and that their body feels beaten up and bruised (like *Arnica*). They feel better when beginning to move (the reverse of *Rhus toxicodendron*), and have to keep moving, rocking and wriggling to obtain momentary relief. They urinate large volumes of urine.

### Baptisia (wild indigo)

Sufferers develop symptoms very quickly, and sink into a stupor at an early stage. They have a dull, red face and appear drugged.

They easily fall asleep while answering a question. This remedy is particularly useful in "gastric flu" (*see* ENTEROCOLITIS, p. 165) where there is a sudden onset of violent diarrhoea and vomiting associated with great prostration. It is also useful in helping the recovery of those with viral pneumonia. In the worst cases, the mouth and throat are foul and the discharges are very offensive (like *Mercurius*). A significant symptom from a homeopathic point of view (and known by homeopaths as a "curious symptom") is that there is a disturbance of body image: sufferers feel as though their limbs are scattered over the bed and cannot be reassembled (a symptom shared with *Petroleum* and *Pyrogenium*).

## *Bryonia* (wild hops)

This remedy suits sufferers whose tongues are white, and who have a great thirst for cold fluids, a preference shared with *Phosphorus*. They find that their symptoms deteriorate after any movement or noise and when they are exposed to a source of dry heat (the reverse of *Nux vomica* and *Gelsemium*). Sufferers wish to lie quite still and be left alone. There may be headache that is made worse on movement and relieved by firm pressure. A cough may develop that can make any pains in the head worse and can lead to PLEURISY or pleuro-PNEUMONIA. Sufferers commonly have dreams of business anxieties. If they go on to develop delirium, there will be a feeling of "wanting to go home". They feel generally irritable.

## *Rhus toxicodendron* (poison ivy)

Sufferers exhibit the typical picture of *Rhus toxicodendron*: stiffness on first moving (the reverse of *Pyrogenium*) that eases off with motion, until the person becomes weak and tired, forcing rest; then the stiffness returns, causing restlessness and a feeling of uneasiness that drives the person to move again. The worst suffering occurs when the person is at rest and motionless (the reverse of *Bryonia*). The symptoms result from cold, damp weather or after the person becomes cold and damp when perspiring (as for *Dulcamara*). Sufferers become anxious and fearful, particularly at night (like *Aconitum*). They therefore show great restlessness, intense fever, thirst and severe aching in their bones (like *Eupatorium*). They also have an unusual mental symptom: a fear of poison.

### *Mercurius solubis* (ammonium nitrate salt of mercury)

The person has a very profuse and offensive-smelling sweat. The throat and mouth generally feel rough and foul (like *Baptisia*). The person salivates profusely, and the saliva also smells offensive. Sufferers get worse, or obtain no relief, from sweating. Their symptoms commonly extend on to the chest.

## Treating immediate post-influenza weakness

Following an attack of influenza, it is common for a person to feel quite weak. To deal with this, it is important to establish antioxidant therapy (*see* POST-VIRAL FATIGUE SYNDROME, p. 24).

In addition to these supplements, there are several homeopathic remedies to consider. The first remedy is *Influenzinum* (a nosode prepared from an influenza virus): give a 30c dose every 12 hours, to a maximum of three doses. If, after a period of one month, there is still no improvement, one of the following remedies should be considered, giving a 30c dose twice a day for one week. The selection of the remedy is decided on the clinical/remedy picture match.

### *Gelsemium* (yellow jasmine)

Sufferers have a marginally elevated fever of about 37.2°C (99°F). They feel chilly, with periodic heats and chills. They have a general weakness and heaviness of their limbs and eyelids. They commonly describe walking as if they are wading through heavy mud.

### Cinchona officinalis (China) (Peruvian bark)

The principal indication of this remedy is weakness following loss of body fluids – in the case of influenza, this is loss through sweat. Sufferers feel chilly, and are sensitive to the cold, to motion and to being touched. They feel worse on alternate days. They also experience a weariness of their limbs, with a beneficial desire to stretch, move or change position.

### Kali phosphoricum (potassium phosphate)

Sufferers are generally weak, with an overall feeling of gloom – that is, a combination of physical and mental depression. They find the least effort a hard task and are very nervous, but they feel better for warmth, rest and good nutrition.

### Arsenicum album (arsenic trioxide)

Sufferers feel extremely anxious and are very restless and full of fear, particularly of dying (this symptom is shared with Aconitum). They feel very cold, so much so that, when they burn up with fever, they feel relieved by the heat. Characteristically they are oversensitive and fastidious. There is a frequent desire for sips of cold water. There are several peculiar (and therefore significant) symptoms: a sensation of pains like red-hot needles going through the body, and a sensation of ice water running through the veins alternating with a sensation of boiling water going through the blood vessels.

### Pulsatilla (wind flower)

Sufferers find external warmth intolerable, and they yearn for fresh air. They feel as if hot water has been thrown over the body, and they feel better when moving slowly (the reverse of Bryonia and Eupatorium). There is a lack of thirst. Sufferers also feel tearful and respond well to a cuddle. Any sweating is worse in the morning. Any cough is dry and occurs at night, and it improves on sitting up, but returns on lying down.

*Sulphur*

Characteristically, sufferers have hot feet at night, and must put them out of the bed clothes to cool them down. They feel worse when washing or taking a bath. They can be contrary, and show an explosive temper that quickly subsides and all is forgotten. They experience frequent hot flashes of heat and are sensitive to the open air and to draughts (the reverse of *Pulsatilla*). They feel hungry, particularly at 11.00 am. They are drowsy by day and restless at night. This restlessness results from a tendency to have frightful dreams.

## Prevention of influenza

An influenza-prevention programme is available from homeopaths. It is advisable for older people and individuals with a chronic illness to be immunized in this way. The remedy is prepared in the traditional homeopathic way, using influenza viruses that have caused previous epidemics. One dose is taken every 12 hours, for three doses.

## *Post-viral fatigue syndrome (PVFS)*

Sometimes the fatigue that occurs with a viral illness continues for several weeks and sometimes months. When this happens, the diagnosis becomes more difficult. A full haematological (blood) work-up is indicated. In many cases, this is normal, and a diagnosis of post-viral fatigue syndrome (PVFS) can be made. The prognosis for this illness is generally good, leading to a full recovery.

The cause of this fatigue is linked to the production of "free radicals" by the body, which results in the formation of rogue oxygen molecules. These get caught up in the body's metabolic pathways, resulting in an inefficient energy supply, thereby causing muscular weakness and general fatigue. The body has natural enzymes to break down these rogue oxygen molecules, and the production of these enzymes can be encouraged by *anti-oxidant therapy* – that is, supplementing the diet with selenium, vitamins C and E, raw carrots (preferably organic), magnesium and zinc – as well as by probiotic therapy (*see* MYALGIC ENCE-PHALOMYELITIS, below). It is also important to take adequate rest during the day and to pace daily activities carefully. People with PVFS have a tendency to overdo things as they recover, to catch up on lost time, but this can lead to a delay in recovery, which causes a lowering of morale.

There are two homeopathic remedies that help stimulate the body to recover. The dose for each is 30c twice a day for five days, reducing to one dose a day for five days, then one dose on alternate days for five days, and finally one dose twice a week until there is an adequate recovery. Look at the clinical pictures of the two remedies shown below, and select the picture that most closely fits the affected person.

### Kali phosphoricum (potassium phosphate)

Sufferers feel a combination of physical weariness and mental depression. They improve minimally by warmth and with good nutritional support.

### Picric acidum (picric acid)

The person has a lack of will power, and shows muscular debility with a heavy, tired feeling, as well as a disinclination to do any mental work.

## Myalgic encephalomyelitis (ME)

This illness was first described in the 1950s as the "Royal Free disease" because of a large outbreak of it among staff at the Royal Free Hospital in London. Ever since, it has caused a lot of controversy within the medical profession as to whether it actually exists or not. It is the author's opinion that it does, and this seems to be supported by a recent survey into all the studies that have been done on ME. One of the conclusions of that survey was that the name for this condition should be changed to "chronic fatigue syndrome (CFS)", but because it is so well known by its present name, the term *myalgic encephalomyelitis (ME)* will be used here.

ME is caused by a number of factors acting together, and it is therefore better classified as a syndrome rather than a disease. The most common feature is for it to be preceded by a viral infection. Indeed, it can be seen as a variation of post-viral fatigue syndrome.

Candidiasis is also considered to be a precipitating factor. Sufferers have repeated infections of the yeast *Candida albicans*, which clings on to the wall of the gastrointestinal tract, releasing its toxins into the bloodstream. Apart from the following diet schedule, the only treatment for this condition is oral nystatin powder, probiotic therapy and colonic irrigation. See box on p. 27 for further details of this diet and treatment.

Some have labelled people with ME as being depressed, hysterical or most certainly neurotic. The characteristic symptoms of ME are great fatigue, muscle pains and vasomotor disturbances (for example, palpitations), and also mental symptoms that include a temporary loss of memory and the wrong selection of words, both when writing and when speaking. All of these symptoms show considerable variability, from hour to hour and day to day. Each of them also varies in intensity within each individual afflicted with ME, so it is impossible to spell out a precise symptom profile for any given person. Instead, all that can be suggested is an overall picture of symptoms consistent with a diagnosis of ME.

The physical examination of a person with ME is unremarkable and produces no diagnostic clues. An electrocardiogram (ECG) is mandatory, especially for those with palpitations as a symptom. Again this investigation gives no diagnostic pointers. Abnormalities in the sweat biochemistry show interesting but non-diagnostic features: low levels of zinc and magnesium are common in this particular analysis. The only abnormalities commonly found in blood tests are a low pyridoxine (vitamin $B_6$) level and a low-to-normal level of thyroxine, the hormone secreted by the thyroid gland (but with a normal level of thyroid-stimulating hormone). The estimations of zinc and magnesium in the blood are not as informative as with the sweat test.

The treatment of a person who is suffering from ME begins with the taking of a detailed medical history to check on any predisposing factors. If the person has had INFLUENZA, 30c *Influenzinum* should be given, one dose every 12 hours, up to a maximum of three doses. If there has been GLANDULAR FEVER, a 30c glandular fever nosode should be taken, one dose every 12 hours, up to a maximum of three doses. If candida is prominent in the history, a special schedule of treatment is indicated, which is described below.

Recently, a blood test has been developed that identifies a group-specific antigen for enteroviruses. Initially, this was thought to be a specific test for ME, as well as for those with a strong history of *Candida* infection, but this has been shown not to be the case. Many patients with classic ME or with a strong history of *Candida* infections do not give a positive result.

---

## Treatment for candidiasis

For those who have had recurrent bouts of *Candida* infection, diet is an important part of therapy. The following should be avoided: all refined sugar, alcohol, refined flour (whole-grain flour products can be used instead), caffeine and artificial flavourings and preservatives.

As part of this strategy, dietary supplements of probiotic granules or tablets are important. *Probiotics* are naturally occurring, beneficial bacteria. These include lactic acid bacteria such as *acidophilus* and effective *bifidobacterium*. They are grown under laboratory conditions, harvested and reconstituted into granules or tablets. These supplements enhance the levels of micro-nutrients that the body needs by restoring the microflora in the bowel so that the nutrients can be more easily absorbed.

After the person has been on the above diet for two weeks, anti-candida drug therapy can be introduced. Nystatin powder is used, which must be obtained from a specialist homeopath supplier (*see* p. 553). It doesn't taste very nice, and the build-up to 5 millilitres twice a day must

---

be made gradually. Occasionally people taking nystatin become inexplicably depressed and fearful. This may be due to the unmasking of a yeast allergy as the yeast load in the gut is reduced. If this happens, the existing dose of the nystatin powder should be doubled. Because of nystatin's unpleasant taste, another anti-*candida* food supplement called caprylic acid, which comes in tablet form, can be used instead. Caprylic acid is derived from coconuts.

For all cases of ME, cognitive psychotherapy is helpful, as this gives a deeper understanding of oneself and the interaction between the body and the mind. As with *Candida*-related ME, diet is important. Most people find it helpful to avoid caffeine, found in coffee, chocolate and cola drinks, and to reduce their consumption of alcohol. Probiotic supplements (*see above*) help boost the immune system and thereby aid recovery. Hypoallergenic multi-mineral and multi-vitamin supplements (to include, particularly, magnesium, zinc, vitamin C and vitamin E – the basis of anti-oxidant therapy) are essential, together with supplements of gamma linoleic acid in the form of evening primrose oil.

As with PVFS, it is important to rest a great deal and ensure that, initially at least, activity is kept to a minimum. People with ME have a tendency to overdo things as improvement occurs, only to relapse and become disheartened. The illness may take many months to disappear. The diet can be relaxed as the person recovers. Individuals must discover which foods suit them best and avoid those that cause symptoms.

The homeopathic remedies mentioned in the section on post-viral fatigue syndrome are also useful in treating myalgic encephalomyelitis – that is, *Picric acidum* and *Kali phosphoricum*. These work in a complementary way with the diet, dietary supplements including probiotic therapy, and psychotherapy.

## Sore throats and tonsillitis

The throat consists of the tongue, hard palate, soft palate (with a small, fleshy protruberance hanging from it, called the uvula), and a tonsillar pad on either side of the soft palate, extending into the pharynx and on to the larynx (voice box). When a person complains of a sore throat, any of these specific areas can be involved. In children particularly, the tonsils are easily and quickly attacked by a virus or bacteria. When this happens, the lymph glands under the jaw become enlarged and tender. For more information on the illness in children, see the section on tonsillitis on p. 453.

The conventional treatment for proven bacterial infections is antibiotic therapy. The conventional treatment for non-bacterial sore throats is paracetamol. It used to be common practice to remove the tonsils and adenoids surgically from young infants to prevent recurring attacks of tonsillitis. However, it is now known that this is not necessary – in fact, the tonsils are an important feature of the immune system.

There are many homeopathic remedies to help in the treatment of both viral and bacterial sore throats, and the following section will describe them and the indications for their use. The dose schedule is: one 30c dose to be given every eight hours for two days, reducing to one 30c dose every 12 hours until the sore throat improves, at which point the remedy may be discontinued. It is important to make sure that the person has adequate rest and eats a proper diet while ill and subsequently when convalescing.

To prevent recurrent attacks of tonsillitis, a specialist homeopath should be consulted to work out the constitutional remedy.

# The common homeopathic remedies for a sore throat and tonsillitis

### Aconitum napellus (monk's-hood)

The person suddenly develops inflammation of the entire visible throat. The uvula feels long and touches the tongue. The throat tingles and burns and, on examination, looks very red. Sufferers feel anxious most of the time, and have a high fever and difficulty in swallowing because the throat feels dry. They also have a great thirst for cold water. All the symptoms are worse at night.

29

### *Belladonna* (deadly nightshade)

The illness develops and progresses rapidly. Sufferers have a bright red face, with widely dilated pupils and a bounding heart. The tongue is bright red, so much so that it is called a "strawberry" tongue; it is also dry and feels as if it is burning. Sufferers have a dislike of fluids (in contradiction to *Aconitum*). Whenever they attempt to swallow liquids or food, spasm develops and the food and/or liquid is ejected through the nose and mouth. Throat feels as if it has a foreign body in it.

### *Nitric acidum* (nitric acid)

Sufferers feel as if there is a fishbone stuck in the throat – swallowing even a small amount of liquid causes severe throat pain, extending to both ears. They feel cold and anxious, and easily become depressed. In health, they enjoy salty and fatty food.

### *Phytolacca* (pokeroot)

The person not only has a sore throat but also, when swallowing saliva or turning the head to the left, a feeling as if a lump is present in the throat. Some people describe this as like a ball of red-hot iron has lodged itself in the throat. The pain, particularly on swallowing, is "referred" to both ears.

### *Kali carbonicum* (potassium carbonate)

Sufferers always seem to be catching a cold that settles on to the throat. There is an associated hoarseness and even possibly voice loss. At the beginning, sufferers feel a non-specific lump in the throat that becomes a "fishbone" sensation as soon as they become cold and as their cold progresses. They feel especially weak.

### *Hepar sulphuris* (Hahnemann's calcium sulphide)

This remedy is of particular use in the later stages of a sore throat. The throat has a sensation of a "fishbone" or "crumb" in it, and the larynx (voice box) is painful and sensitive to the touch and also when food passes behind it. The person can get easily angered and abusive. An unusual symptom is that both the pain in the larynx and the cough worsen when a hand is placed outside the bed clothes. Any exposure to a cold, dry wind will make all the symptoms worse.

### Ignatia (St Ignatius' bean)

The person feels as though there is a plug in the throat, a sensation that becomes worse when swallowing. The tonsils are studded with ulcers, giving a feeling of constriction and of a feather being present in the larynx. This produces a tickly cough that is made worse by coughing.

### Sepia (inky juice of cuttlefish)

This remedy produces left-sided symptoms and signs, so that it is the left tonsil that is inflamed although it is not particularly red. There is a sensation of a lump in the throat, and this can present as a symptom at night by waking sufferers who feel as though they have swallowed something in their sleep. Sufferers that this remedy suits are chilly and indifferent to the people around them and prefer their own space.

# Less common remedies with differing symptom presentation

### Cinnabaris (mercuric sulphide)

The person has a red, sore throat but also has the unusual symptom of pressure on the nose, as if there were a very heavy pair of spectacles pressing on it.

### Capsicum annuum (cayenne pepper)

Sufferers' throats feel constricted and spasmodically closed. Those whom this remedy suits are probably fat and flabby, look red but feel cold, and are worse when uncovered. This is the sore throat of "smokers and drinkers".

### *Lycopodium* (club moss)

This remedy causes a sore throat that mainly affects the right side. There is also a specific deterioration of symptoms between 4.00 and 8.00 pm. The symptoms are generally improved by the swallowing of warm fluids.

### *Lachesis* (bushmaster snake venom)

This remedy causes a sore throat that mainly affects the left side. The symptoms are better after swallowing solid food rather than liquids. They are worse on awakening.

### *Pyrogenium* (artificial sepsin)

With this remedy, the main characteristic is the sensation of the mouth being full of pus. The breath also smells foul. The pulse rate is much higher than would be expected from the temperature.

## Extreme pustular tonsillitis

### *Mercurius solubis* (ammonium nitrate salt of mercury)

This remedy suits the person with the classic form of tonsillitis: a high fever, red throat and pus on the tonsils. The glands under the jaw are swollen and tender. The tongue is furred and has teeth marks on it.

# *Glandular fever (infectious mononucleosis)*

This illness can initially present as a sore throat. There is occasionally a fine rash on the trunk of the body. When pressed gently, the lymph glands in the neck can be felt, and so, often, can the spleen. The person feels extremely fatigued. The diagnosis is established by a blood test and a throat swab to exclude a streptococcal infection. Bed rest is advised, as is the avoidance of contact sports until the spleen is no longer enlarged.

The homeopathic treatment includes the above general advice for sore throats, together with the following remedies.

*Ailanthus glandulosa* (Chinese sumach) is the first remedy of choice for the sore throat of glandular fever. The throat is red and swollen, and the neck is swollen because of glandular enlargement. The remedy picture also describes a fine skin rash, a husky voice and general drowsiness with a frontal headache. Using the 30c potency, give one dose twice a day for two days, followed by one dose of 6c potency three times a day for five days.

During convalescence, the fatigue continues in some people despite improvements in the sore throat and glandular enlargement. In these cases, the remedy to use is *Glandular fever nosode* 30c, one dose to be taken every 12 hours for a maximum of three doses. In addition, the diet should include the antioxidant supplements (*see* MYALGIC ENCEPHALOMYELITIS).

If it is important that catching glandular fever be prevented – for example, if a person has been in contact (kissing is said to be required!) with someone who has or has recently had glandular fever, then giving *Glandular fever nosode* 30c, one dose every 12 hours up to a maximum of three doses, will act as a preventive measure.

# Coughs

A cough is caused by an irritation of the larynx (voice box) or trachea (windpipe). Coughs can be either "wet" or "dry" – that is, they do or do not produce sputum – and may or may not be spasmodic. The modern definition of ASTHMA (*see* p. 94) is a continuing cough, and not necessarily one associated with wheezing. For information on asthma in children, see p. 441.

Smoking is a common irritant to the trachea, by either active or passive smoking. Because the smoke destroys the cilia, the hair-like structures lining the trachea, mucus can drip down it to the lungs, where it can cause an infection. When smoking is stopped, the cilia regrow, a process that takes about two weeks. This is an important fact, not only for the active smoker but also for passive smokers, many of whom are members of a smoker's family; it explains why the cough of a smoker (or of a passive smoker) worsens immediately after the smoking is stopped. As the cilia regrow, they begin to prevent the mucus from reaching the lungs, allowing the lungs to clear.

The remedies that follow are divided into three sections: those for a dry cough, those for a wet cough and those for a spasmodic cough, along with their remedy pictures. The remedies should be taken at a 30c potency, one dose every eight hours for two days, then one every 12 hours for one day, and finally one dose a day for five days.

From the remedy pictures, it will be seen that certain environmental situations are beneficial to certain individuals and their coughs. It is obvious that these conditions should be met to provide the most favourable conditions for recovery. As well as these environment factors, smoking must be avoided by both active and passive smokers.

# Dry coughs

### *Aconitum napellus* (monk's-hood)

The cough comes on suddenly after exposure to cold, dry winds. It is a constant, short, dry cough producing a feeling of suffocation that can lead to CROUP. Sufferers feel anxious and fearful, and are restless and worsen at night. They feel better when lying on their back.

### *Belladonna* (deadly nightshade)

The source of this dry cough is from a dry and painful larynx (voice-box); the person often clutches their larynx before coughing as though there was a speck of something on it. The cough comes

34

in spasms, the person gets red in the face, and there may well be an inspiratory whoop (this remedy is useful for whooping cough).

### *Bryonia* (wild hops)

The dry, hacking cough stems from a tickle in the throat. The symptoms are improved by keeping still and by pressure on the sternum (breast bone). They are made worse by movement, deep breathing and by lying in bed – the person has to sit up.

### *Nux vomica* (poison-nut)

The dry cough makes the person's chest very sore. The cough is spasmodic and may cause retching, a severe headache as though the skull will burst, and a bruised feeling in the abdomen as if it had been lacerated. The person is hypersensitive, both mentally and physically, and is easily offended.

### *Tuberculinum* (nucleo-protein from tubercular abscess)

The person experiences a hard, dry cough. Night sweats are common. The person feels suffocated in a warm room and craves fresh air (like *Pulsatilla*) and particularly cold winds. This remedy is particularly useful in clearing up coughs in those who have a family history of tuberculosis.

## Wet coughs

### *Calcarea carbonica* (calcium carbonate)

The person has a tickling cough that produces sputum that contains pus and is sour in taste and offensive in smell. The person sweats from the head and neck and has cold, damp feet.

### *Pulsatilla* (wind flower)

The cough produces much yellow-green sputum, which is worse

in the evening and, notably, when the person lies down at any time of the day. It is also made worse by heat of any form, and the person feels better with fresh air coming into the room from an open window. The cough has a tendency to become spasmodic in the evening, when sputum production diminishes. Sharp pains are sometimes felt in the chest, particularly on the left side. The person is not at all thirsty, and has to be encouraged to drink.

### *Hepar sulphuris* (Hahnemann's calcium sulphide)

The dry cough is made worse when the person is exposed to cold, dry weather, and improves in warm, moist conditions. Cold in any form causes a deterioration in the symptom picture – for example, when any part of the body becomes exposed, such as by putting an arm out of bed. The cough can deteriorate into a suffocating coughing attack. This is CROUP (*see* p. 407).

### *Causticum* (Hahnemann's mixture of quicklime (calcium oxide) and potassium bisulphate)

The cough is raw, giving a sore feeling through the chest, and seems to come from the back of the throat. The larynx (voice box) is hoarse and at its worst in the morning. The symptoms are made worse in dry, cold winds when there is a possible frost on the ground. They are also made worse when the person lies down, sings or talks. They are improved by drinking cold water. There is a small amount of a thick mucus that is difficult to cough up; when it is finally produced into the throat, it slips back and is swallowed. There is commonly a leakage of urine during bouts of coughing (like *Rumex crispus*), particularly in older people.

### *Phosphorus*

The cough is dry, tickling: an irritation in the larynx extending to below the sternum. At times, it can be violent, causing such pain in the chest that sufferers are obliged to hold their chest wall. This compression feels as if a great weight is on the chest. When there is severe coughing, sufferers may experience involuntary anal leakage. They feel cold, have a thirst for cold drinks, like salt, and become sensitive and nervous in the dark. There is a particular fear of thunder. In the later stages of a *Phosphorus* cough, there is sputum production that is worse in the morning and the sputum may become yellow-green in colour and finally blood-stained.

# Spasmodic coughs

### *Drosera* (sundew)

The person feels a crawling sensation in the larynx, which provokes coughing. This cough is violently spasmodic, causing retching with vomiting. One coughing bout follows another in rapid succession so that sufferers find it very difficult to catch their breath. The cough is worse at night, because this symptom is made worse by lying down. This is the classic cough of WHOOPING COUGH (p. 429).

### *Rumex crispus* (yellow dock)

Sufferers notice that the cough changes when they move from room to room and particularly when they breathe cold air (like *Phosphorus*) – that is, the cough is provoked by changing from a warm environment to a cooler one. It is common for urine leakage to occur during a bout of spasmodic coughing (like *Causticum*). The cough is worse at night, when sufferers are lying down (like *Drosera*). It is dry to start with but finally produces much tough mucus in the larynx, with a constant desire to spit it out. However, the sputum is so sticky that it is impossible to get out, so sufferers swallow it instead. This gives temporary relief, but the cycle of sputum production then returns, with the constant desire to clear the throat and ultimately swallowing the sputum.

### *Ipecacuanha* (ipecac root)

The person has a spasmodic/asthmatic cough, and the chest feels full of sputum, but coughing does not really produce much. Sufferers feel nauseated, but this feeling is unrelieved by vomiting. Coughing makes them short of breath, and they may vomit without feeling nauseated beforehand.

### Arsenicum album (arsenic trioxide)

Sufferers feel very cold and are extremely anxious. The cough is suffocative and asthmatic and makes them feel very ill. The catarrh spreads downwards from the nose to the larynx and then on to the chest. The symptoms get worse at the middle of the night. Sufferers are very restless, and despite the illness, they maintain a very neat and tidy appearance and ensure that there is enough space around them.

### Kali carbonicum (potassium carbonate)

Sufferers' coughing is worse at 3.00 am, and the sputum takes the form of small, round lumps of blood-streaked mucus. The cough is of an asthmatic nature, and sufferers find relief by leaning forward so that their head is on their knees. The cough causes cutting or stitching pains in the chest.

### Spongia tosta (roasted sponge)

This is a classic CROUP remedy (*see* p. 407).The person's chest is dry, with no wheezing or cough. The breathing sounds like a saw being driven through a board. It is made worse by trying to talk and lying with the head low.

# Ear Problems

The ear has two actions: to act as a hearing sensor, and to act as a balancing sensor.

The visible part of the ear is called the pinna. It contains the entrance to a canal that leads to the eardrum (tympanic membrane). Beyond this is the middle ear, which contains the ossicles, a series of three bones that turn the vibrations of the eardrum into a nervous impulse for the auditory nerve. The inner ear – called the labyrinth – houses the mechanism for translating this nervous impulse, as well as the nerve endings that are responsible for balance, which reside in three semicircular canals. The air pressure in the middle ear is equalized with the pressure in the outside world via the Eustachian tube, a canal linking the middle ear with the nose.

## Barotrauma

If the Eustachian tube is blocked by mucus from a cold and the outer air pressure falls – which usually happens in pressurized aircraft – the eardrum is pushed in towards the middle ear. This causes pain and partial deafness that can last for two to three days.

This *barotrauma* can be alleviated if sufferers breathe out through their nose while pinching their nostrils tight so that air cannot escape. It also helps to swallow repeatedly and suck a sweet on takeoff and on descent. The following homeopathic remedy is also useful.

### *Borax* (sodium borate)

This remedy picture shows sufferers who react adversely to downward motion and whose ears are particularly sensitive to sound. Any smoke also causes distress. Using the 30c potency, take one dose when the pilot signals that the aircraft is about to descend.

# Earache (*otitis media*)

This is a very painful condition because the eardrum is very sensitive. Younger people are more likely to have this than older people (*see* p. 410 for the section on ear infections in children). It must always be assessed by a medical practitioner, in order to establish the correct diagnosis. If earache follows a cold, an infection of the middle ear (*otitis media*) is very probable. A discharge of blood and/or pus confirms the presence of such an infection. The conventional treatment is with antibiotics.

Homeopathy can be used with success. For those children who suffer recurrent attacks of *otitis media*, a specialist homeopath should be consulted to establish the constitutional remedy. If this consultation is not possible, the following homeopathic remedies can be used, giving the 6c potency at a rate of one dose every 30 minutes. Select the remedy from the following remedy pictures, matching the picture with the physical symptoms.

### *Belladonna* (deadly nightshade)

This remedy picture describes sufferers with a tearing, throbbing pain deep in the ear. They are very sensitive to loud noises, have a flushed face and probably a fever that may make them delirious. The pain is made worse from any warm application.

### *Chamomilla* (camomile)

The remedy picture is of an earache that causes sufferers to become frantic – if they are mild, calm and gentle, this is the wrong remedy. Characteristically, one cheek is red while the other is pale. If the person is a child, he or she can only be consoled by being carried around.

### *Hepar sulphuris* (Hahnemann's calcium sulphide)

This remedy picture describes an earache that is improved by warmth and by wrapping up the head, covering the ear. The ear may already be discharging pus.

### *Pulsatilla* (wind flower)

This remedy picture describes an earache in which some pressure within the middle ear appears to be forcing the eardrum outwards. Sufferers find it difficult to hear, as if the ear is stuffed up. The external ear may be swollen and red in colour. All the symptoms are worse at night.

# Sinusitis

The sinuses are air spaces within the bones around the nose. The maxillary sinus, beneath the cheekbone, drains into the nose, as do the frontal sinus underneath the eyebrows and the ethmoid sinus just behind the bridge of the nose. All of these sinuses are lined by a mucous membrane that can become infected by certain viruses and bacteria. The resulting infection causes a build-up of pus that cannot drain into the nose and so causes pain and possibly a fever. The person feels bunged up and unwell.

The initial treatment is pain relief – paracetamol is a suitable pain-relieving tablet – and a programme of decongestion: breathing in through the nose rather than the mouth, and breathing in steam from a large bowl of hot water with a towel draped over both head and bowl. Conventional treatment will include antibiotics and surgical drainage if necessary.

Some people have an allergy or intolerance to dairy products from cows, and this can cause repeated upper respiratory infections. If this is the case, all dairy products made from cows' milk should be avoided. Soya products, goats' milk and goats' dairy products are suitable alternatives. This applies to both children and adults. The complementary therapy of reflexology is very helpful and successful in treating acute attacks of sinusitis and preventing them from recurring.

Homeopathic treatment, too, can be started initially and used for two days. If there is no sign of improvement, seek medical advice. Consultation with a specialist homeopath will provide a constitutional remedy to help with recurrent attacks of sinusitis.

If this is not possible, the following remedies may be used. Select the appropriate remedy by matching its remedy picture with the physical symptoms. Using the 6c potency, give one dose four times a day, for as long as necessary.

### *Belladonna* (deadly nightshade)

This remedy picture describes sufferers with sore, swollen and red noses. They imagine that there are certain odours in the room when there are none. Any nasal catarrh consists of mucus mixed with blood. The mouth is dry, and the tongue is strawberry-coloured, swollen and painful. Sufferers have a tendency to grind their teeth, and their gums throb with pain.

### *Hepar sulphuris* (Hahnemann's calcium sulphide)

This remedy picture describes soreness of the nostrils with catarrh that is thick and offensive-smelling (like old cheese). Sufferers are very sensitive to cold, dry winds, which cause sneezing every time they go into that environment. They can feel dejected and sad, particularly in the evening and at night. They are easily irritated by the most trivial of matters.

### *Kali bichromium* (potassium bichromate)

This remedy picture describes people who feel pressure and pain at the root of their noses. The nasal septum becomes ulcerated, and the nasal discharge is thick, ropey and greenish-yellow in colour. The characteristic feature of this remedy is that the discharge comes out in long, tough elastic plugs from the nose.

### *Pulsatilla* (wind flower)

This remedy picture describes stitching pains in the face that wander about but seem to start in the right side. The pains involve all the sinuses, producing a yellow-coloured catarrh. Sufferers have a tendency to weep, but now the tears can start to scald. They and their symptoms are better in the fresh air and feel worse in a stuffy atmosphere. They may have already suffered a frontal headache from overwork.

### *Silicea* (pure flint)

This remedy picture describes a person whose facial bones around the nose feel very sensitive. The tip of the nose is itchy, and the nasal discharge forms hard crusts that, when removed, cause bleeding from the nasal septum.

# Earwax problems

Wax is a natural substance that usually flows out of the ear's external canal to the outside without causing any symptoms. Occasionally, it can build up in the canal leading up to the eardrum, when it can cause difficulty in hearing, itchiness and a buzzing noise in the ear known as *tinnitus*.

The wax can be gently softened by dropping into the ear canal olive or almond oil that has been warmed to slightly more than room temperature. This will lead to the escape of the wax from the ear canal in the normal way. **On no account should the wax be removed manually with cotton buds or any other object, as this can cause damage to the eardrum.** If this doesn't work, the wax can be syringed out by a nurse or medical practitioner.

There are two homeopathic remedies that have in their remedy pictures the ability to help the problem of earwax. The 6c potency is used and is given as one dose twice a day for at least one week. However, either of the remedies can be continued for a much longer period of time if necessary.

### *Causticum* (Hahnemann's mixture of quicklime (calcium oxide) and potassium bisulphate)

The remedy picture describes a ringing, roaring and pulsating sensation in sufferers' ears, leading to deafness. They find that words echo in their ears and that there is an accumulation of wax in the outer ear canal.

*Lachesis* (bushmaster snake venom)

This remedy has the ability to resolve hard wax. Its distinguishing feature is that the person it will suit is very talkative and dislikes anything wrapped around their throats.


# Glue ear (*serous otitis media*)

This condition is caused by an accumulation of a thick gluey fluid in the middle ear. It happens when the Eustachian tube fails to allow this fluid to drain away. The main symptom is deafness, which can lead to educational difficulties in children.

The principal cause of this problem, which mainly affects children (*see* p. 410 for more information on such infections in the young), is unknown. It may be due to the overprescribing of antibiotics in treating middle ear infections (*otitis media*) in children. Drinking cows' milk and eating dairy products from cows have also been implicated, as the protein in these products causes the body to over-react, resulting in an "allergic" reaction and the formation of this sticky fluid. Therefore, part of the treatment is to avoid cows' milk and all dairy products from cows and substitute with soya preparations or goats' milk and goats' milk dairy products.

Conventional treatment may include long-term antibiotic therapy or the surgical insertion of grommet tubes into the eardrums to help the fluid drain away.

There are several homeopathic remedies that can be used to help the body remove this gluey fluid. Select the remedy from the following remedy pictures, and using the 6c potency, give one dose twice a day, every day for at least three months. It is important to check the progress of the condition of the ear on a monthly basis.


### Kali muriaticum (potassium chloride)

This remedy picture describes a long-term catarrhal condition of the middle ear. The person is aware of snapping noises in the ear.

In addition, the lymph glands become swollen around the ear and under the jaw.

### Lycopodium (club moss)

This remedy picture describes a humming and roaring sound in the ears associated with difficulty in hearing. The person is aware that every sound causes a peculiar echo in the ear. There may be a rash (eczema) on or behind the ear lobe. If this condition follows an infection of mild scarlet fever (SCARLATINA), then a ringing sound (tinnitus) may be present in the ear.

### Mercurius dulcis (calomel)

This particular remedy has a marked influence on catarrhal conditions of the middle ear, particularly when the Eustachian tube is blocked. The person tends to have offensive-smelling breath, with a constant flow of saliva that is dark in colour and also offensive in odour. The tongue is usually black in colour.

### Pulsatilla (wind flower)

This remedy picture shows a diminution in hearing with an aching pain in the ear, particularly at night in the affected ear.

## Labyrinthitis

This is a viral infection of the labyrinth, the part of the middle ear responsible for maintaining balance. It relates the position of the body relative to the outside world, both in real terms and in perceived terms (the eyes may tell the body one thing, but the body itself may feel something else). When this part of the ear is infected, the wrong information is given to the brain, resulting in giddiness (also known as vertigo) that may cause the person to fall down and possibly also cause nausea with vomiting. Untreated, this condition will last for about one month.

The conventional treatment is to give a specific sedative drug so that the labyrinth is quietened.

There are several homeopathic remedies that will help treat this condition. Using the 6c potency, give one dose four times a day until the symptoms begin to improve, which will be in less than one month.

### Aurum metallicum (gold)

This remedy picture describes labyrinthitis in a person who has a past medical history of an illness involving a stroke (cerebrovascular accident). This person is seriously depressed.

### Belladonna (deadly nightshade)

This remedy picture describes sufferers who lose their balance and either fall to the left or backwards. They develop a headache that is better when they sit down.

### Borax (sodium borate)

This remedy picture describes giddiness with nausea and vomiting, all brought on by downward motion. This includes any rocking movement, being carried downstairs and being laid face down in bed for fear of falling. In this state, the person's hearing is very sensitive to the slightest noise but is not disturbed as much with louder noises.

### Bryonia (wild hops)

This remedy picture describes sufferers who develop giddiness, nausea and vomiting whenever they look up. Aware of roaring and buzzing noises in their ears, they feel better when lying down, but whenever they attempt to stand up they develop giddiness – a symptom that is shared with Phosphorus.

### Calcarea carbonica (calcium carbonate)

This remedy describes giddiness brought on when sufferers look up. They feel cold, and are particularly sensitive to the cold around their ears and neck. Those whom this remedy suits will be obstinate, have a tendency to be constipated and sweat easily around the head.

### Cinchona officinalis (China) (Peruvian bark)

This remedy picture describes giddiness brought on by the loss of body fluids (vomiting, diarrhoea, profuse sweating, blood loss).

### Conium (poison hemlock)

This remedy picture describes sufferers who develop giddiness made worse when they lie down and move their head from side to side. The giddiness is also made worse with any mental strain.

### Gelsemium (yellow jasmine)

This remedy picture describes giddiness in sufferers who have a tired look about their face and who also have blurred vision. The facial muscles are contracted, especially around the mouth, and the lower jaw tends to droop.

### Natrum salicylicum (sodium salicylate)

This remedy picture describes a buzzing sound (tinnitus) in the ear, deafness and a feeling of giddiness (vertigo).

### Phosphorus

This remedy picture describes older people who develop giddiness whenever they get out of bed or whenever they change from a lying to a standing position. (This is a symptom that is shared with *Bryonia*.) These people are sensitive, have a fear of thunderstorms and benefit from short periods of sleep.

### Salicylicum acidum (salicylic acid)

This remedy picture describes giddiness where sufferers have a tendency to fall over to their left side. They also develop a head-ache and a feeling of confusion whenever they stand up suddenly.

### *Silicea* (pure flint)

This remedy picture describes giddiness when looking up. Suf-ferers feel more comfortable with their head wrapped up warmly and when lying on their left side. Any headache starts in the back of the head and spreads over the scalp, settling over the eyes.

## Ménière's disease

This illness represents a combination of giddiness (vertigo) with deafness. The giddiness may also cause nausea with vomiting, and the deafness may be associated with persistent noises in the ear (tinnitus).

Diagnosis must be made by a specialist after tests on auditory function. The conventional treatment is with drugs that alter fluid retention in the body.

Acute attacks of giddiness can be treated with an appropriate remedy described in the section on labyrinthitis (*see above*). Using the 6c potency, give one dose every four hours until the giddiness settles.

There are several homeopathic remedies that can be used to help treat Ménière's disease. Using the 6c potency, one dose can be given every eight hours for several weeks if necessary.

### *Carboneum sulphuratum* (carbon bisulphide)

This remedy picture describes sufferers with impaired hearing and who are aware of a buzzing and singing noise in their ears, as if a harp were playing. These sufferers may have abused alcohol in the past or may be currently abusing alcohol.

### *Chenopodium anthelminticum* (Jerusalem oak)

This remedy picture describes a distorted hearing pattern in which the hearing is improved with high-pitched sounds and there is a comparative deafness to the spoken voice. The picture also describes a buzzing sound in the ears and the occasional bout of giddiness. A characteristic feature of this remedy is a significant pain in the shoulder blade (scapula).

### Chininum sulphuricum (quinine sulphite)

This remedy picture describes violent ringing, buzzing and roaring in the ears associated with deafness. Sufferers find standing upright difficult and are always falling over. They find that symptoms are worse when they are lying on their left side.

### Pilocarpine muriaticum (pilocarpine chloride)

This remedy picture describes tinnitus and deafness, with profuse sweating.

## Otosclerosis

This is a type of deafness that occurs primarily in older people. The three ossicles in the middle ear, which translate the vibrations of the eardrum into nervous impulses that register meaningful sound, become fixed together. In the older person, the deafness comes on slowly but progressively. This condition can also occur in younger people, when the deafness happens more rapidly.

Conventional treatment would be a consultation with a specialist who may recommend surgery.

Homeopathic treatment involves one of the two following remedies, selected because they most closely fit the physical symptoms. Using the 6c potency, take one dose twice a day as a long-term therapy. The treatment can be stopped as the hearing improves.

### Calcarea fluorica (calcium fluoride)

This remedy picture shows an ability to dissolve hard stony material in any part of the body. It is particularly applicable in treating the hardened material around the ossicles of the middle ear.

### *Graphites* (black lead)

This remedy picture describes deafness that is improved with background noise. Sufferers are aware of a cracking sound in their ears when they are eating. They may also notice a moist skin eruption behind their ears. When the eardrum is examined, a thin, white, scaly membrane is seen to be covering it.

## Otitis externa

This is an infection of the outer ear canal. It may result in a moist discharge of clear fluid, pus or blood. The skin of this outer canal is very sensitive and should not be scraped in any way.

The conventional treatment will probably include antibiotic drops or tablets, with a possibility of drops containing a steroid drug.

There are several homeopathic remedies that are applicable to this condition. Using the 6c potency, give one dose every four hours until the condition is seen to be improving.

### *Aconitum napellus* (monk's-hood)

This remedy picture describes an illness that comes on very suddenly. The symptoms include a red, hot, painful and swollen outer ear. The person is very sensitive to noise and finds music particularly unbearable. This remedy is short-acting and can be given as a 6c potency every 30 minutes for a maximum of 12 doses. If there is no improvement, proceed to *Belladonna*, using the dosage schedule at the beginning of this section on *otitis externa*.

### *Belladonna* (deadly nightshade)

This remedy picture describes a condition where there is a tearing pain in the outer ear. The person's face is flushed and he or she will probably have a fever.

### *Graphites* (black lead)

This remedy picture describes not so much an acute (sudden) picture but more of a continuing problem where there is itchiness of the outer ear canal with only a suggestion of a discharge.

### *Mercurius solubis* (black oxide of mercury)

This remedy picture describes an acute infection of the outer ear canal, with pain and a discharge that contains pus and possibly blood.

# Tinnitus

This condition describes a persistent buzzing, humming or ringing sound in the ears. Some conventional drugs can cause this – for example, aspirin – and impacted ear wax can also result in this symptom. The sound can be masked by listening to an alternative sound through headphones.

There are several homeopathic remedies that can also be used to help alleviate this symptom. Using the 6c potency range, take one dose four times a day.

### *Antipyrine* (coal tar derivative)

This remedy picture describes pain as well as a buzzing sensation in the ears. Sufferers are prone to attacks of profuse perspiration. They may also have hallucinations that they are losing their sight and hearing.

### *Cannabis indica* (hashish)

This remedy picture describes throbbing, buzzing and ringing noises in the ear, as if water is being boiled in it. The person becomes extremely sensitive to any noise.

### *Carboneum sulphuratum* (carbon bisulphide)

This remedy picture describes a buzzing and singing noise in the ear, like the playing of a harp. Sufferers may have abused or may still be abusing alcohol. They have muscular wasting and are very sensitive to the cold.

### *Cinchona officinalis (China)* (Peruvian bark)

This remedy picture describes a situation where sufferers are aware of ringing in their ears, and their hearing is sensitive to noise. The external ear is sensitive to the touch and the earlobe is red and swollen.

### *Salicylicum acidum* (salicylic acid)

This remedy picture describes a sensation of roaring and buzzing in the ears, associated with deafness and giddiness.

# Mouth and Dental Problems

This section includes disorders of the mouth, tongue, teeth and gums. For information on and types of treatments for disorders that occur specifically in children such as teething, turn to p. 435 in the special section devoted to this age group.

## Bad breath (halitosis)

This condition can cause a lot of worry. People find it difficult to be sure themselves whether or not they suffer from bad breath, and the only way to find out is to ask someone else.

It is often caused by bad dental hygiene leading to gingivitis (*see later*) or chronic periodontitis (pyorrhoea). However, it can also be due to recurrent sore throats (see p. 28), the eating of certain food such as garlic, curry and onions, drinking alcohol and smoking tobacco, and certain gut disorders such as REFLUX OESOPHAGITIS.

The immediate treatment is to correct any of these causative factors. Chewing parsley leaves or a clove can help to alleviate the odour of bad breath.

There are several homeopathic remedies that are applicable for specific indications. Their physical pictures are described below, and the appropriate one should be selected by matching its picture with the presenting symptoms. Using the 6c potency, give one dose four times a day for up to seven days.

### *Arnica* (leopard's bane)

This remedy picture describes a fetid breath odour, particularly after an injury to the jaw where there is stale blood in the mouth. Sufferer's mouths are dry and they are thirsty and have a taste in their mouths that is like bad eggs.

### Aurum metallicum (gold)

This remedy is particularly applicable to young girls at puberty, but it need not be limited exclusively to this group. The breath smells foul and bitter, and the gums are ulcerated.

### Carbolicum acidum (carbolic acid)

This remedy picture describes CONSTIPATION associated with bad breath. Sufferers probably have a craving for tobacco and also have indigestion, giving a bad taste in their mouths. Their sense of smell is very sensitive, and there is a burning sensation in their mouths that goes down into the stomach. They find that fluids are easily and painlessly vomited.

### Graphites (black lead)

This remedy picture describes breath that smells of urine. The person tends to be overweight, and may also have skin problems that ooze a honey-like exudate (see ECZEMA, p. 267).

### Mercurius corrosivus (corrosive sublimate of mercury)

In addition to breath that is so foul that the whole room is permeated with the smell, this remedy picture describes bleeding gums that are swollen and spongy; as a result, the teeth are loose and several will have fallen out. The tongue is swollen and so furred that the teeth leave an imprint around the edges. There is a profuse flow of saliva, and the person has a salty, bitter taste in the mouth.

### Mezereum (spurge olive)

This remedy picture describes breath that smells of rotten cheese. Sufferers may have a desire for the fat from ham. Their mouths tend to water easily, and their tongues tend to have a burning sensation that extends down into the stomach. They may well have a gastric ulcer.

### Nux vomica (poison-nut)

This remedy picture describes breath that smells foul particularly following a stomach upset, probably brought on by the over-consumption of alcohol. The symptoms are worse in the morning, when the person is left with a feeling of nausea. This remedy is useful as a "hangover" remedy.

### Petroleum (crude rock oil)

This remedy picture describes sufferers who give out an odour of garlic (a symptom shared with *Tellurium*). They are ravenously hungry because they have a persistent stomach ache when their stomachs are empty. They even have to get out of bed at night in order to have something to eat (this symptom is shared with *Psorinum*).

### Phosphorus

This remedy picture describes swollen, ulcerated gums that bleed easily. Any tooth extraction bleeds for a long time afterwards. This bleeding gives the breath a stale, sour odour. Sufferers have a fear of thunderstorms.

### Psorinum (scabies vesicle)

This remedy picture describes an ulcerated tongue and gums, producing a foul-tasting, tough mucus that sticks to the soft palate. Sufferers are very hungry and need to get out of bed at night in order to satisfy their hunger (a symptom shared with *Petroleum*). They have flatulence that smells of bad eggs. They are cold and are therefore very sensitive to cold weather.

### Quercus (acorn kernel)

This remedy picture describes breath that smells of faeces. The remedy is an antidote to the effects of alcohol, and is therefore useful in the treatment of alcoholics where the craving for alcohol has to be removed.

### Rheum (rhubarb)

This remedy picture describes a mouth that produces a lot of saliva, teeth that have a sensation of coolness in them, and saliva that thickens overnight, causing bad breath.

### Sinapis nigra (black mustard)

This remedy picture describes breath smelling of onions. The person commonly has hayfever.

### Spigelia (pinkroot)

This remedy picture describes a person with bad breath who also has a heart problem, usually palpitations.

### Tellurium

This remedy picture describes breath that smells of garlic. The person usually has a craving for apples.

## Cold sores

Cold sores are the result of a specific viral infection – HERPES SIMPLEX – initially causing blisters in the mouth and on the tongue and subsequently on the face, which then go on to form ulcers. This virus is very infectious and can spread to the genital area of the same person, causing genital herpes, or to the eyes, causing corneal ulcers.

The conventional treatment is to use antiviral applications or antiviral tablets. Untreated, the condition will last for one to two weeks.

Homeopathic treatment is best obtained by consulting a specialist homeopath, particularly if the person suffers from recurrent cold sores. If this is not possible, the following homeopathic remedies can be used instead of the conventional medication. Using the 6c potency, give one dose four times a day for up to two weeks, or use the mother tincture where indicated in the remedy picture profile, placing one drop on the sore daily.

Select the remedy from the following pictures, matching the remedy picture with the physical symptoms.

### Capsicum annuum (cayenne pepper)

This remedy describes sufferers who have cracks in the corner of their mouths, a burning pain on the tips of their tongues, and foul-smelling breath. They have ulcers on their tongue and probably an itchy, blister-type rash on their faces, particularly on their chins.

### Natrum muriaticum (sodium chloride)

This remedy picture describes sufferers who cannot bear any fuss being made of them. They have a desire for salty foods and a dislike of extremes of temperature (hot or cold), and they bear grudges. Their lips and the corners of their mouths are cracked; in particular, the lower lip has a deep crack in its centre. There are blisters like pearls on their lips and chins, and blisters on their tongues give a sensation as though there were a hair on each one.

### Rhus toxicodendron (poison ivy)

This remedy picture describes a swollen face covered in a blister rash. The cheekbones are sensitive to the touch, and the face develops a neuralgic pain that is associated with a chilly feeling, a sensation that is worse in the evening. The corners of the mouth are ulcerated, and blisters, like pearls, form around the mouth and also on the chin (a symptom shared with *Natrum muriaticum*).

### Sempervivum tectorum (house-leek)

This remedy picture describes ulcers in the mouth (*see* MOUTH [APHTHOUS] ULCERS, p. 125) and on the tongue, which bleed very easily, especially at night. The tongue feels very sore and has stabbing pains going through it. The skin around the mouth also has many blisters.

# Dental decay (dental caries)

Tooth decay is the result of a diet rich in refined sugar. Fluoride either in toothpaste or in drinking water reduces the amount of dental caries. However, it is arguable whether it is wise to put fluoride into drinking water as an excess of this mineral can lead to symptoms or side-effects. Flossing and mechanical water irrigation can both be beneficial.

The following homeopathic remedies will also help. Select the remedy from the picture described, matching the picture to the physical symptoms. The dosage schedule is given with each remedy.

In addition to the selected remedy, a dose of 30c *Bacillinum* (macerated tuberculous lung) should also be given once a month. It is important, however, not to give *Bacillinum* to a person who has a history of asthma.

### *Calcarea carbonica* (calcium carbonate)

This remedy picture describes short, squat people whose scalps tend to sweat a lot and who have a tendency to obesity. They also have a flat hard palate, with white, square front teeth, wide dental arches and an absence of overcrowding. Using the 30c potency, give one dose twice a week but not on consecutive days.

### *Calcarea fluorica* (calcium fluoride)

This remedy picture describes people who have an obvious facial asymmetry with asymmetric dental arches, scoliosis (twisting) of the spine, and very flexible joints with a tendency to suffer from recurrent sprains and dislocations. Their teeth tend to be over-crowded and the enamel on them is poor in quality and grey in colour. Using the 30c potency, give a single dose once a week.

### *Calcarea phosphorica* (calcium phosphate)

This remedy picture describes a person who is tall, has a narrow face and a well-arched palate with yellowish front teeth that have a tendency to become overcrowded. Using the 30c potency, give a single dose twice a week but not on consecutive days.

### *Kreosotum* (beechwood kreosote)

This remedy describes a picture of early and rapid decay of the first teeth of a child – deciduous dentition (milk teeth). The dose is using the 30c potency to be given twice a week (but not on consecutive days).

# Dry (infected) tooth socket

This condition will need dental advice and may require tooth extraction or antibiotic therapy. Mouthwash therapy can be used immediately (*see* MOUTH [APHTHOUS] ULCERS, p. 125) to help alleviate the discomfort. A remedy picture that describes teeth that ache and are sensitive and sore to the touch can benefit from a local application in the form of a dressing impregnated with *Plantago major* (plantain) mother tincture.

While dental advice is being obtained, the following homeopathic remedies can be given in addition to the local application and the use of mouthwashes. Select the remedy from the following remedy pictures; the dosage schedule will be described with each one.

### *Belladonna* (deadly nightshade)

This remedy picture describes throbbing toothache in a person who has a red face, a rapid heart rate and widely dilated pupils. Using the 30c potency, give one dose every hour until dental help is available.

### *Coffea cruda* (unroasted coffee)

This remedy picture describes such unbearable pains that sufferers toss themselves around in anguish, obtaining relief only by holding cold water in the mouth. Using the 30c potency, give one dose every 15 minutes until dental help is available.

### *Hepar sulphuris* (Hahnemann's calcium sulphide)

This remedy is useful following a tooth extraction. Using the 6c potency, give one dose every four hours for five days.

### *Silicea* (pure flint)

This remedy is useful in expelling any residual tooth fragments following a tooth extraction. The remedy picture describes a person who has sweaty, smelly feet. Using the 6c potency, give one dose twice a day for three weeks.

# Fear of dentists and dental procedures

This section deals with the undue nervousness experienced by some people when going to see the dentist and having to cope with certain dental procedures. The following remedies are applicable only to adults. For information on remedies for children with this problem, see p. 408.

### *Aconitum napellus* (monk's-hood)

This remedy picture describes great fear (to the extent that sufferers feel that they will die) and generalized anxiety with no other specific symptoms. Using the 30c potency, give one dose hourly as required.

### *Argentum nitricum* (silver nitrate)

This remedy picture describes anxiety associated with agitation, producing diarrhoea and hurried speech. Sufferers that this remedy will suit have a particular fear of heights and of crowds. They like sweet foods and salt. Using the 30c potency, give one dose the evening before the appointment at the dentist's, one dose early in the morning on the day of the appointment, and one dose one hour before the procedure.

### *Gelsemium* (yellow jasmine)

This remedy picture describes anxiety associated with feelings of drowsiness and of muscular weakness (at the knees in particular, so that the person "goes weak at the knees") and an apparent lack of memory. Using the 30c potency, give one dose in the evening before the appointment, one dose early in the morning of the day of the appointment and one dose an hour before the appointment.

### *Silicea* (pure flint)

This remedy picture specifically describes a fear of needles (injections) and is clearly indicated where the dentist is proposing to use a local anaesthetic injection. Using the 30c potency give one dose the night before the dental appointment, and one dose on the morning of the appointment and one dose one hour before the appointment.

It is also recommended that *Arnica* (leopard's bane) is given after any dental procedure. Using the 30c potency, give one dose every three hours for a maximum of ten doses. However if an injection is to be made by the dentist, *Arnica* should not be given beforehand. This is because the pain of a dental procedure is made worse if *Arnica* precedes it.

# Gingivitis

This is an infection of the gums between the gum margin and the tooth, where bacteria grow in food particles that get caught. Eventually the infection causes the gums to retract and the teeth to fall out.

Both conventional and homeopathic treatment is to maintain dental health (see p. 58). If the infection is acute, further conventional treatment would be to cut the gum, which then regrows. If treatment is not carried out, the teeth will have to be removed and a set of false teeth prescribed.

The homeopathic treatment consists of rinsing the mouth with the mouthwashes described in the section on mouth (aphthous) ulcers (*see* p. 125), and to combine this with one of the following remedies. Match the physical symptoms with the remedy picture. Using the 6c potency, give one dose twice a day for two weeks.

### *Antimonium crudum* (black sulphide of antimony)

This remedy picture describes gums that are detached from the teeth. They bleed easily and the teeth ache. Sufferers develop cracks in the corners of their mouths, and their lips are dry with a saltish taste in their mouths.

### *Borax* (sodium borate)

This remedy picture describes painful gumboils and a bitter taste in the mouth.

### *Carbo vegetabilis* (vegetable charcoal)

This remedy picture describes blood oozing from the gums when sufferers clean their teeth. Their breath smells, and their gums, which may turn black, are painful whenever they chew. The teeth are painful, particularly when eating anything very hot or very cold.

### *Kreosotum* (beechwood kreosote)

This remedy picture describes bluish, spongey, bleeding gums. Teeth are very painful, develop black spots on them and rapidly decay. Sufferers have bad breath.

### *Mercurius solubis* (black oxide of mercury)

This remedy picture describes painful, swollen, bleeding gums. Gumboils are common. Sufferers have bad breath, and their teeth feel painful, particularly at night, and are worse when anything very hot or very cold is consumed. They have an increase in the amount of saliva they produce.

### Natrum muriaticum (sodium chloride)

This remedy picture describes gumboils and bleeding gums. The particular symptom of this remedy is that the tongue is mapped with teeth impressions. The person commonly has a crack in the middle of the lower lip.

### Phosphorus

This remedy picture describes bleeding gums with soreness, particularly behind the front of the lower teeth. The tongue is dry, smooth and red. Sufferers feel that their palates itch.

### Silicea (pure flint)

This remedy picture describes gums that are sensitive to cold air and cold water and have gumboils. The teeth lose their enamel, become rough and finally break down. Sufferers feel as if their teeth are too big for their mouths. Their tongues are brown and have a peculiar symptom: a feeling that there is a hair on the back of the tongue.

### Staphysagria (stavesacre)

This remedy picture describes teeth that have become loose and are black and crumbling. Sufferers have toothache, bleeding gums and bad breath.

## Glossitis

In this condition, the tongue feels sore and as if it is burning. Its surface is flat because the taste buds (papillae) have wasted away (atrophied). The cause is usually a lack of a mineral or vitamin –

iron, vitamin B12, nicotinic acid or folic acid – and correction of the deficiency will improve the condition. However, this will take a few weeks, and in the meantime, the following homeopathic remedies can be given to help improve symptoms. For all these remedies, the dosage schedule is one dose four times a day for two weeks, using the 6c potency.

### *Arsenicum album* (arsenic trioxide)

This remedy picture describes a tongue that is dry, clean and red in colour, particularly as a central streak. The symptoms are made worse by drinking cold water and improved by drinking warm liquids. The symptoms worsen towards midnight.

### *Belladonna* (deadly nightshade)

This remedy picture describes a tongue that is dry, red in colour (slightly more so on the right side) and very shiny as if glazed. Sufferers have a great thirst for cold water. Characteristically those whom this remedy will suit have red faces, widely dilated pupils and a rapid heart rate. They may well have a fever.

### *Phosphorus*

This remedy picture describes a tongue that is dry and smooth and which may be red or white in colour. The gums are swollen and bleed easily, and the whole mouth has a burning sensation that goes down into the gullet (oesophagus). Sufferers are thirsty for cold liquids, and those whom this remedy will suit have a fear of thunderstorms.

### *Sulphur*

This remedy picture describes a tongue that is white with a red tip and red around its borders. There is a bitter taste in the mouth, which generally feels sore. The lips are dry. This remedy will suit those people who are laid back, enjoy alcohol and a joke and have a definite point of view.

# Mouth (apthous) ulcers

*See* GASTROINTESTINAL TRACT DISORDERS, p. 125.

# Salivary gland inflammation and stone formation

The salivary glands secrete fluid into the mouth, which contains enzymes that help break down food and so start digestion. The parotid salivary gland drains into the inside of the cheek. The submandibular salivary gland drains into the mouth under the tongue.

These glands can become infected either by a virus (as in MUMPS) or by bacteria (which need treating, or else the infection may become quite serious), giving symptoms of pain, swelling and fever; with a bacterial infection, the saliva may develop a putrid taste. The progress of a viral infection is two to three weeks; the only conventional treatment that may be needed is pain relief. The conventional treatment for a bacterial infection is antibiotic therapy with or without pain relief.

Occasionally, a stone can become lodged in the duct (tube) that drains the salivary gland. This causes pain, particularly when the person is about to eat a meal and salivates at the prospect. It is also common for the gland to develop a secondary bacterial infection. The conventional treatment is to remove the stone surgically. Sucking a lemon may also help: the juice stimulates the gland to create more saliva, which can flush out the stone.

Homeopathic treatment is also available. Select a remedy from the following, choosing one that matches the physical symptoms. A dosage schedule is given with each remedy.

### *Belladonna* (deadly nightshade)

This remedy picture describes sufferers with swollen salivary glands who have flushed, red faces, bounding heart rates and throbbing pains in their glands. Using a 6c potency, give one dose every two hours for a maximum of 12 doses, reducing to one every six hours until the gland improves.

### *Calcarea carbonica* (calcium carbonate)

This remedy picture describes a dry mouth in which stone formation in the salivary glands – particularly the submandibular glands – is common. Using the 6c potency, give one dose every hour for a maximum of six doses while awaiting medical attention.

### *Ipecacuanha* (ipecac root)

This remedy picture describes inflamed salivary glands associated with nausea. Using a 6c potency, give one dose every six hours for three days.

### *Iris versicolor* (blue flag)

This remedy picture describes swollen, tender salivary glands, associated with a profuse flow of saliva. Sufferers commonly have a headache in the front of the head, which they describe as a "sick headache" and which comes on with rest. Using a 6c potency, give one dose every four hours for a maximum of 12 doses.

### *Mercurius corrosivus* (corrosive sublimate of mercury)

This remedy picture describes putrid-tasting saliva that increases in volume, especially at night. The gums are usually swollen and sore. Using a 6c potency, give one dose every two hours for a maximum of 12 doses. If there is no improvement after this time, get medical help.

### *Nitric acidum* (nitric acid)

This remedy picture describes swollen salivary glands associated with aphthous ulcers. The characteristic pains of this remedy are splinter-like. Using the 6c potency give one dose every four hours for a maximum of twelve doses.

### *Phytolacca* (poke root)

This remedy picture describes submandibular salivary glands that are as hard as bone. The person may also find them tender to the touch, and the pain is commonly referred up to the ears. The saliva is usually sticky. Using the 6c potency, give one dose every four hours for one day, reducing to one dose every six hours for a further two days, and then one dose twice a day until the glands improve.

### *Pilocarpin muriaticum* (pilocarpine chloride)

This remedy picture describes swollen salivary glands, particularly the parotid, and is the characteristic remedy for MUMPS (*see* p. 422). The saliva is sticky. Using the 6c potency, give one dose every four hours on the first day, reducing to one dose every six hours for a further two or three days as required.

## Oral thrush

This is caused by a fungus called *Candida albicans*. White-coloured plaques form in the mouth, which when scratched leave a raw sensitive area that bleeds easily. This condition occurs commonly in newborn babies, in older people and in others who have low resistance to infection. This can happen in certain diseases, and if a person is stressed, has received antibiotics for another condition or is taking a steroid (corticosteroid) drug. However, it is important not to stop a steroid drug without consulting the medical practitioner who prescribed them.

The conventional treatment is to give anti-fungal drops. Older people who use dentures should also be careful to sterilize them regularly. Both refined sugar and alcohol encourage *Candida albicans* to grow in a person with low resistance to infection, so a look at the diet to ensure that it is nutritious enough is an important first step.

Homeopathically, the treatment is to correct the diet and reduce stress if necessary and consider taking one of the following remedies. The dosage schedule for all of them is to use the 6c potency and give one dose four times a day until the condition starts to improve, at which point the remedy can be stopped.

### Borax (sodium borate)

This remedy picture describes white fungal-like growths in the mouth, which bleed when touched and when the person eats. They taste bitter and of a "cellar mould". The mouth is hot and tender. This remedy should be used as soon as the condition is first noticed.

### Candida albicans

This is a homeopathic remedy made from the actual fungus that causes the illness. It should be used by those who suffer from recurrent attacks of oral thrush. After taking Borax for an acute attack, using the dosage schedule given at the beginning of this section, proceed with the 6c potency of Candida albicans once a day for many months.

# Teeth grinding (bruxism and bruxomania)

Grinding the teeth is usually due to nervous tension. If it occurs during the day, it is called bruxomania; if it only occurs during the night, it is called bruxism. One way to reduce nervous tension naturally is by stopping drinking or eating to excess anything containing caffeine. Those who are addicted to sweet foods can become tense if food is delayed, so they should try to eat at regular intervals, avoiding refined carbohydrates and indulging their sweet tooth on fruit containing natural sugars. A supplement of 50 milligrams of vitamin $B_6$ (pyridoxine) twice a day can be helpful, especially in women who are taking the oral contraceptive pill or who suffer from premenstrual syndrome (PMS).

The following homeopathic remedies are applicable for the specific indications mentioned with each one. The recommended dosage schedule is described with the remedy.

### *Cina* (worm seed)

This remedy picture is most suitable for children. They show irritability and even convulsions associated with screams and violent jerking of their hands and feet. Their skin is sensitive to the touch, and they feel hungry and want to be rocked. They have a tendency to grind their teeth at night. They have intestinal irritation and may have a problem with threadworms. Using the 30c potency, one dose should be taken an hour before going to bed. This can be repeated for ten doses.

### *Nux vomica* (poison-nut)

This remedy picture describes overworked business people who have a tendency to overindulge in alcohol, coffee and tobacco. Tense and unable to relax, they are highly strung, are perfectionists and are inclined to tackle too many jobs at the same time. They also have a tendency to have gastric upsets. Using the 30c potency, take one dose twice a day for two weeks.

## Toothache

This condition requires urgent dental assessment as it probably indicates an infection of the tooth socket that, if untreated, could lead to abscess formation.

The following homeopathic remedies can be used as an initial treatment, prior to seeing the dental practitioner.

### *Chamomilla* (camomile)

This remedy picture describes pain that is completely intolerable. The characteristic feature is one red cheek while the other is normal. Using the 200c potency, give one dose every 30 minutes for a maximum of five doses.

### Sepia (inky juice of cuttlefish)

This remedy picture describes toothache occurring during pregnancy. Using the 6c potency, give one dose every four hours.

### Plantago major (plantain)

This remedy picture describes a toothache that is made worse by anything cold. Using the 6c potency, give one dose every 15 minutes until the person is seen by the dentist.

### Staphysagria (stavesacre)

This remedy picture describes a toothache occurring in a person whose teeth are generally in poor condition, black and crumbling. Using the 30c potency, give one dose every hour until the person is seen by the dentist.

# Wisdom tooth eruption and extraction

In adults, the eruption of wisdom teeth can be extremely painful, especially when they become impacted. For this reason, wisdom teeth are often extracted as a preventative measure (prophylactic dental extraction), even if they have not caused any trouble.

If there is pain in the wisdom tooth area and the wisdom teeth have not been extracted, the probable cause of the pain is from an infection. The treatment needs to be supervised by a dentist who will probably prescribe antibiotic therapy before surgery.

Homeopathic treatment can be carried out while a person is waiting to see the dentist.

### Salvia officinalis (sage)

Make up a mouthwash using this (see MOUTH [APHTHOUS] ULCERS, p. 125, for instructions) and give it several times during the day as required.

### Belladonna (deadly nightshade)

This remedy picture describes throbbing pain in the wisdom tooth area. Using the 30c potency, give one dose every two hours until the dentist has been consulted.

### Hepar sulphuris (Hahnemann's calcium sulphide)

This remedy helps promote the expulsion of pus from the infected wisdom tooth. Using the 6c potency, give one dose three times a day.

If the wisdom teeth are being extracted under a general anaesthetic, the homeopathic treatment is to use a 30c potency of both *Arnica* (leopard's bane) and *Hypericum* (St John's wort). Give one dose an hour before the procedure, and repeat both remedies twice a day for two days.

If the wisdom teeth are being extracted under a local anaesthetic, it is wise to not use *Arnica* as this will make the pains worse. *Hypericum* 30c can be given one hour before the procedure and repeated twice a day for two days. This will help the gums to heal.

# Nose Problems

## Hayfever and allergic rhinitis

These related conditions cause an irritation to the mucous lining of the nose, leading to stuffiness, nasal discharge and repeated sneezing attacks. In hayfever, there are also symptoms affecting the eyes – itchiness with profuse tear production.

Hayfever occurs seasonally. This is because the primary irritants (allergens) are air borne, grass and tree pollen or grass cuttings in the spring and early summer or mosses and mould spores in the winter. Allergic rhinitis continues throughout the year, and the cause may not be immediately obvious. Tree moulds, animal fur, house dust mites and certain foods are all possibilities.

As well as a personal medical history, a family history is taken, and this usually shows a significant number of relatives who have suffered from allergies. ASTHMA and ECZEMA are both often connected with hayfever and allergic rhinitis.

The conventional approach may well include skin patch testing. In this, tiny amounts of various potential irritants are injected just under the skin. If the person is allergic to one or more of these substances, the skin will become red at the point where they were injected. Having obtained this result, it is possible to desensitize people against their allergies by giving a further series of injections of decreasing dilutions of the implicated substances, so that in the end they are able to tolerate the undiluted allergens. The desensitization process can produce side-effects. These are usually mild, such as itching, swelling and/or rashes, but it can also cause more serious side-effects, such as bronchospasm (when the airways in the lungs close up) and even life-threatening anaphylatic shock. It is because of these serious possible consequences that desensitization should only be carried out where adequate emergency care is available.

The other method of conventional therapy is with drugs. Steroid nasal inhalers suppress the nasal symptoms, and antihistamine medication stops the cells in the nose from discharging histamine, the chemical responsible for producing allergic symptoms. The major side-effect of many antihistamines is drowsiness, and for that reason, those using them should not drive motor vehicles or use machinery. A new generation of this type of medication is emerging that does not have drowsiness as a side-effect.

Homeopathically, the occurrence of hayfever or allergic rhinitis is considered as evidence of a deeper problem and not simply a collection of local symptoms. It is best to consult a specialist homeopath who will be able to prescribe a remedy based not only on the specific problem but also on the general profile of the person as a whole. If this is not possible, follow the instructions given below.

If you have a strong family and/or personal history of allergies, the following nosode should be used.

### Psorinum (scabies vesicle)

The remedy picture of this particular remedy is not as important as when selecting other remedies. This remedy is used on the principle established by Hahnemann of a *miasm* (*see* ASTHMA, p. 94). As such, it wipes the slate clean as far as the "allergic" history is concerned, so further homeopathic prescriptions will work better. Using the 30c potency, give one dose every 12 hours for a maximum of three doses. This schedule can be repeated every month according to the response of the person.

It is possible to make a homeopathic potency of a specific allergen: animal fur (cat, dog, guinea pig or horse), a specific pollen (but if uncertain as to which pollen is the cause, a mixed pollen potency is available), house dust mite, and tree moulds (particularly for symptoms occurring in autumn and winter). It can be used as a 6c potency and given as a single dose two or three times every day. This schedule can be used in conjunction with *Psorinum* as mentioned above.

The following remedies can be used (with *Psorinum*) if the allergen is uncertain. The dosage schedule is the same as the one used for a specific allergen remedy.

### *Allium cepa* (red onion)

This remedy picture describes a person whose eyes water greatly and who has much clear nasal discharge that burns the skin in and around the nose. (This is the reverse of *Euphrasia* where the nasal discharge is bland and the tears are burning in quality). There is a lot of sneezing that becomes worse when the person enters a warm room.

### *Ambrosia* (ragweed)

This remedy picture describes eyes that burn and smart and produce a profuse amount of tears, as well as an intolerable itching of the eyelids. The nose has a stuffed-up feeling, and there is usually a watery nasal discharge that is associated with many sneezing attacks.

### *Arsenicum album* (arsenic trioxide)

This remedy picture describes sufferers who have an unquenchable thirst and are very restless, anxious and exceedingly neat and tidy. All of their symptoms are worse at midnight. They are very sensitive to the cold and feel better in the warmth, as do all of their symptoms. Their eyes are burning, their tears produce a burning sensation on the skin, and their eyelids are red, swollen, scaly and granulated. Their eyes are very sensitive to the light, a symptom that is improved by external warmth. The nose produces a thin, watery discharge that burns the ends of the nostrils. Sneezing occurs seemingly without relief, except that it is better indoors than outdoors.

### *Arsenicum iodatum* (arsenic iodide)

The characteristic feature of this remedy picture is a persistent, irritating and corrosive nasal discharge with tears that also cause the person's skin around the eyes to feel burned. The rest of the skin is dry and itchy. In certain areas of it, the superficial layer scales off, leaving a raw surface. The symptoms of this remedy are made better by any form of heat.

### *Arundo* (reed)

This remedy picture describes sneezing attacks that are preceded by a burning and itching sensation on the hard palate of the mouth as well as the conjunctiva, the membranes lining the eyelids. This is a particularly useful remedy for the early spring or autumn/winter hayfever season.

### *Cuprum aceticum* (copper acetate)

This remedy picture describes tears and sneezing with a nasal discharge, all of which cause a burning sensation on the skin. Coughing produces a thick sputum that causes the person to fear suffocation. These symptoms are associated with a spasmodic cough that can become asthmatic and can also lead to an attack of ANGINA PECTORIS in those who already have heart disease.

### *Dulcamara* (bittersweet)

This remedy picture describes the association of symptoms with damp conditions and the deterioration of symptoms in these conditions. The nose becomes stuffed up whenever there is cold rain. For this reason, sufferers choose to keep their noses warm because they know that any cold, damp air will block them up completely. The eyes are affected as well, causing them to produce a profuse watery discharge.

### *Euphrasia* (eyebright)

This remedy picture describes a marked reaction of the mucous membranes of the nose and particularly the eyes. A profuse, flowing and non-irritant nasal discharge is produced, as is a great quantity of tears that burn the skin (the reverse of *Allium cepa*, where the tears are non-irritant and the nasal discharge is burning in quality). The eyelids are swollen and the person has a frequent desire to blink. The tears have a tendency to form a sticky mucus on the surface of the eye (cornea), and the person blinks to remove this.

### *Linum usitatissimum* (common flax)

The important feature of this remedy picture in treating hay fever and allergic rhinitis is its widespread irritative reaction on other organs. It causes asthma, allergic skin reactions (urticaria or hives) and paralysis of the tongue.

### *Naphthaline* (coal tar derivative)

While this remedy picture describes profuse sneezing attacks, its significant feature is the symptoms of the eyes, which become red and the retina may become detached. Chest symptoms may develop into asthma; if this happens, the person feels more comfortable in the open air.

### *Nux vomica* (poison-nut)

This remedy describes a picture where the eyes are sensitive to light (photophobia), a symptom that is worse in the morning and causes smarting, which leads to much watering. The nose is stuffed up, particularly at night, and sufferers have a tendency to snuffle all the time. The snuffles are especially common when they are exposed to a dry, cold atmosphere and are made worse on entering a warm room. The "stuffed-up-ness" alternates between the two nostrils, so one nostril can be clear while the other is blocked. The outer ear canal is itchy, and sufferers are usually irritable. They are also ambitious workaholics and tend to over-indulge in tobacco, caffeine and alcohol.

### *Psorinum* (scabies vesicle)

This remedy may have already been used as an initial treatment for a strong personal and/or family history of allergies. This doesn't matter as it can be used separately as a local/specific remedy. Its remedy picture describes a very cold person whose eyelids become chronically swollen and red (a condition known as *blepharitis*). The nasal discharge is variable, ranging from nothing more than a sensation of stuffiness to a profuse, bland discharge. Commonly, those whom this remedy will suit also have asthma. Breathing is easier when sufferers lie down with their arms spread wide apart, and is worse when they sit up.

### *Pulsatilla* (wind flower)

This remedy picture describes a yellow-coloured discharge from the eyes and nose. The latter is stuffed up, particularly the right nostril. The symptoms of the nose and eyes are made worse in a warm room and are improved by being outside in the fresh air. The person that this remedy suits is probably of a tearful disposition, has fair hair, dislikes warm environments, prefers fresh air and dislikes fatty food.

### *Rosa damascena* (damask rose)

This remedy picture describes a non-irritant, watery discharge from both the eyes and the nose. The significant feature of this remedy is that the Eustachian tube is involved, causing difficulty in hearing and TINNITUS.

### *Sabadilla* (cevadilla seed)

This remedy picture describes spasmodic sneezing attacks, producing a runny nose with severe frontal (above the eyes) headaches, and an associated watering of the eyes. The eyelids are red and swollen. The person feels worse in the cold, and is nervous, timid and easily startled.

### *Sanguinaria* (blood root)

This remedy picture describes a profuse nasal discharge that is offensive in smell and yellow in colour. The eye discharge is bland and non-irritant. The person may well have NASAL POLYPS (*see below*). The face is usually red, and the cheeks have a burning sensation.

### *Silicea* (pure flint)

This remedy picture describes sufferers who have sneezing attacks in the morning. They have lost their sense of smell, and the bones around their noses are sensitive to the touch. A peculiar symptom is the itchiness right at the tip of the nose. The tear ducts are swollen, and sufferers' eyes are sensitive to light (photophobia).

### *Wyethia* (poison weed)

The characteristic feature of this remedy picture is an irritation and itching sensation at the back of the nose with a stuffed-up feeling in it that is not relieved by clearing the throat or by blowing.

## Nasal polyps

Persistent irritation of the mucous membrane lining the nose, from hay fever and allergic rhinitis, can cause the membrane to protrude and form visible polyps. These can cause obstruction to breathing through the nostrils and a reduction in the sense of smell, and can block the entrance to the sinuses, leading to attacks of sinusitis.

Conventional treatment is the correct approach and involves minor surgery.

The following homeopathic remedies are applicable in treating nasal polyps. However, they should only be taken while awaiting surgery, or as a preventive following the operation to prevent the recurrence of polyps. While awaiting surgery, use the 6c potency and give one dose four times a day. As a preventive, use the 30c potency and give one dose once a week.

## Calcarea carbonica (calcium carbonate)

This remedy picture describes a situation where sufferers develop a cold every time the weather changes. Their nostrils feel sore and easily become ulcerated. There is an offensive odour coming from the nose, which is seen to contain polyps. The catarrhal symptoms seem to worsen when sufferers are hungry.

## Lemna minor (duckweed)

In a healthy subject, this remedy acts especially on the nostrils, causing a pain as if a string is being pulled between the nostrils and the ears. A putrid odour emerges from the nostrils in which nasal polyps may be seen.

## Phosphorus

This remedy picture describes a nose that is oversensitive to odours and can sense imaginary ones. Sufferers have a continuous catarrhal nasal discharge so that they always keep plenty of tissues handy. Nasal polyps are a frequent occurrence, and they have a tendency to bleed easily.

## Sanguinaria (blood root)

This remedy picture describes a nose that has a profuse yellowish discharge that smells offensive. Nasal polyps are a common feature. It is common for diarrhoea to follow a cold that produces a nasal discharge.

## Teucrium marum (cat thyme)

This remedy picture is one in which the nasal and rectal symptoms are marked. There is a continuous nasal discharge from both the front of the nostrils and the back of the nose into the mouth. There is a crawling sensation in each nostril associated with much tear production and sneezing attacks. Nasal polyps are a very common feature. The rectal symptoms include a constant irritation and itching around the anus, particularly in the evening when in bed.

### *Thuja occidentalis* (arbor vitae)

This remedy picture describes a nasal discharge consisting of thick, green mucus that contains blood and pus. On blowing their noses, sufferers feel pain in their teeth. Nasal polyps are commonly found.

# Vasomotor rhinitis

This condition causes a stuffed-up feeling in the nose that can occur at any time of the year and is due to the blood vessels in the nostrils becoming swollen (vasodilated). This may be due to a continuing allergic reaction or a rebound reaction to overuse of nasal sprays, paradoxically employed to help alleviate the nasal stuffiness.

This is a condition that conventional therapy can do little to help.

Homeopathic treatment is best obtained through consultation with a specialist homeopath who will be able to consider sufferers' symptoms with their general profile. If this is not possible, the following two remedies can be used. Select the one whose remedy picture matches the current physical symptoms. The 6c potency should be given as one dose four times a day for two weeks, reducing to one dose twice a day until the symptoms abate.

### *Lycopodium* (club moss)

The characteristic feature in this remedy picture is an unstable circulatory system, so that the person may have one red ear while the other is of normal colour or one foot that is hot while the the other is cold. Similarly the nose can become blocked without any obvious reason. The symptoms tend to be worse between 4.00 and 8.00 pm, and sufferers' noses tend to be more blocked on the right side than the left. They have a preference for sweet, warm foods, become anxious in anticipation of important events and don't like being left on their own.

### Sanguinaria (blood root)

This remedy picture has for its main features vasomotor disturbances, as seen in flushing of the face and periodic burning of the
soles of the feet and palms of the hands. Similarly the nose can
become periodically blocked up. This remedy particularly suits a
woman who is going through the menopause.

If neither of these remedies match the physical symptoms of
the person, the remedies described in the section on hayfever and
allergic rhinitis may be considered, using the dosage schedule
given at the beginning of this section on vasomotor rhinitis.

# Eye Problems

T he eyes consist of an outer, relatively hard exterior – the eyeball – over which lies a thin membrane (the conjunctiva). The front part of the eyeball is the translucent cornea, through which light passes, going on to strike the light-sensitive receivers of the retina at the back of the eyeball, which translate the light energy into nervous impulses. These travel via the optic nerve to the brain, where the impulses are "seen".

It is important to treat any illness of the eyes. If there is pain with blurring of vision, an immediate consultation with a medical practitioner is indicated.

The following section deals with eye problems for which homeopathy can be used as a method of therapy. The dosage schedules are described with each remedy.

## Black eye and other eye injuries

Black eyes are caused by direct trauma so that the soft skin tissue around the eye socket becomes bruised.

The following homeopathic remedies are applicable to this condition.

### *Arnica* (leopard's bane)

This remedy picture describes bruising on any part of the body. Using the 30c potency, give one dose immediately, followed by a second dose 30 minutes later. Then, using the 6c potency, continue the treatment by giving the remedy every four hours for one day, reducing the frequency to one dose of 6c potency four times a day until the bruising settles.

If the bruising is more extensive, involving the eyelid and possibly the conjunctiva, use the following remedies, selecting the right one by matching the remedy picture with the physical symptoms. Use the same dosage schedule as for *Arnica*.

### *Hypericum* (St John's wort)

This remedy picture describes a situation where the remedy is useful for controlling pain from nerves crushed through injury. It is a useful pain-killer that can be given after the medical practitioner has treated the injury. Using the 30c potency, give one dose twice a day for one week, reducing to one dose on alternate days until the pain subsides.

### *Ledum* (marsh tea)

Appropriate where there is bruising of the eyelids and the conjunctiva. The injury feels better when a cold compress is applied. Using the 30c potency, give one dose twice a day for one week, reducing to one dose on alternate days until the pain subsides.

If the eyeball itself has become injured, it is important to seek medical attention. The above remedies can be used as an immediate first aid therapy, but the following one can also be considered.

### *Symphytum* (comfrey)

This remedy picture describes pain following a blunt, penetrating injury to the eye. Using the 6c potency, give one dose four times a day until the medical practitioner has diagnosed the nature of the problem. The remedy can be continued after the medical practitioner has done this, being given until the pain from the injury has subsided. It can be safely used as a complementary therapy with whatever conventional treatment is offered.

## Blepharitis

This is an inflammation of the eyelids, caused by bacterial infection or as part of an allergic reaction. The conventional treatment is with antibiotic tablets, an antibiotic steroid ointment or drops.

Homeopathic treatment is, using the 6c potency, to give one dose of one of the following remedies every two hours for a maximum of 12 doses. If there is no improvement, consult a medical practitioner. If the condition is long-lasting, use the 30c potency and give one dose on alternate days for three weeks.

### *Apis mellifica* (honey bee)

This remedy picture describes eyelids that are swollen, red and burn and sting. The inflammation can turn into a localized collection of pus called a STYE (*see below*).

### *Graphites* (black lead)

This remedy picture describes eyelids that are red and swollen. The skin on them is dry and may show eczema producing a honey-coloured discharge. The eyes have a tendency to ache, particularly when the person looks into artificial light.

### *Mercurius-hydrargyrum* (quicksilver)

This remedy picture shows red, thick and swollen eyelids. They feel as if they are burning, and there is a discharge of pus. This condition is commonly caused by exposure to the glare of a fire or an arc-welding operation.

### *Pulsatilla* (wind flower)

This remedy picture describes red, swollen eyelids that may show an accumulation of pus, forming a stye; there is a yellow-coloured discharge. If the blepharitis is a continuing problem and the person also notices indigestion, this remedy will suit him or her. The symptoms are made worse in a warm room.

## Cataract

When the lens of the eye begins to alter its make-up – in old age, through illnesses such as DIABETES MELLITUS, in newborn babies who have been exposed to a too high concentration of oxygen – the vision starts to become misty. If it advances to a degree that the person is unable to see, surgical removal of the lens is the correct approach. Usually one eye is affected more than the other, so that the surgical removal is made one at a time.

Several homeopathic remedies can be used in the early stages of cataract formation, and certainly when the vision has deteriorated to the extent that an operation has become necessary.

### *Calcarea carbonica* (calcium carbonate)

This remedy picture describes a dimness of vision as if looking through a mist. The pupils are permanently dilated and the eyes are consequently very sensitive to light (photophobia). The general profile of this person will help point to this remedy: cold, sweats easily from the head, obstinate and tends to be constipated. Using the 6c potency, give one dose four times a day for two weeks, reducing to twice a day until vision improves.

### *Calcarea fluorica* (calcium fluoride)

The remedy picture describes flickering of the eyes with sparks appearing in front of them. Granular spots are to be found on the white of the eyes, and cataracts are commonly found. This remedy is very good at dissolving hard, stony lumps. Using the 6c potency, give one dose four times a day for two weeks, reducing to twice a day until the vision begins to improve.

### *Cineraria* (dusty miller)

This remedy picture describes a cataract together with corneal opacities. This remedy is particularly useful following any trauma. Using the mother tincture, place one drop into the affected eye four times a day for several months.

## *Ledum* (marsh tea)

This remedy picture describes cataract formation in a person who also suffers from gout, although the gout is not the cause of cataract formation. Using the 6c potency, give one dose four times a day for two weeks, reducing to twice a day until the vision begins to improve.

## *Naphthaline* (coal tar derivative)

This remedy picture describes a person who may suffer from hayfever, and eye symptoms that include cataract formation with possible corneal opacities. The person may have a past medical history of a detached retina. Using the 6c potency, give one dose four times a day for two weeks, reducing to twice a day until the vision begins to improve.

## *Phosphorus*

This remedy picture describes a sensation as if a veil had been pulled over the eyes, or a mist or dust has appeared in front of the visual field. Black objects seem to float in sufferers' visual fields, and they find that these are improved if they shield their eyes with a hand held to one side. Candlelight appears to be surrounded by a green halo, and black letters appear red in colour. Sufferers develop tired eyes and a headache without having used their eyes very much. Those whom this remedy suits also have a fear of thunderstorms. Using the 6c potency, give one dose four times a day for two weeks, reducing to twice a day until the vision begins to improve.

## *Quassia* (quassia wood)

This remedy picture describes a marked action on the eyes and gastric organs. It causes cataract formation in healthy people, who will also have flatulence and acid reflux. Using the 6c potency, give one dose four times a day for two weeks, reducing to twice a day until the vision begins to improve.

### *Silicea* (pure flint)

This remedy picture describes sufferers who have an aversion to light (photophobia), especially daylight, which causes a dazzling, sharp pain that goes right through the eyes so that they are tender to the touch, particularly when closed. Vision is confused so that letters appear to run into one another. Those for whom this remedy will be particularly suitable tend to have sweaty feet that smell. Using the 6c potency, give one dose twice a day for six months, and then one dose daily thereafter.

# Conjunctivitis

This is an inflammation of the conjunctiva covering the eyeballs and lining the eyelids, caused by an infection or an allergy. If the person wakes up with a yellow discharge from the eyes, this usually means that the cause is a bacterial infection. This is a common illness in newborn babies. An allergy generally makes the person feel as if there is grit in the eyes; there is no discharge, but the whites of their eyes become red. The conventional treatment is to use antibiotic drops.

Homeopathic remedies can treat both allergic and bacterial conjunctivitis. If it is due to an allergy, it is important to identify the relevant allergen and remove or avoid it. Using the 6c potency, give one dose of one of the following remedies every one hour for a maximum of 12 doses. If there is no improvement, seek medical advice.

### *Aconitum napellus* (monk's-hood)

This remedy picture describes conjunctivitis that has been brought on by accidental injury or from exposure to cold, windy weather. The remedy is associated with anxiety and fear of death.

### *Argentum nitricum* (silver nitrate)

This remedy picture describes eyes that have a profuse, purulent discharge from the conjunctiva. The eyelids are sore, red and swollen. The eyes become easily strained when doing close, detailed work, a symptom that is made worse in a warm room. This remedy is associated with fear of heights and of crowds. The person likes both salt and sugar.

### *Euphrasia* (eyebright)

This remedy picture describes an eye discharge that is non-purulent and profuse.

### *Pulsatilla* (wind flower)

This remedy picture describes eyes that are itchy and burning. The eyelids are inflamed, and the discharge coming from the eyes is profuse and yellow. The person may suffer from indigestion at the same time. All the symptoms are made worse in a hot atmosphere. The general picture of the person that this remedy will particularly suit weeps easily and often, prefers fresh air and dislikes arguments and fatty foods.

# Detached retina

The retina usually detaches itself from the back of the eye as a result of trauma. The initial symptoms are flashing lights and black, floating shapes like a cobweb in the eye, followed by a loss of vision, first in the peripheral visual field, then in the central part.

Detached retina usually occurs in one eye only and needs emergency medical treatment. The retina can be reattached to the back of the eye through laser therapy.

Homeopathic treatment is only applicable while awaiting medical attention, and as a preventative against a recurrence or against the same problem occurring in the other eye (more likely to occur in someone who has already had a detached retina).

For the immediate treatment, use the 6c potency and give one dose every 30 minutes until the medical practitioner has assessed the problem. As a preventative, use the 30c potency and give one dose twice a week.

### Gelsemium (yellow jasmine)

This remedy picture describes sufferers whose eyelids feel so heavy that they can hardly be lifted open. Their vision is not particularly good, and they may well be suffering from GLAUCOMA (see below). They are likely to develop a detached retina. Those whom this remedy particularly suits tend to suffer from anxiety, as if they were always about to take an examination.

### Naphthaline (coal tar derivative)

This remedy picture describes a marked affinity for the eye and includes detachment of the retina. It also describes cataract formation and opacities in the cornea. The person may well have hayfever and an irritation in any part of the urinary system.

## Glaucoma

This condition is the result of a build-up of pressure in the front chamber of the eye caused by a blockage in the normal flow of fluid between the front and rear chambers, due to a problem with the muscular iris, which usually regulates the flow. This pressure build-up leads to a breakdown of the retina, the visually sensitive part of the eye, and can lead to blindness. For this reason, conventional treatment is absolutely necessary. This may include eyedrops to control the muscle of iris, to keep it constricted, as well as an operation to create a new passage between the front and back of the eye. There is usually a family history of glaucoma, and if this is the case, regular eye checks are important to assess eye pressure. Homeopathy plays a very small part in therapy.

The early symptom of glaucoma is redness of the cornea, particularly at night when the pupil of the eye is widely dilated. As the pressure increases, the cornea becomes cloudy and the eyeball tender to the touch. The person may begin to vomit and feel tired.

In this situation, it is important to seek medical advice. While awaiting this, one of the following remedies can be used. Using the 6c potency, give one dose every 15 minutes for a maximum of 12 doses, reducing to one dose every hour for a maximum of 12 doses, then further reducing to one dose every four hours until medical advice is received.

### Aconitum napellus (monk's-hood)

This remedy picture describes eyes that feel dry as if there is sand in them. The person may notice shooting pains in them and be uncomfortable when looking at objects that have sun reflected off them. Their eyes have a staring quality to them.

### Belladonna (deadly nightshade)

The eye symptoms of this remedy include a throbbing pain deep in the eyes, which is worse when the person lies down and when he or she looks at the light (photophobia). The eyes are red and they feel swollen. The vision becomes blurred.

### Colocynthis (bitter cucumber)

This remedy picture describes violent pains within the eye before sufferers develop glaucoma. As the eyes become stony hard, they notice their eyelids twitching and becoming painful.

### Phosphorus

This describes distortions of vision with flashes of light and the appearance of red, green and black haloes around objects. These haloes are made more apparent when the person shades his or her eyes. The general profile of the person, which will help in the selection of this remedy, includes a fear of thunderstorms.

### Physostigma (calabar bean)

This remedy picture describes the onset of glaucoma following an injury to the eye.

# Stye

This is an infection at the root of an eyelash, which can lead to a boil. The conventional treatment is to prescribe an antibiotic as well as investigating illnesses, such as DIABETES MELLITUS, that could predispose a person to this type of infection.

Both homeopathically and conventionally, it is important for sufferers from styes to boost their immune systems by taking extra vitamin C – at least one gram a day – and not rub their eyes with dirty fingers. Homeopathic treatment is best obtained by consultation with a specialist homeopath who will be able to not only treat the particular problem but also the person as a whole. If such a consultation is not possible, the following homeopathic remedies can be considered. Using the 6c potency, give one dose four times a day until the stye begins to resolve.

### *Pulsatilla* (wind flower)

This remedy picture describes eyelids that are inflamed, leading to stye formation. The person may suffer from indigestion and feels much worse exposed to heat. The general profile of the person that this remedy will particularly suit is that he or she prefers fresh air and dislikes a warm atmosphere and fatty foods.

### *Staphysagria* (stavesacre)

This remedy picture describes recurrent stye formation. The eyeballs appear sunken and surrounded by blue rings, and are so hot that any spectacles that are worn become misted over. The eyelids are itchy. This picture also describes a person who feels indignant.

# Twitching eyelids

In the absence of other symptoms and signs of eye problems, the cause of this twitching is nervous tension, fatigue or anxiety.

Conventional treatment is to discover and eradicate the basic cause of this tension, fatigue or anxiety.

The homeopathic treatment is best obtained through consultation with a specialist homeopath, but the following remedies may be used as a basic therapy. Using the 6c potency, give one dose every four hours for a maximum of ten doses.

### *Agaricus muscarius* (toadstool)

This remedy describes twitching of many muscle groups. The eye symptoms include not only twitching of the eyelids but also the whole eyeball, so that the person finds that print moves up and down.

### *Codeinum* (alkaloid of opium)

This picture describes twitching and trembling of the whole body. These twitches are associated with sensations of itchiness and warmth. The eyelids have a marked involuntary twitch.

### *Zincum metallicum* (zinc)

This remedy picture describes a worn-out person who has multiple twitches in his or her body including in the eyelids. The person feels better when eating a meal and worse when touched.

# Lower Respiratory Tract Illnesses

This section deals with the treatment of the following illnesses: asthma, bronchitis, laryngitis, pleurisy and pneumonia.

Before antibiotics and bronchodilators were discovered, homeopathy was the only method of therapy available for treating these conditions and as such, it was successful. However, in today's medical climate, it is important to obtain a conventional medical opinion on these illnesses as they are potentially serious and even life-threatening, and on the decision whether antibiotic and bronchodilator therapy should always be considered the best therapeutic option.

If it is decided to use conventional therapy, a homeopathic remedy can still be used alongside it. Homeopathy is able to work as a complementary form of therapy and not necessarily as a strictly alternative therapy. The homeopathic remedy does not interfere with conventional medical therapy, nor do the vast majority of conventional medicines interfere with homeopathic remedies. In fact, prednisolone and codeine are the only two conventional drugs that have a diminishing effect on the action of homeopathic remedies.

Prednisolone is a valuable drug used in the treatment of asthma and should not be withdrawn without first obtaining medical advice. By using homeopathic remedies with this drug, it is possible that the amount of prednisolone needed to maintain respiratory health can be reduced. However, any reduction must be planned with the medical practitioner.

When using homeopathy to treat chest illnesses, the "layer principle" applies. This means that, as the person's condition changes, so the choice of remedy will need to be amended.

When selecting an initial remedy or indeed a subsequent one (when the person's condition has changed), check the remedy pictures given below, matching the remedy that suits the person's symptoms most closely and remembering the importance of the "similar principle" in homeopathy – that "like cures like".

# Asthma

Asthma is defined as chronic, reversible obstructive airways disease. Physically, this means wheezy breathing, although nowadays the term "asthma" is also used to describe an unremitting cough. Therefore, asthma must be considered as a possible diagnosis when a person has a persistent cough with or without a noticeable wheeze. Asthma is a serious disease for which medical opinion must be sought, as it is possible for the person to have complete respiratory failure. (For information on treating asthma in children, see p. 441.)

Asthma can be due to several factors: allergy, infection or some inherited predisposition. If it is obvious what the allergic cause of the asthma is, this obviously has to be avoided. Pet fur is a common culprit, and staying away from the causative pet is essential. However, the identified pet can also be "made" into a homeopathic remedy: cat or dog hair can be turned into a remedy of a potency of 6c, which can be taken as one dose twice a day every day until the symptoms are under control. The house dust mite is another common allergen, and similarly this can be made into a 6c potency remedy to be given as one dose twice a day. In both of these examples, it is important to remove these initiating factors in the person's environment as completely as possible.

The use of homeopathy in treating asthma is quite complicated and therefore is best treated by a specialist homeopath. If this is not possible, the following remedies can be used to help treat asthma, but **the conventional drug therapy must not be discontinued**.

# Hahnemann's miasm theory

The homeopath regards asthma as a deep-seated illness that has arisen as a result of the suppression of a more superficial illness. An example is the treatment of ECZEMA with steroid creams, the skin disease being regarded as the superficial condition and the lung disease as the deeper problem. This means that the homeopath's approach differs from the conventional approach.

Hahnemann was the first to see the link between superficial illness and deep-seated illness. Skin diseases represent superficial illnesses that, if suppressed and not cured at a deep, fundamental level by using homeopathy, will produce other illnesses such as asthma. Therefore, when treating one illness homeopathically, another related illness may be revealed during the process of curing. So, when treating asthma, eczema can occur or recur.

This suppression of chronic illness and its importance in treating deep-seated illness led Hahnemann to consider the term *miasm* (from the Greek for "pollution"). In his time, chronic illness was believed to be caused by one of three things: syphilis, gonorrhoea and itchy skin problems like scabies. Hahnemann reclassified these three illnesses as miasms and gave two of them new names: gonorrhoea became "sycosis" and scabies became "psora". For these new miasms, he prepared a new type of homeopathic remedy made from the diseases themselves. This is called a *nosode*, and from these illnesses, Hahnemann produced three specific remedies: respectively, *Syphilinum, Medorhinum* and *Psorinum*.

In the homeopathic treatment of chronic asthma (and indeed all chronic illnesses), the initial assessment of an individual must include an assessment of that person's miasmic state. This by no means suggests that a person has had syphilis, gonorrhoea or scabies, nor any of their immediate family. However, since Hahnemann's time, a more modern interpretation of his theories has emerged so that today it is possible to relate modern illnesses to the old miasms.

In addition, since Hahnemann came up with his theories, it has been recognized that a number of other diseases cause chronic, suppressed illness and should be included as miasms. These diseases (and their appropriate nosode preparations) are: glandular fever (*Glandular fever nosode*), measles (*Morbillinum*), tuberculosis (*Tuberculinum*) and cancer (*Carcinosin*).

## Finding and taking the correct nosode

When treating an individual for a condition such as asthma, the person's personal history and family history will be taken, and from these facts, all the above conditions will be embraced and from this, a single miasm will emerge as a significant feature. The appropriate nosode is then selected and used at the start of any long-term treatment. Using the 30c potency, give one dose daily for three days. No further homeopathic remedy should be given for at least two weeks following this initial schedule. The nosode can then be repeated after a period of one month if the symptoms have not improved.

After the two weeks from the initial dose of the miasmic nosode, an appropriate homeopathic remedy relevant to the overall physical picture can be given. This is selected in the usual way by matching the physical presentation with the remedy pictures given below. The suggested dosage schedule – for babies, older children and adults – is, using the 30c potency, give one dose daily for three days and then work out the minimum dose needed to keep the symptoms at bay.

An appropriate nosode in the 30c potency can also be given as a single dose in an acute asthma attack, and then repeated every four hours to a maximum of three doses or, if a 6c potency is used, every 15 minutes to a maximum of six doses (see the end of this section on asthma for emergency treatment).

The remedy pictures of the nosodes follow. Five other remedies are included that are not nosodes but are regarded as deep-acting remedies.

### *Glandular fever nosode* (gland from a person who has suffered from glandular fever)

This remedy picture describes a person who develops asthma following an attack of GLANDULAR FEVER or has a significant family history of that illness.

### *Medorhinum* (gonorrhoeal bacteria)

This remedy picture describes people who feel better lying on their stomachs when not having an asthma attack; when having an attack, they feel better with their knees supporting the body and leaning on their elbows. The asthma is improved when sufferers are by the seaside, but symptoms are worse during the day. These people also develop anxiety in anticipation of forthcoming events.

### *Psorinum* (scabies vesicle)

This remedy picture describes people whose asthma returns every time the weather turns colder, and who develop hayfever at the appropriate time of the year. Their breathing is easier when they lie flat with their arms spread wide apart, and is made worse in the open air. They feel sad and that death is on the horizon or that they will have a personal business failure. In homeopathic jargon, such an individual is a "chilly type of *Sulphur*".

### *Syphilinum* (syphilitic chancre)

This remedy picture describes symptoms that are characteristically worse at night, on lying down and during a thunderstorm. They are aggravated from sunset to sunrise (the night is a dreadful time). The person notices a peculiar sensation as if the sternum (breastbone) is being drawn down into the vertebrae of the spine.

### *Tuberculinum* (nucleo-protein from tubercular abscess)

This remedy picture is selected for a person with asthma who has a strong personal or family history of tuberculosis (but it should not be given in cases where the person has active tuberculosis). The person seems to take a cold every time fresh air is inhaled and yet paradoxically the person craves for fresh air. The person has a fear of animals, dogs in particular.

### *Drosera* (sundew)

This remedy picture is indicated for asthma following an attack of WHOOPING COUGH and also, but not essentially, for those with a personal or family history of TUBERCULOSIS. The wheeziness is brought on by the spasmodic cough and whenever the person begins to talk. The symptoms are worse when he or she is lying down and, of course, when the person goes to bed – the asthma is at its worst particularly late at night.

### *Pulsatilla* (wind flower)

This remedy picture describes symptoms that show great variability and which come and go very quickly. The cough is worse in the evening and at night, when sufferers feel a need to sit up in bed to get relief from this irritating symptom. They also feel a sensation of firm pressure on their chests and stomachs. All the symptoms are made worse with heat of any form, and sufferers feel better for – and therefore feel an overwhelming need for – fresh air. They also respond well to physical and emotional support and positively dislike disharmony, going to great lengths to avoid arguments. They strongly dislike fatty food, and probably weep easily and often. The *Pulsatilla* person has a lack of thirst and has to be strongly encouraged to take fluids.

## Silicea (pure flint)

This remedy picture has a characteristic feature in that the remedy suits those people with sweaty feet and who find an improvement in their symptoms by wrapping up their heads. Their coughing becomes violent when they lie down and is improved in wet and/or humid conditions. They have a fear of needles.

—

## Sulphur

This remedy picture describes people who feel better with the windows flung wide open. They feel as if there is a heavy load on their chests, with pain going through to their backs that is made worse when they lie on their backs and is improved when they sit up. The chest rattles with mucus, particularly at 11.00 am. The shortness of breath is worse in the small hours of the morning. These individuals find that every cold turns into asthma (a symptom shared with *Dulcamara*, but the latter is an acute remedy while *Sulphur* is a deeper-acting remedy that will probably be used after *Dulcamara*). *Sulphur* individuals are, in an holistic way, warm physically and hungry, often crave fatty food and tend to kick off the bed clothes in order to cool down their overheated feet. In homeopathic jargon, the *Sulphur* person is a "ragged philosopher" – a person who has an instant opinion on every subject, is always good for a laugh, hates criticism but is emotionally very demonstrative.

## Thuja occidentalis (arbor vitae)

This remedy picture has a characteristic feature in that the illness follows on from a recent immunization. A peculiar symptom is that the person only sweats on the uncovered parts of their body. The symptoms are worse at 3.00 am and in cold, damp situations. It is a left-sided remedy in that other symptoms tend to occur on the left side. The person commonly dreams of falling from a height.

---

## Emergency treatment for the acute asthma attack

**If someone suffers an acute asthma attack, medical treatment must be obtained as a matter of urgency.** The following homeopathic schedule can be followed while waiting for medical attention. It is designed to give symptomatic relief and not a long-term cure, so ignore Hahnemann's miasmic theories at this critical stage.

Just give the appropriate remedy that matches the physical picture (using the "like cures like" principle) in a 6c potency. One dose can be given every 15 minutes for a maximum of six doses. The remedy can be given in liquid or powder form. In liquid form, one dose is one drop for babies and two drops for older children and adults.

---

## After an asthma attack

Once an asthma attack has been satisfactorily treated, a longer-term strategy can be devised, using miasmic theories to obtain a fundamental cure of the underlying problem. The dosage schedule is as mentioned at the beginning of this section: a 30c potency, one dose to be given daily for three days. The aim is to match the individual requirement with the minimum amount of homeopathic remedy, and the dosage schedule is ultimately decided by the individual's reaction to the remedy. This will differ from person to person, so it is impossible to make hard-and-fast rules about dosage schedules. Therefore, only broad guidelines will be given here. If the remedy picture fits, but the timings below do not, you should still choose that remedy.

*Remedy pictures according to the time when symptoms are at their worst*

11.00 pm
*Aralia racemosa* (American spikenard)

This remedy picture describes a person's asthma that develops when they lie down to go to sleep. It starts as a spasmodic cough usually at 11.00 pm, and there is a feeling of a lump in the throat. Unusually the least current of air causes sneezing with a copious nasal discharge. The sputum tastes salty; this is an unusual but distinctive symptom.

## 1.00–2.00 am
### Arsenicum album (arsenic trioxide)

This remedy picture describes chest symptoms that are at their worst between 1.00 and 2.00 am. They are made better by sufferers leaning forward and from gentle rocking movements. Sufferers feel worse when subjected to cold air and better when heat in any form is applied. Therefore they feel worse when given ice cream and better for hot drinks. They find lying in bed physically uncomfortable, are extremely anxious and are full of fears, particularly of dying. The *Arsenicum* person is very restless and finds it difficult to keep still.

## 2.00–4.00 am
### Kali carbonicum (potassium carbonate)

This remedy picture describes people who have asthma attacks that are worse in the middle of the night and in the cold and particularly when they are subjected to a draught. The infection affects mainly the lower right chest. Sufferers notice stabbing pains in their chests, which occur independently of breathing. Coughing and breathing are made easier when they sit up and lean forward with their heads on their knees or on a table. They also find breathing easier when they make rocking movements of their whole body. They find it impossible to lie on their backs and difficult to lie on their right sides (the *Bryonia* person prefers lying on the affected side or on the back).

## 3.00 am
### Cuprum metallicum (copper)

This remedy picture describes asthma that is characterized by violent spasmodic coughing lasting one to three hours and which then suddenly stops. The person feels a strong sense of suffocation. The attacks are worse at 3.00 am and are usually accompanied by vomiting and spasms of the whole body. An unusual symptom (and therefore of great significance) is a strong metallic taste in the mouth.

## 4.00 am
### Natrum sulphuricum (sodium sulphate)

This remedy picture describes asthma symptoms that affect the lower lobe of the left lung. The chest symptoms are associated with wheezing and are made worse in damp weather and damp conditions. All the symptoms are worse between 4.00 and 5.00 am. Every cold seems to bring on an asthma attack in people of a susceptible disposition.

### Nux vomica (poison-nut)

This remedy picture describes asthma that comes on with every stomach upset: having gone to bed, sufferers wake up with a feeling that something has disagreed with them; they sit up and the asthma attack starts, usually at 4.00 am. They crave stimulants such as alcohol and caffeine, something to brace the person as a whole. They tend to be perfectionists and are very ambitious.

## 4.00–8.00 pm
### Lycopodium (club moss)

This remedy picture describes chest symptoms that are worse in the late afternoon, between 4.00 and 8.00 pm, and are associated with abdominal distension, with a slow and disordered digestion. Sufferers feel more comfortable when they have their clothes loosened. They tend to have a frown on their forehead, as though they are carrying the worries of the world. They do not like being left on their own, particularly at sundown.

*Remedies that are indicated when certain atmospheric conditions make symptoms worse*

## Damp, wet, cold
### *Dulcamara* (bittersweet)

This remedy picture describes chest symptoms that are brought on by cold, wet and damp conditions, and are made worse by physical exertion. These symptoms are relieved by the application of warmth and by the person moving about.

## Cold, dry
### *Aconitum napellus* (monk's-hood)

This remedy picture describes chest symptoms that come on suddenly and violently, causing sufferers to become very anxious and fearful, particularly of dying. The symptoms result from being exposed to cold, dry winds and from fright, shock and overall worries. *Aconitum* is never indicated when sufferers are patient and calm. Their emotions are like a great storm that sweeps over everyone and then passes away. They feel better in a warm room and at night. See also *Spongia tosta* below.

### *Antimonium tartaricum* (antimonium tartrate)

This remedy picture describes a chest that sounds very rattly as though it is full of mucus, but coughing produces very little sputum. The coughing makes sufferers feel very weak and exhausted, and they feel better sitting up and by being supported in this position. They become uninterested in eating or drinking, and are irritable, not wanting to be touched or disturbed. The symptoms are worse in damp and cold weather, but can also feel worse from warmth.

### *Hepar sulphuris* (Hahnemann's calcium sulphide)

This remedy picture describes people who have a croaky cough and voice. Any cough is worse in the morning, and they feel that they have to bend their head backwards. They can become quite depressed, even contemplating suicide. They feel more comfortable in a warm and moist atmosphere.

### Spongia tosta (roasted sponge)

This remedy picture describes people who have fears and anxieties similar to the remedy picture of *Aconitum*. The physical difference between the two pictures is that *Spongia* has more severe spasm of the larynx (voice box) than *Aconitum*. The sputum is white and difficult to expectorate and has to be swallowed. These people feel more comfortable in a warm, moist atmosphere.

### Warm, wet
### Carbo vegetabilis (vegetable charcoal)

This remedy picture describes asthma that is associated with a lot of flatulence and stomach distension. Sufferers feel a desperate need for cool air to be fanned over their faces. They collapse and feel exhausted. These attacks come on in damp conditions.

### Lachesis (bushmaster snake venom)

This remedy picture describes an asthma attack that may well start in the middle of the night while sufferers are asleep or as they wake up. They feel better bending forward and worse when covering their mouths or touching their larynxes (voice boxes). They feel uncomfortable when wearing anything tight around their neck, when moving their arms and after talking. The sort of person that *Lachesis* suits well has a purple complexion, is suspicious and a chatter-box.

*Several remedies that have their own separate, distinctive features*

### Ambra grisea (ambergis, a secretion of the whale)

This remedy picture describes people who are nervous and whose asthmatic symptoms are much worse in the presence of other people. The coughing is associated with much flatulence. The sufferers and their symptoms are made worse by listening to music and anything out of the normal routine. The asthmatic symptoms come on with only the minimum of exercise.

### Bromium (bromine)

This remedy picture describes sufferers who notice a cold sensation in their chests whenever they inhale. The associated cough is spasmodic, and the asthmatic symptoms are improved when at sea. This remedy, therefore, is of particular use to sailors who develop asthma when they return to land duties – they feel a sensation as if smoke is filling their lungs. A peculiar symptom (and therefore of great significance) is that their larynx feels cold. It is a useful remedy to follow *Pulsatilla*, as *Bromium* shares many of the same general profile symptoms.

### Kali nitricum (potassium nitrate)

This remedy picture describes sufferers with asthma who, apart from breathlessness, also feel stitches in their chests. The breathlessness is such that they are unable to drink properly and can only manage a sip at a time. This drinking of sips of water makes them feel better and is a distinctive feature of this remedy.

### Lobelia inflata (Indian tobacco)

This remedy picture describes an asthma attack that is preceded by a pricking sensation all over the body, including the fingers and toes. The shortness of breath is accompanied by a sensation of constriction in the chest. There is also a sensation of pressure on the chest that is made easier by walking quickly. The person's urine is coloured a deep red and contains a lot of red sediment.

### Naja tripudians (cobra venom)

This remedy picture describes a person who feels constriction in the chest and throat. It is commonly associated with people with heart conditions. They commonly wake up gasping and choking (like *Lachesis*), and find it difficult to lie on their left side.

# Bronchitis

This is an infection of the smaller airways of the lungs, descending from the main windpipe (trachea). It can affect the young child as well as the older person. The cause is either viral or bacterial, and it is commonly preceded by a cold. This illness is classified as either acute (a sudden one-off illness during which the person usually has a fever) or chronic (a continuing illness).

The evolution of bronchitis from acute to chronic is made "easier" if the person smokes (either actively or "passively") or is overweight. As prevention is better than cure, it is important to pay attention to these two causative factors. If the chronic bronchitis continues for a long time, the lung tissue becomes permanently destroyed and a more serious condition called emphysema ensues.

If the person becomes feverish with chronic bronchitis or emphysema, and/or he or she begins to expectorate yellow or green sputum, medical advice should be sought, as antibiotic therapy might be the appropriate therapy.

However, homeopathy can be used alongside this approach. Use the remedy pictures below to select the appropriate remedy, matching the picture with the physical symptoms. Using the 30c potency, give one dose every six hours for the first day, reducing by one dose each day until a maintenance schedule of one dose a day is reached. This schedule is continued for a maximum of ten doses.

*Acute bronchitis*
## Aconitum napellus (monk's-hood)

This remedy is useful for any of the chest illnesses that are characterized by a very sudden onset of symptoms, particularly when sufferers have been chilled by cold but dry weather. They have a hard, dry, painful cough, their breathing rate is increased and their lungs feel congested and tight. They find it more comfortable to sit in an upright position. The larynx feels tender, and they are often found to be grasping it. Their throats feel dry and have a burning sensation. The sufferers themselves feel restless, anxious and fearful.

### Belladonna (deadly nightshade)

This remedy picture describes sufferers who not only have acute bronchitis but also have the characteristic features which will help select this remedy: a flushed face, fast heart rate, widely dilated pupils and possibly a delirious state of mind. They are often heard to moan with every breath.

### Bryonia (wild hops)

This remedy follows *Aconitum napellus* well. The person's cough is hard and painful, and the expectoration has now become thicker. Sufferers' lips and tongue are dry, and they are thirsty for large quantities of fluid. Each breath is painful, and breathing is, therefore, short and rapid as deep breathing causes so much pain. Sufferers prefer to lie perfectly still and on the painful side. The pains feel like stitches and are improved by the application of firm pressure.

### Ferrum phosphoricum (iron phosphate)

This remedy is to be used as the first choice in the treatment of the first stage of all inflammatory chest illnesses. The remedy picture describes people who have a short cough that is dry and painful. Their chests feel sore and they will almost certainly have a fever. This remedy is given as a single dose of the 30c potency. It can then be followed by one or more of the remedies below (matching the remedy picture to the physical symptoms), using the dosage schedule described at the beginning of this section.

## *Ipecacuanha* (ipecac root)

This remedy picture describes bronchitis in all age groups but is particularly useful in the treatment of the young and very young (i.e. babies). It is especially good at treating bronchitis during infancy: these children have a spasmodic cough, their chests rattling with supposed sputum but little is produced. However, sufferers can feel nauseated and indeed vomit. The remedy is not exclusively used for children: the key indication is coughing with nausea and vomiting.

## *Phosphorus*

Sufferers have a tight chest and a tickly cough that is quite dry. They are anxious and respond well to and need a lot of reassurance. They take a lot of sips of cold water, feel worse lying on their left side and are frightened in thunderstorms.

## *Pyrogenium* (artificial sepsin)

This remedy picture describes sufferers who have a fever and who sweat but the sweating does not bring down the body temperature. This oscillates rapidly, and the pulse rate can be out of proportion to the temperature. The tongue is fiery red and smooth. The person can become delirious and, in this state, develops a dual personality, during which time there is a struggle to put the apparently disorganized body together again. Sufferers often complain that the bed feels too hard.

### *Chronic bronchitis*

When this is diagnosed, it is important to treat any infection as quickly as possible since the person can easily develop PNEUMONIA and respiratory failure. It is important to seek medical opinion, as an antibiotic has to be a considered option.

Homeopathy can be used either on its own or with any conventional treatment in a complementary way. The following remedies can be considered, choosing the picture that most closely fits the person's particular symptoms. The remedies for the treatment of acute bronchitis should be considered in the initial stages of treatment of an infection, with the same dosage schedule. The following remedies can be used at a later stage when the infection has resolved. In this case, a dose of 6c three times a day will be helpful.

### *Antimonium tartaricum* (antimonium tartrate)

This remedy picture describes sufferers who have a very rattly chest that sounds as though it is full of mucus, but despite this, they find it very difficult to expectorate anything. They have short, rapid breathing that causes them to feel as if suffocation is not very far away. They are more comfortable in the sitting position. They feel dizzy when coughing, and coughing attacks alternate with gasping. Their pulse is weak and rapid.

### *Capsicum annuum* (cayenne pepper)

This remedy picture describes people who have an explosive cough that synchronously releases foul-smelling wind. Their faces are probably fat and flabby and certainly red but cold (the reverse of *Belladonna* which has a red and hot face).

### *Hippozaenium* (gladerine-allein and farcine)

This remedy picture describes noisy breathing that is short and irregular. Those it suits are older persons with chronic bronchitis who feel that suffocation is imminent.

### *Lachesis* (bushmaster snake venom)

This remedy picture describes sufferers whose larynxes are very sensitive to the touch and they dislike them being covered. All the symptoms are worse after sleep. The chest symptoms are improved by sufferers sitting up and, particularly, bending forward (a symptom shared with *Kali carbonicum*); they are made worse with pressure (the reverse of *Bryonia*). The cough can sometimes be an annoying tickle, as though food has gone down the wrong way. Generally the symptoms of *Lachesis* tend to be left-sided.

## *Lycopodium* (club moss)

This remedy picture describes a bronchitis where there is a constricting pain in the chest whenever sufferers cough. Their sputum is thick, commonly contains blood and has a salty taste. The general profile of sufferers will help select this remedy. Their foreheads tend to be frowning, and their symptoms deteriorate between 4.00 and 8.00 pm. They dislike cold food and drink, preferring warm. Holistically, they do not like being left alone, their symptoms tend to be right-sided and they probably have a history of urinary or digestive difficulties.

## *Phosphorus*

This remedy picture describes people whose chest symptoms include the feeling of a great weight on the chest, followed by the expectoration of bright-red blood and sputum that is rust-coloured and pus-filled, tastes sweet and salty and is cold. The chest infection is mainly on the lower lobe of the right lung. Sufferers notice stitching pains in their chests, particularly on the left side, but they are more comfortable lying on their right side. All the symptoms are made worse during thunderstorms. They feel thirsty for cold water (a symptom shared with *Bryonia*). They feel better after sleeping (the reverse of *Lachesis*), and they desire company as they fear being alone. The typical profile of the person that *Phosphorus* suits in a holistic way is tall and slender and has an artistic temperament.

## *Ranunculus bulbosus* (buttercup)

This remedy picture describes a person who may have a problem with alcohol. In a chest infection, the chest feels very sore, bruised and sensitive to the touch. These sore spots persist even after the infection has resolved. The person has bright red cheeks and a clean tongue.

### *Rhus toxicodendron* (poison ivy)

This remedy picture describes sufferers who have pain in the whole of their bodies that is worse at rest (the reverse of *Bryonia*). Their tongues are dry and have a red line down the centre (a sign shared with *Veratrum viride*). They may notice a leakage of urine and faeces. They have a tickling cough behind their breastbones (sternums), which occurs mainly during the night. It commonly produces blood (haemoptysis). Sufferers increasingly find it difficult to catch their breath.

### *Senega* (snakewort)

This remedy picture describes sufferers who have a lot of catarrh in the chest, which makes the chest sound rattly. The sputum is so thick that it is difficult to expectorate. Sufferers have hoarse voices and find it difficult to talk. They are probably elderly, and feel as though their chests are being forced inwards and backwards towards the spine. They feel better when bending the head backwards.

### *Veratrum album* (white hellebore)

This remedy picture describes coldness and extreme weakness. Sufferers usually have cold perspiration on their foreheads. Their chests are usually rattling with mucus, which they find difficult to cough up. The coughing is made worse when they move from a warm room to a cold one. This remedy particularly suits the chronic bronchitis of older people.

## Laryngitis

The major symptom of acute laryngitis is a croaky voice. It can be caused by several factors: viruses, bacteria or physical overuse (found in singers, public speakers and sporting coaches, for example). In babies, it causes CROUP (*see* p. 407). The conventional treatment is a physical examination of the larynx (voice box), a possible swab test and probably antibiotic therapy. If the laryngitis has been caused by overuse, rest of the voice is obvious and essential for recovery with no need for antibiotics. If the illness is due to an infection (and it is quite likely that a close friend or family member has already had the infection), it is still important to rest the larynx as much as possible as well as seeking medical treatment.

*Remedies to be used when the voice has been overused*
The dosage schedule for the homeopathic treatment in these cases is to use the 6c potency and give one dose every hour for a maximum of six doses, then to reduce to one dose every four hours until the voice improves. This will take one to two days.

### *Arum triphyllum* (Jack-in-the-pulpit)

This remedy picture describes a throat that feels sore and a voice that is uncertain. It has become known as "clergyman's sore throat". The glands under the neck are enlarged, and the raw feeling of the throat extends to the root of the mouth.

### *Lachesis* (bushmaster snake venom)

This remedy picture describes a throat that feels generally sore, more so on the left side. Sufferers feel that the soreness will never get any better. Physical examination reveals no abnormality (much to the surprise of sufferers), despite the fact that they are experiencing so many symptoms. They are certain that a foreign object is present at the back of their throats, as a result of which they have a persistent feeling that their throats are swollen and that this object has to be swallowed. However, paradoxically, swallowing saliva or liquids makes the symptom worse. The discomfort causes pain to be referred to the ear, mainly the left one. Sufferers also feel a need to loosen clothing around their necks, as if they will be choked unless they do so. They tend to be very talkative.

## *Wyethia* (poisonweed)

This remedy picture describes a laryngitis from overuse and is therefore of particular use for singers and public speakers. The larynx feels dry, the uvula (the long, fleshy part at the back of the throat) feels elongated, whereas it is not normally felt, and the person feels a need to constantly swallow saliva.

### Acute infective laryngitis

For acute infective laryngitis, the dose schedule is to use the 6c potency and give one dose every two hours for a maximum of six doses, then reduce to one dose every four hours for one day, finally reducing to one dose four times a day until the symptoms improve, at which point the remedy can be discontinued.

## *Aconitum napellus* (monk's-hood)

This remedy picture describes a person who has a sore, red throat with a painful, hoarse larynx. The symptoms come on very quickly, and the person feels unduly frightened and anxious, so much so that they fear death. The symptoms are improved in the open air but not in a cold wind.

## *Causticum* (Hahnemann's mixture of quick lime [calcium oxide] and potassium bisulphate)

This remedy picture describes a sore throat giving catarrh and a hacking cough that causes the person to hold their breastbone (sternum) as the cough releases a tearing pain. Sufferers' symptoms are worse in the evening, giving them sleepless nights. The symptoms commonly follow a cold, and sufferers may find their speech indistinct due to paralysis of the tongue. The inside of the cheek is bitten for the same reason. The symptoms are improved by warmth and a humid atmosphere.

### *Ferrum phosphoricum* (iron phosphate)

This remedy picture describes sufferers who feel that their larynx is sore and their voice is definitely hoarse. Commonly, their throats are sore and red as well. The picture also describes people who have developed a fever.

### *Hepar sulphuris* (Hahnemann's calcium sulphide)

This remedy picture describes sufferers whose voices are obviously croupy and their throats sore with the sensation that there are splinters in them. It is this sensation that causes pain to be referred into the ears when swallowing. These symptoms are improved in warm, moist conditions.

### *Phosphorus*

This remedy picture describes a throat that feels sore and dry. Sufferers' symptoms are worse in the evening. They have a preference for and feel better by drinking sips of cold water, and become frightened in thunderstorms. The picture also describes a tickly cough.

### *Spongia tosta* (roasted sponge)

This remedy picture describes a voice that has a definite squeaky quality. This remedy is particularly useful for treating CROUP in children. The voice becomes unrecognizable as the child squeaks in order to make words. This is a potentially serious condition, requiring medical attention.

## Pleurisy

Pleurisy is an inflammation of the lining of the lungs (the pleurae). It can be caused by an infection (bacterial or, less commonly, viral) involving the lungs directly (PNEUMONIA) or through injury. Pleurisy can affect children as well as adults.

The illness reveals itself by severe pain, usually on one side of the lungs, whenever the person breathes in. In this instance, it is important to seek medical advice as the correct diagnosis is important and the appropriate conventional treatment started.

There are certain specific homeopathic remedies that can be used alongside conventional medicines for both children and adults.

Using the 6c potency, initially give one dose every hour, for a maximum of 12 doses. This schedule can then be reduced to one dose three times a day for two days and finally to one a day until the symptoms improve. Select the remedy by matching its picture with the physical symptoms.

### Aconitum napellus (monk's-hood)

The characteristic feature of this remedy picture is the suddenness of the onset of all symptoms. A common precipitating factor is exposure to cold and dry winds. The person feels unduly anxious and is fearful of dying.

### Belladonna (deadly nightshade)

This remedy picture shows sufferers with red faces, dilated pupils and congested eyes; the skin is dry and hot. They show great nervousness, and they may become delirious, during which state, they hallucinate, seeing frightening images. At other times, they feel sleepy and yet find sleep difficult. This remedy is useful in treating BRONCHITIS where there is a dry, hard cough that comes in paroxysms and is spasmodic. It is also useful in treating pleurisy, particularly the right-sided variety, which causes great pain on breathing that is made worse when the bed is jarred and when sufferers lie on their sore side. (This is the reverse of Bryonia in which the pain is improved by lying on the painful side.)

### Bryonia (wild hops)

This remedy picture has a characteristic feature: any movement causes pain, which is relieved by rest. The person also finds relief from the symptoms by lying on the painful lung. He or she has an irritable nature.

### *Cantharis* (Spanish fly)

This remedy picture describes chest pains that are burning in quality and a cough that is dry and comes on frequently. The person's heart rate is rapid and irregular.

### *Chelidonium majus* (celandine)

The remedy picture describes sufferers with right-sided chest symptoms. Pleurisy is generally present and causes such severe pain on movement that sufferers feel as though a knife has sliced right through them. Transfixed by this pain, they have to sit up. (This is like *Bryonia*, but whereas *Bryonia* must lie still, *Chelidonium* must sit up.) The characteristic symptom of this remedy is pain in the lower angle of the right shoulder blade, which passes from the outer chest wall and into the right armpit. The cough is loose and rattling, but sufferers find it difficult to expectorate. Their tongues are furred and tooth-notched (a symptom shared with *Mercurius*).

### *Hepar sulphuris* (Hahnemann's calcium sulphide)

This remedy picture describes the treatment of pleurisy that is reserved for those cases that are taking a longer than expected time to heal. Coughing is made worse whenever any part of the body becomes cold or is uncovered. When the person is physically examined, it is common to find that fluid has accumulated on the lung affected by the pleurisy.

### *Squilla* (sea-onion)

The characteristic features of this remedy relevant to the chest are the stitching pains in the chest, associated with painful contractions of the abdominal muscles. There is a furious coughing coupled with sneezing. The cough is provoked by taking a deep breath, from exertion and by moving from a warm room to a cooler one.

## Sulphur

The picture of this remedy relevant to the chest is one of stitching pains in the chest, which radiate through to the back and are made worse by lying on the back and by breathing deeply. The pulse rate is commonly faster in the morning than in the evening. The breath becomes shorter in the middle of the night, and this symptom is improved by sitting up. The overall picture of these people as a whole is particularly relevant in choosing this particular remedy. They are generally untidy, enjoy fatty and sweet foods, tend to have early morning diarrhoea and are intolerant of wearing clothes, particularly footwear as their bodies overheat. To this extent, their feet tend to drift out of the bedclothes.

# Pneumonia

Pneumonia is an inflammation of the lungs, usually caused by the same viruses that cause the COMMON COLD or INFLUENZA. However, specific bacteria, the *Pneumococci*, can also cause this disease. This is a serious infection that needs medical attention. The conventional treatment for viral pneumonia is, as with all illnesses caused by viruses, simply the relief of symptoms, but penicillin can be prescribed for pneumococcal pneumonia.

Homeopathic treatment is best obtained through a consultation with a specialist homeopath.

The following homeopathic remedies should only be used in exceptional circumstances on their own; ordinarily they should be used in a complementary way with conventional antibiotic therapy.

The homeopathic remedies are listed below, with their physical pictures. Select the one that fits the physical symptoms most closely. This applies to children of all ages and to adults. Using a

30c potency, give one dose every four hours for two days, reducing to one dose once a day until satisfactory improvement has occurred.

### *Aconitum napellus* (monk's-hood)

The characteristic feature of this remedy picture is the sudden onset of symptoms, particularly when associated with dry, cold winds. There are diffuse chest pains, and anxiety with an overwhelming fear of dying. This remedy is probably only useful for a short time, and a second remedy will generally be needed to complete the healing process. The dosage schedule of this second remedy follows that of the first.

### *Baptisia* (wild indigo)

This remedy picture is particularly useful for pneumonia following INFLUENZA. Sufferers' lungs feel compressed, and as a result, they find breathing difficult. Their tongues are dry and coloured brown down the centre. They hesitate about going to sleep for fear of suffocation and nightmares. The symptoms are made worse in humid and hot atmospheres.

### *Bryonia* (wild hops)

This remedy picture describes a cough that is made worse on entering a warm room and produces a brick-coloured sputum. The sharp chest pains are made easier when sufferers lie on the worst affected side. They may feel a heaviness beneath their sternum (breastbone), and this discomfort radiates to the right shoulder.

### *Ferrum phosphoricum* (iron phosphate)

This remedy picture describes the early inflammatory conditions before the physical signs of pneumonia have become prominent. Breathing is short and panting, and sufferers may even expectorate pure blood. However, they are not restless or anxious. The symptoms are worse at night, particularly between 4.00 and 6.00 am.

### Chelidonium majus (celandine)

This remedy is particularly useful for the person who already has liver disease. The right lung is most commonly affected, and deep breathing causes a pain that radiates into the right shoulder blade.

### Gelsemium (yellow jasmine)

This remedy suits the person who develops a chest infection following INFLUENZA. Sufferers lack thirst to a remarkable degree, and feel heavy in mind as well as body. They have a congestive headache that causes muscular soreness, extending from the head to the neck and shoulders. The symptoms are worse in damp, foggy weather and particularly before a thunderstorm, and are made better by leaning forward and by profuse urination.

### Mercurius solubis (ammonium nitrate salt of mercury)

One of the key features of the *Mercurius* remedy picture is a furred tongue with teeth marks notched in its surface. The person sweats profusely without getting any relief of symptoms; the more sweat, the worse he or she feels. The medical situation for which this remedy must be considered is pneumonia with excessive and offensive sweat, and offensive-smelling mouth and breath with equally offensive sputum.

### Nitric acidum (nitric acid)

This remedy picture suits those people who are generally browneyed, chilly, intolerant of fuss (a symptom that is shared with *Natrum muriaticum*) and who love fatty food and salt. Their chests feel oppressed, a symptom that becomes worse when they bend backwards. The sputum sticks like glue, is yellow in colour and tastes bitter and salty; later on, it can be found to contain black coagulated blood. Sufferers, who experience stitch-like pains in the right chest, fear death and are obviously anxious about their illness (a symptom shared with *Aconitum*).

### Phosphorus

This remedy picture describes a cough that is associated with the production of a rust-coloured sputum, with the whole body trembling with the coughing. The symptoms and the person feels worse when lying on their left side.

### Sanguinaria (blood root)

The main features of this remedy are the production of a rust-coloured sputum and the fact that sufferers feel better lying on their backs, although coughing forces them to sit up. They commonly feel discomfort in the right side of their chests, with the pain going through to their right shoulders. This remedy suits the pneumonia that may follow INFLUENZA and WHOOPING COUGH.

### Veratrum viride (white American hellebore)

This remedy picture suits those who develop a sudden congestion of the lungs. They look bloated, and have bloodshot eyes and a red face. Breathing is slow and heavy, and sufferers feel the need to sit up even though this makes them feel faint. Unusually their tongues have a dry, red streak along their centres. The body temperature is very high and rapidly oscillates, and is associated with much sweating.

## Tuberculosis

This illness is caused by an unusual bacterium and is spread by tiny droplets from the mouth or nose of an infected person or by drinking milk that has not been properly tested for tubercular infection. It most commonly affects the lungs, but it can occasionally affect the brain, kidneys or bones. Those most likely to get this infection eat a poor diet, exercise little and are subjected to much stress. In recent times, tuberculosis has become unfortunately more common in the West as a more virulent bacterial strain has emerged.

The conventional treatment – and this is the recommended form of therapy – consists of a combination of antibiotic therapy (to be continued for at least one year), rest and a proper diet. Babies and other people considered at risk from catching the disease can be preventatively immunized.

Homeopathic treatment must take second place and is best supervised by a specialist homeopath. If this is not possible, the following homeopathic remedies can be considered.

The homeopathic remedy *Tuberculinum*, a nucleo-protein from a tubercular abscess, can be used as a preventative or as a part of a miasmic treatment package (*see* p. 95) in cases where the person has a past medical history of tuberculosis. In both of these situations, the potency to use is 30c, one dose to be given every 12 hours for a maximum of three doses.

*Drosera* (sundew) is another remedy that can be used as preventative treatment. It is of particular use if the person has had a past medical history of WHOOPING COUGH. In this respect, it can also be used as a miasm. The dosage schedule is as for *Tuberculinum*.

The following homeopathic remedies are indicated in treating tuberculosis and can be used as a complementary form of therapy with conventional treatment. Using the 6c potency, give one dose twice a day for as long as the conventional treatment lasts.

### Arsenicum iodatum (arsenic iodide)

The remedy picture describes a person who has an insistant cough but is unable to bring up much phlegm. Sometimes he or she loses the ability to talk.

### Baryta carbonicum (barium carbonate)

This remedy picture suits children in particular. The children it describes tend to be slow and shy of strangers, and they tend to catch every cold that's doing the rounds. This remedy shares with *Silicea* the fact that sufferers' feet are cold and produce a foul-smelling sweat. The neck glands become enlarged with tubercular infection, and can sometimes suppurate.

### *Bromium* (bromine)

The characteristic feature of this remedy picture is the appearance of enlarged neck glands, particularly in children. These glands never suppurate, although they become hard. As a generalisation, this remedy picture describes a person who feels better at sea, and the remedy seems to suit blond-headed people with blue eyes in particular.

### *Calcarea carbonica* (calcium carbonate)

This remedy picture describes sufferers who have a tickly cough that is worse at night when they are unable to cough up phlegm. During the day, the cough is much more productive and may contain blood. Sufferers tend to have night sweats, particularly on their heads.

### *Cistus canadensis* (rock rose)

This remedy picture describes a person with glandular swellings and who is extremely sensitive to the cold. The glands that are most frequently affected are those in the neck. This remedy has a peculiar symptom in that the person has a craving for cheese.

### *Drosera* (sundew)

The characteristic feature of this remedy is a spasmodic cough that is worse when lying down. It is of particular use in the breakdown of old tubercular glands. If this remedy is selected, use the 30c potency and give one dose every 12 hours for a maximum of three doses; repeat this schedule at monthly intervals.

### Iodum (iodine)

This remedy picture describes sufferers who have a rapid metabolism and who lose weight despite a good appetite. They are very easily fatigued, and the slightest effort causes marked perspiration. There is an enlargement of many glands, which can be tubercular; the breasts, however, lose their size and waste away in both men and women. This remedy suits people with dark hair and dark complexions, compared with *Bromium*, which suits fairheaded people with blue eyes.

### Phellandrium (water-dropwort)

This remedy picture describes a persistent cough that can cause a sticking pain through the right breast and breastbone (sternum). This pain extends through to the back close to the shoulders.

### Phosphorus

This remedy picture shows that this remedy has a direct effect in the treatment of tuberculosis, particularly where the illness has spread into the bones, causing destruction (necrosis) of the bone itself. It suits young children, particularly those who are slender and are growing very rapidly.

### Sepia (inky juice from cuttlefish)

This remedy picture describes tuberculosis of bones, particularly those of the fingers. The type of person that this remedy suits is indifferent to loved ones, feels over burdened, hates noise and wants to get away from it all and be alone and quiet.

### Silicea (pure flint)

This remedy picture describes hard glands, especially around the neck, that have become affected with tuberculosis. The person's feet sweat profusely and with a foul smell, and he or she prefers warm, wet weather.

## *Theridion* (orange spider)

This remedy picture shows that the remedy has an affinity for the tubercle bacteria no matter which part of the body it affects. Therefore, the personal picture is important in selecting it. This describes hypersensitive individuals who react unfavourably to noise, with shrill sounds penetrating into their teeth. They become nauseous from motion (either in a motor vehicle or a boat), and this is much worse when they close their eyes.

# Gastrointestinal Tract Disorders

This section deals with ailments of the gastrointestinal tract – from the mouth to the anus. These include problems of the liver (hepatitis, jaundice), the gall bladder (cholecystitis) and the pancreas, all of which secrete substances into the gastrointestinal tract. In addition, there are problems with the small intestine (including the appendix and the caecum) and large intestine (including adhesion formation), and constipation and haemorrhoids (piles) are also discussed. Finally, anorexia nervosa, binge eating and bulimia nervosa will be covered – homeopathic remedies can be useful in the treatment of these difficult problems.

## Mouth problems

Most of these disorders are discussed on pp. 53–7. Here we will deal solely with *aphthous ulcers*.

These painful sores, commonly called "mouth ulcers", occur mainly on the inside of the cheeks. There is no known cause, although there are some links with stress. Thus it is important for individuals to look at their own stress situation critically in terms of sleep, diet, work and relationships.

The conventional treatment is with steroid-based tablets placed over the ulcer.

### Homeopathic mouthwash

The homeopathic treatment is initially with a homeopathic mouthwash made from 30 drops of a combination of mother tinctures (*described below*) placed in 250 millilitres (8.5 fl. oz) of water and swilling 20 millilitres (approximately 0.5 fl. oz) around in the mouth several times a day (the mouth wash should not be swallowed). This mouthwash can be used in any condition – not only those involving the inside of the cheeks but also dental problems.

The following are the basic mother tinctures that are used in the preparation of the mouthwash:

- *Calendula officinalis* (marigold): this promotes healing of the apthous ulcer.
- *Hydrastis* (golden seal): this not only promotes healing of apthous ulcers but also reduces the pain they cause.
- *Salvia oficinalis* (sage): this can be used to reduce pain, swelling and inflammation of any disorder in the mouth or dental area.

# Other remedies

The following homeopathic remedies can be used in addition to the mouthwash. Select the remedy according to its remedy picture, matching it with the physical symptoms. Using the 6c potency, give one dose every two hours for a maximum of ten doses, and then reduce to one dose four times a day until the apthous ulcers resolve.

### *Borox* (sodium borate)

This is the remedy of choice to treat apthous ulcers. The taste sensation in this remedy picture is peculiar, describing a bitter taste reminiscent of mould. However, to choose this remedy, it is not absolutely essential to have this particular symptom. Another one is that the person feels worse with downward motion (e.g. going down in a lift, or coming into land in an aircraft). He or she also tends to be nervous and dislikes loud noises.

### Hydrastis (golden seal)

This remedy picture describes apthous ulcers associated with a tongue that is white in colour, swollen and ulcerated and shows the imprint of the teeth on it. The saliva is thick, and the breath is offensive.

### Kali bichromium (potassium bichromium)

This remedy picture describes apthous ulcers with yellow or yellow-green bases. The back of the throat (uvula) is swollen.

### Nitric acidum (nitric acid)

This remedy picture describes apthous ulcers that bleed easily and which have splinter-like or sticking pains associated with them.

### Nux vomica (poison-nut)

This remedy picture describes not only mouth ulcers but also saliva that is usually bloodstained. The back part of the tongue is covered with thick "fur" – that is, it is coloured white or yellow – and has cracked edges, yet the front part is quite clean. The gums are usually swollen and bleed easily. The teeth ache, and this sensation is made worse when cold liquids are swallowed. The general profile of the person will help in the selection of this remedy rather than simply the presence of mouth ulcers. He or she is hard-working and ambitious and seeks perfection in everything attempted. There is also a tendency to smoke and consume caffeine and alcohol in excess.

### Sempervivum tectorum (house-leek)

This remedy picture describes much ulceration in the mouth and tongue, giving stinging pains and, in particular, making the tongue feel very sore. The ulcers bleed easily, especially at night.

### Sulphuricum acidum (sulphuric acid)

This remedy picture describes apthous ulcers, gums that bleed easily and breath that smells foul. The characteristic symptom is of an underlying debility that gives sufferers a tremor and generalized weakness. They also crave stimulants including alcohol. This remedy picture applies particularly to women who have just given birth and are breast-feeding.

# Oesophagus problems

This section looks at three problems that can affect the oesophagus, commonly known as the gullet. *Reflux oesophagitis* occurs when acid from the stomach ascends into the oesophagus, inflaming it and giving a burning sensation just below the breastbone (sternum) – "heartburn" – and a bitter taste in the mouth. This often happens when there is *hiatus hernia*: the opening (hiatus) in the diaphragm, the muscular sheet that separates the chest and abdomen, becomes weakened and permits the upper stomach and its acidic contents to slide into the chest and so reach the oesophagus. Finally, there is *globus hystericus*, a distressing feeling of an obstruction in the throat that, sufferers believe, prevents food and/or liquid going down into the oesophagus – or even prevents air from reaching the lungs – even though, in fact, there is no obstruction. All these symptoms are made worse when sufferers lie flat, are overweight and/or eat spicy foods. Correction of these factors will help alleviate some of the symptoms.

The conventional treatment is with antacid liquid therapy and certain drugs to help heal the ulceration caused by the stomach acid.

Homeopathic treatment involves the use of one of the following remedies. Select one by matching its picture with the physical symptoms. Using the 6c potency, give one dose four times a day until the symptoms improve.

### Asafoetida (gum of the stinkasand)

This remedy picture describes a person who is suffering from *globus hystericus*. The sensation is as if the normal action of the muscles that move food from the mouth to the stomach have gone into reverse. There is much flatulence, giving a bitter taste in the mouth. It is, above all, a very "windy" remedy – in fact, the person is left wondering where all the wind is coming from. The belched wind smells offensive and emerges as if a pop-gun is going off every second.

## *Lycopodium* (club moss)

This remedy picture describes nervous indigestion that is worse between the hours of 4.00 and 8.00 pm and is associated with a "hunger headache". Sufferers have anticipatory anxiety (i.e. become anxious in advance of certain events), want to be alone and yet like company to be close at hand. They also like warm and sweet foods, and tend to loosen their clothing as their stomachs become full and they experience flatulence and discomfort. They feel that they must be very careful not to put any pressure on their bloated stomachs in case they make their indigestion worse.

## *Nux vomica* (poison-nut)

The remedy describes indigestion resulting from a turbulent stomach that becomes easily distended and is tender to the touch. There is much flatulence, and stomach acid comes into the oesophagus, causing burning and giving a bitter taste in the mouth. The general profile of the person as a whole will help in the selection of this remedy: ambitious, hard-working and something of a perfectionist, and over-indulgent in alcohol, coffee and cigarettes.

## *Robinia* (yellow locust)

The description of this remedy picture makes Robinia a great heartburn remedy, with acidity as a key symptom. The symptoms are at their worst at night when the person lies down. There is distension of the stomach and bowels, with the latter having a colicky pain. A specific indication is that sometimes children can smell sour, and indeed this is a remedy that suits children well.

# Stomach disorders

Three different conditions are dealt with in this section. *Gastritis* is the inflammation of the mucous membrane that lines the stomach, caused by alcohol, certain drugs (most commonly aspirin), infection by *Helicobacter pylori* bacteria or extreme stress; symptoms include discomfort in the upper abdomen, nausea and vomiting. Ulcers in the stomach (*gastric ulcers*) or the duodenum (*duodenal ulcers*), the first part of the small intestine, are raw patches where stomach acid has eaten through the lining; the primary symptom is a gnawing pain in the abdomen when the stomach is empty. It is now known that almost all ulcers are the result of infection by *H. pylori* bacteria. The symptoms for both gastritis and gastric and duodenal ulcers are made worse by smoking, drinking alcohol, coffee and tea, and taking aspirin. Finally, *motion/travel sickness* will be discussed.

It is important to get a medical opinion if a gastric or duodenal ulcer is suspected because both need full conventional investigation. This will include endoscopy (a technique that enables the doctor to look directly into the stomach through a fibreoptic telescope) and possibly barium X-rays. Conventional treatment is with specific drugs to heal the ulceration by reducing gastric acid secretion.

If homeopathic treatment is desired, the best option is to see a specialist homeopath who will be able to make an overall assessment of the person as a whole together with the specific problem. If this is not possible, the following homeopathic remedies will work alongside conventional treatment in a truly complementary manner. Select the remedy by matching its picture with the physical symptoms. Using the 6c potency, give one dose four times a day until the symptoms resolve.

### *Antimonium crudum* (black sulphide of antimony)

The characteristic feature of this remedy is excessive irritability together with a thickly coated white tongue (the tongue symptom is similar to *Bryonia*). The stomach symptoms are characterized by a loss of appetite but a desire for acidic foods including pickles (although vinegar disagrees). Sufferers feel bloated after eating, are nauseous and will probably vomit. Constantly belching, they feel worse in the evening and particularly in hot weather. They generally display a sentimental temperament, are peevish and dislike being touched or looked at.

### Argentum nitricum (silver nitrate)

The remedy picture describes flatulent indigestion (dyspepsia) that occurs after every meal, giving a sensation as though the stomach will burst. The belching is initially difficult, with the air finally rushing out with a great noise and violence. Physically it suits the gastritis of an alcoholic. Sufferers have a characteristic craving for refined sugar and sweets. They are generally apprehensive, showing an anticipatory anxiety even to the point of having diarrhoea. They dislike crowds and have a fear of heights.

### Bryonia (wild hops)

The remedy picture describes symptoms of indigestion after eating as if sufferers' stomachs have a stone lying in them, which makes these individuals angry and cross. Their mouths are dry, their tongues are coloured white and there is a considerable thirst for large volumes of liquid. They cannot tolerate disturbance of any sort, either mental or physical. They are better when lying quite still and prefer to be left alone. They cannot sit up in bed as this movement makes them feel sick and faint.

### Chamomilla (camomile)

The characteristic features of this remedy picture are emotional peevishness and restlessness, as well as gastrointestinal symptoms. It is common for one cheek to be red and the other a normal colour. The stomach is painful, as though there is a stone in it, and there is marked flatulence that may also be associated with bilious vomiting. The stomach pains are made worse by the belching. The person is hypersensitive to pain, reacting violently to it. A child is comforted by being held and carried around the room.

### *Graphites* (black lead)

The characteristic feature of this remedy picture is that sufferers have an aversion to meat and sweets make them nauseous. The gnawing pain in the stomach is made better by eating; lying down also helps. Relief is also obtained from eating hot food and drinking hot fluids. This remedy is particularly suitable for those with duodenal ulcers.

### *Ipecacuanha* (ipecac root)

This remedy picture describes a person who feels continually nauseous, with much belching and salivating; above all, there is a great deal of vomiting, which relieves the nausea. The tongue is usually clean, and with the strong flow of saliva, the mouth is usually moist. The person feels as though the stomach is hanging down and relaxed.

### *Natrum carbonicum* (sodium carbonate)

The characteristic feature of this remedy picture is the great debility caused by summer heat and the chronic effects of sunstroke. The stomach is swollen and sensitive. Sufferers feel particularly hungry at 5.00 am and have to get out of bed to have something to eat. The slightest error in the diet causes stomach upset, characterized by distension and much belching. The stomach symptoms are improved by eating soda biscuits. Affected individuals suffer from fatigue and weakness in both mind and body: there is nervous exhaustion and confusion, with sufferers ending up thoroughly bad-tempered. Starchy food causes a looseness of bowel activity, which also can occur from drinking milk (to which sufferers anyway have an aversion) and when they want to enjoy their own space. They dislike sympathy and any fuss being made of them.

## *Nux vomica* (poison-nut)

The picture of this remedy describes nausea that occurs in the morning and after eating. The appetite is depressed, and somewhat surprisingly, sufferers also come to dislike their accustomed smoking, alcohol and coffee. There is a contractive stomach ache with an inclination to vomit, as well as marked flatulence causing stomach distension and tenderness, particularly under the ribs. These symptoms are worse after eating or drinking. If vomiting does occur, it is foul-tasting and sour-smelling. Constipation commonly occurs, from the infrequent use of the toilet, or sufferers pass only a small amount with each attempt, with a feeling that their rectums have not properly emptied.

## *Ornithogallum umbellatum* (Star of Bethlehem)

This remedy picture is of particular help in treating gastric ulcers. It describes a coated tongue, loss of appetite and a painful feeling over the stomach. This pain becomes agonizing when food or wind passes through the pylorus (the outlet from the stomach into the duodenum). The stomach becomes distended, and there is frequent foul-smelling belching. There is also vomiting of old blood, which looks like coffee grounds, and of fresh blood.

## *Phosphorus*

This remedy picture describes a burning feeling in the stomach, an excessive thirst for cold water, nausea with empty belching, and finally vomiting of blood (old or fresh). The preference for drinking cold water is such that warm fluids cause nausea and vomiting. Paradoxically, even when cold fluid is drunk, as it warms in the stomach it is vomited back up. The burning stomach pains are eased with cold food and ice cream, both of which are well tolerated without being vomited. The picture also describes sufferers who have profuse painless diarrhoea with blood in their stools. They also have a fear of thunderstorms, are sociable, needing company, and can tire easily but respond well to

133

short naps. This remedy will help those with bleeding duodenal and gastric ulcers.

## Pulsatilla (wind flower)

This remedy picture describes indigestion brought on by the eating of fatty foods. This remedy is selected by looking at the general profile of the sufferers, who tend to have mild, gentle, yielding dispositions. Tears come easily, and they yearn for and respond well to tactile support. They dislike warm environments, butter, cream and, in fact, all fats. Their gastrointestinal symptoms can be summarized as a lack of hunger, thirst and constipation. They commonly pass wind with cutting abdominal pain in the morning, with colicky abdominal pain developing in the evening. There is a frequent urge to use the toilet, which produces a soft stool with mucus and a little blood.

## Sepia (inky juice of cuttlefish)

The characteristic feature of this remedy is morning nausea and possibly vomiting with bile. This is the classic remedy for the early morning sickness of pregnancy, in which state the person also has an aversion to meat, fat and bread; the sight and smell of food can cause nausea. A guiding picture in selecting this remedy is of the person as a whole, who is indifferent to those loved ones occupying their "space", preferring their own company.

## Sulphur

This remedy picture describes sufferers who feel a burning in their stomach, which is relieved by drinking cold liquids and eating ice cream. They feel weak and empty at 11.00 am and crave for food at that time. They desire sweets, fat and alcohol in the form of beer and ale. They are intolerant of wearing too many clothes, as they feel hot – in fact, they prefer walking barefoot to cool down their bodies. They also prefer to kick their bedclothes off so that their feet can stick out and cool down. This remedy will help those people who have duodenal ulcers.

# Motion/travel sickness

This condition occurs in certain individuals whenever they travel in a car or on a boat.

The conventional treatment is with antihistamine drugs or with tranquillizers.

Homeopathic treatment will involve one of the following remedies. Using the 30c potency, give one dose the night before the planned journey, one on the morning before setting out and, if it is a long journey, one again in the middle of the trip. Select the remedy by matching its picture with the physical symptoms.

### *Bryonia* (wild hops)

This remedy picture describes feelings of nausea and faintness whenever sufferers move. Their stomachs are sensitive to the touch, and they feel pressure there, as if there is a stone in their stomachs. They feel hungry, yet whenever they eat, they vomit immediately. Similarly they are thirsty for large volumes of fluid, yet this too is quickly vomited.

### *Cocculus* (Indian cockle)

This remedy picture describes nausea whenever sufferers travel, and this generally leads to vomiting. They can feel nauseous just by looking at a boat in motion. These symptoms are worse in cold weather and when sufferers have a cold. There is a metallic taste in their mouths, and they dislike any food or drink.

### *Kali carbonicum* (potassium carbonate)

This remedy picture describes sufferers who easily become nauseous whenever they move, feeling better when they lie down. They feel anxious in their stomach, which is sensitive to the touch and has a constant feeling as if it is full of water. They generally feel weak and are very sensitive to the cold.

### *Petroleum* (crude rock oil)

This remedy picture describes sufferers who feel nauseated on any movement, particularly after they have eaten cabbage. They also notice that, as soon as they feel nauseated, saliva accumulates in their mouths.

### *Phosphorus*

This remedy picture describes individuals who become nauseous, possibly resulting in vomiting, whenever they smell cigarette smoke. This is therefore not primarily a motion/travel sickness remedy, but one to be used by those who know that, when travelling, they are likely to come into contact with cigarette smoke. The general profile of the person, which will also help in the selection of this remedy, includes a noticeable fear of thunderstorms.

### *Tabacum* (tobacco)

This remedy picture describes people who vomit at the slightest movement. The vomit occasionally contains faecal matter. The preceding nausea is made worse whenever they smell tobacco smoke. This remedy suits those travelling in vehicles run on diesel.

# *Liver problems*

The liver is the detoxifying organ of the body, in which all waste products and poisonous substances in the blood are filtered out into the bile, a greenish-brown liquid. Bile drains, first, into the gall bladder and then into the small intestine via the common bile duct. The liver itself can become infected by viruses such as those responsible for GLANDULAR FEVER and yellow fever, and it can also be damaged by certain drugs. Because of this, it is **always worth checking with your medical practitioner the side-effects of the medicines that he or she prescribes, to** ensure that you are not being given any that, together, will damage the liver.

However, in this section we will be concentrating on the serious viral illnesses hepatitis A, B and C, all of which involve liver inflammation with the damage or death of liver cells. All forms of hepatitis require medical supervision.

*Hepatitis A* develops suddenly, although the incubation period – from the time that the virus enters the body until symptoms are felt – can be as long as three months. The virus responsible for it enters the body via the mouth through food that has been contaminated by the infected faeces of another person.

It is of vital importance, therefore, that strict hygiene is maintained while the person is ill (and, of course, at all other times) so that the virus is not transmitted to others.

The first symptoms are very similar to those of INFLUENZA, followed by jaundice, a yellowing of the skin, eyes and urine and pale-coloured stools which indicate that the bile is not leaving the body in the normal way. Sufferers lose their appetites, and if they smoke, they cannot tolerate smoking. The illness spontaneously starts to improve after two or three weeks, during which time sufferers should have plenty of bed rest and eat a light, nourishing diet; they must also avoid alcohol for six months.

*Hepatitis B* produces similar symptoms to hepatitis A, but the incubation period is longer at six months. This virus is present in the blood and can be transmitted to others by the sharing of hypodermic needles, sexual contact and contaminated blood products.

People who regularly travel to high-risk areas are advised to take their own sterile needles with them as an emergency precaution should they need a blood transfusion or an injection.

This illness is more serious than hepatitis A as it can lead to chronic hepatitis and even liver failure.

There are no specific conventional treatments for hepatitis A or B, but there are, however, vaccines available to protect against them. Less than complete protection for both is afforded by an intramuscular injection of immunoglobulin. The vaccine specifically designed to thwart hepatitis A should be considered by those who travel frequently to high-risk parts of the world or if there is an epidemic of hepatitis A. There is also an active vaccine against hepatitis B that is available for those in high-risk occupations (e.g. health professionals) and those who behave in ways that leave them at risk of contracting hepatitis B (e.g. male homosexuals and drug addicts).

*Hepatitis C* is a recently discovered viral illness. It is transmitted via the blood, and has infected those given contaminated blood products, such as those suffering from haemophilia. Cases are even known to have resulted from contact with blood on paper, such as bank notes and papers used to snort cocaine. It can also rarely be contracted via sexual contact.

The symptoms only appear after a very long period – up to 20 years. The person develops muscular pains, painful headaches and severe bouts of fatigue. This is potentially the most serious form of hepatitis, leading to destruction of the liver (cirrhosis) and a significantly high incidence of primary liver cancer. At the moment, the conventional treatment is experimental, involving the drugs interferon and ribavirin.

The initial homeopathic treatment for hepatitis C is similar to that indicated for MYALGIC ENCEPHALOMYELITIS (including anti-oxidant and probiotic therapy). These supplements can be used at the same time as the homeopathic remedies given below.

There are certain homeopathic remedies that can help alleviate the symptoms of hepatitis A, B and C. The remedy pictures are described below. Choose the picture that most suits the physical symptoms; using the 6c potency, give one dose twice a day.

### Aconitum napellus (monk's-hood)

This is the first remedy to use when an attack of hepatitis is diagnosed. The remedy picture describes tearing pains in the region of the liver, and a very anxious person who has a fear of dying.

### Belladonna (deadly nightshade)

This remedy picture describes severe pains in the right upper abdomen or in a small spot near the tummy button (umbilicus), which is made worse by lying on the right side, firm pressure and any jarring movements. Sufferers have a desire for lemons or lemonade, which help alleviate the symptoms, and they have characteristically red faces with widely dilated pupils and fast heart rates.

### *Bryonia* (wild hops)

This remedy picture describes inflammation of the liver that is made painful by any movement. When sufferers cough, they feel as if their livers will burst (a symptom that is shared with *Natrum sulphuricum*).

### *Chelidonium majus* (celandine)

This remedy, which has a particular affinity for the liver, suits all disorders of this organ and is therefore an important first choice. The liver area is tender to the touch, and peculiarly, the pain is referred through to the back and to the right shoulder blade. Eating temporarily relieves these symptoms, sufferers preferring hot food and drinks. Their abdomens are distended and feel constricted, as if they are tied round with string.

### *Cornus circinata* (round-leafed dogwood)

This remedy is useful in treating hepatitis that has progressed into the chronic form (chronic active hepatitis). Sufferers are probably jaundiced, their bowels are generally overactive and they feel as if they will break in two at the waist.

### *Hydrastis* (golden seal)

This remedy picture describes a tender and swollen liver, and an action on the mucous membranes that results in the production of a thick, yellowish and ropey secretion. This can be anywhere but more usually in the upper respiratory tract.

### *Lachesis* (bushmaster snake venom)

In this remedy picture, the liver area is tender to the touch, and the abdomen is swollen, painful and, if gently tapped, has a tympanic sound. The person cannot tolerate anything around the waist.

### *Magnesia muriaticum* (magnesium chloride)

This remedy describes a pressing pain in the liver when walking or when touching the liver area. The person feels more pain when lying on the right side. The person eats frequently in order to ease the gnawing discomfort in the stomach. Physical examination of the person shows that the liver is enlarged and that there is fluid within the abdominal cavity (ascites).

### *Nux vomica* (poison-nut)

This remedy picture describes constrictive pains in the liver area, which extend into the right shoulder. Physical examination reveals that the liver is enlarged and is sensitive to any pressure so that sufferers loosen their clothing. They may be jaundiced, and they long for alcohol and fatty food, both of which disagree with them. They have an aversion to meat, tobacco and coffee (all of which they normally like) and water.

## *Gall-bladder problems*

The gall-bladder is a small pouch situated under the right lower rib margin, which collects the bile produced by the liver from waste products from the blood. In the gall-bladder, the bile is concentrated and then travels down the cystic duct and the common bile duct to be secreted into the duodenum (the first part of the small intestine), where it helps to promote the absorption of certain foods. It is bile that gives the stools their brown colour.

However, sometimes the bile becomes so concentrated in the gall-bladder that it solidifies into stones.

These can either have calcium in them – in which case, they are radio-opaque and will show up on X-rays – or they consist of cholesterol and so will not be radio-opaque. However, both types will be seen during ultrasound scanning.

A high percentage of people over the age of 60 have gallstones that produce no symptoms at all. Sometimes, however, the gall-bladder can become inflamed, a condition known as *cholecystitis*, which produces severe constant pain in the right side of the abdomen, just under the ribs; there is also fever and, occasionally, jaundice. Another risk with gallstones is that one or more will move out of the gall-bladder and block the cystic duct. This causes a severe colicky pain – *gallstone colic.*

If the stones do not move out of the duct, they will cause an obstructive jaundice.

In all of these situations, medical advice is needed.

The conventional treatment for cholecystitis is antibiotic therapy with painkillers, and for gallstone colic, painkillers alone. In both cases, surgery is sometimes indicated.

Homeopathic remedies for the treatment of cholecystitis or gallstone colic can be given while awaiting medical attention, and when this occurs, they can be used in a complementary way with the conventional therapy. Select the remedy from the remedy pictures given below matching the latter with the physical symptoms.

If the person hasn't got a fever and is showing signs of gallstone colic, the recommended potency is 6c with one dose given every 30 minutes for a maximum of ten doses. If symptoms persist and the person doesn't develop a fever, give one 6c potency dose every four to six hours until the symptoms have abated.

If the person has a fever, the recommended potency is 30c given every hour for a maximum of four doses, reducing to one dose four times a day for one day, and further reducing by one dose a day to a maintenance dose of one a day until the person has improved.

The following are the homeopathic remedies for the treatment of cholecystitis and gallstone colic before any operation has been recommended.

### *Aconitum napellus* (monk's-hood)

This remedy picture describes a hot, tense swelling under the right lower ribs, causing pain so intense that sufferers have to sit upright and have breathing difficulties. They also sweat with anxiety and are particularly fearful of dying.

### *Apis mellifica* (honey bee)

This remedy picture describes severe burning and stinging pains on the left as well as the right side of the gall-bladder area.

### *Baptisia* (wild indigo)

This remedy picture describes pain in the liver area (the right upper abdomen) that is made worse from walking and from drinking beer. The person quickly becomes drowsy and goes to bed.

### *Belladonna* (deadly nightshade)

This remedy picture describes extreme sensitivity especially to anything that jars the body; this will worsen the pains in the gall bladder considerably. It is because of this sensitivity symptom that this remedy is indicated. The usual features of *Belladonna* – a red, hot face, widely dilated pupils and a bounding heart rate – need not necessarily be present.

### *Berberis vulgaris* (barberry)

This remedy picture describes pain in the region of the gall bladder extending into the stomach. The pain is made worse from pressure and when the person stands up.

### *Bryonia* (wild hops)

This remedy picture describes pain that is made much worse from movement of any sort. It also describes pain in the right upper abdomen (liver) such that, when sufferers cough, they feel as if their livers will burst (a symptom shared with *Natrum sulphuricum*). Features of the person as a whole will help in selecting this remedy: a thirst for large volumes of cold drink, a white tongue, constipation and irritability.

## *Calcarea carbonica* (calcium carbonate)

This remedy picture describes colicky pains that radiate from the left side of the stomach to the right (the reverse of *Ipecacuanha*). These pains are associated with profuse sweating, particularly on the head, hands and feet. The sweat is cold although the rest of the body is warm. The pains are relieved by bending double. The person is sensitive to cold, wet weather and has a desire for eggs, particularly boiled eggs.

## *Carduus marianus* (St Mary's thistle)

This remedy picture describes gallstone colic associated with a peculiar symptom: a feeling as if a pea is crawling through a narrow canal on the underside of the liver and on to the stomach (a symptom shared with *Natrum sulphuricum*). The tongue is an unusual colour: a white centre with red indented edges (the reverse of *Iris versicolor*).

## *Chelidonium majus* (celandine)

This remedy picture describes a person who is usually jaundiced and has pain of the gallstone variety (colic). The abdomen is distended and feels constricted as though a string is tightly tied across it. The colicky pain is referred to the back and, specifically, to the right shoulder blade.

## *Cinchona officinalis (China)* (Peruvian bark)

This remedy picture describes gallstone colic that is made worse from the slightest touch or soft direct pressure over the gall bladder area (just beneath the right lower ribs), and from movement of any sort and from cold air. It is improved when the person bends double or exerts *firm* pressure over the area. The symptoms recur at regular intervals every day or every night at a specific time. The person may experience drenching night sweats.

### Colocynthis (bitter cucumber)

The guiding features of this remedy picture are neuralgic pains associated with a personality that can be easily angered. The agonizing pains from the gallstone colic are eased by bending double and from firm pressure on the painful area.

### Dioscorea villosa (wild yam)

This remedy picture describes sufferers with weak digestion that results in rumbling noises with the passage of a great deal of wind. They can suddenly develop gallstone colic, and the symptoms worsen when they bend double. They feel better standing erect or bending backwards. The sharp pains of the colic in this remedy picture are referred towards the right nipple.

### Ipecacuanha (ipecac root)

This remedy picture describes pains in the stomach that pass from left to right (the reverse of *Calcarea carbonica*). The symptoms are associated with nausea and a clean tongue, and the pain is relieved by vomiting. The person develops a cold sweat on the forehead, has no thirst and probably has an itchy skin.

### Iris versicolor (blue flag)

This remedy picture describes cutting pains in the region of the gall bladder, which are improved by movement. Sufferers are aware of a burning in their stomachs, and their tongues are dry and coated on each side, with a red streak in their centres (the reverse of *Carduus marianus*).

### Kali bichromium (potassium bichromate)

This remedy picture describes a pinpoint pain in the liver area, which becomes a sharp stitch on sudden movement after sitting down. These pains are also made worse by drinking beer (a symptom shared with *Baptisia*). During the evening, the person can be seized with a violent aching in the region of the liver and extending up to the shoulders. This ache can last for several hours and is made easier when the person undresses.

### Kali carbonicum (potassium carbonate)

The picture of this remedy describes pain with a stitching quality in the region of the liver. The person may or may not be jaundiced, will almost certainly feel weak, will have wind and a desire for eating sweets. All people that this picture will suit show an intolerance to cold weather and an early morning (3.00 am) deterioration of symptoms. The pain is also aggravated after the eating of fatty food.

### Lithium carbonicum (lithium carbonate)

This remedy picture describes violent pains in the liver area, typical of gallstone colic. This is associated with pains in the bladder, and the person tends to have a red nose.

### Magnesium phosphoricum (magnesium phosphate)

The guiding feature of this remedy picture is that the colicky pains are eased by the application of local warmth rather than pressure. There is a lot of wind, which they seem to be constantly passing, but belching gives no relief. The abdomen is swollen so that sufferers feel more comfortable when their clothes are loosened.

### Mercurius solubis (black oxide of mercury)

This remedy picture describes pressing pains in the liver area so that the person is unable to lie on their right side. The symptoms are worse at night particularly in the warmth of the bed, and are worse for the sweating that the person has. The person has a craving for bread and butter.

### *Natrum sulphuricum* (sodium sulphate)

This remedy picture describes symptoms similar to those of gallstone colic. This is eased by sufferers rubbing the skin over the gall bladder, and when they lie on their left side. They notice a peculiar symptom: as if a pea is crawling through a narrow canal to underneath the liver, extending into the stomach. All symptoms have a tendency to become worse at about 4.00 am.

### *Nux vomica* (poison-nut)

This remedy picture describes gallstone colic associated with spasms of the abdominal muscles that give stitching pains in the liver. The skin over the liver is sensitive and sufferers cannot bear tight clothing for this reason. Constipation is usually a problem, with ineffectual urging to defecate. This remedy picture shows that the remedy attempts to relax the muscles of the cystic duct, enabling the stone to pass out into the gastrointestinal tract.

# Remedies for those undergoing gall-bladder surgery

If a conventional operation is recommended, the following homeopathic remedies should be considered:

- *Arnica* (leopard's bane): 6c four times a day for five days or until any bruising begins to subside. To be given with ...
- *Hypericum* (St John's wort): 6c four times a day, with the *Arnica*, for three to five days to help the skin incision heal. When this happens, this remedy can be discontinued.

"Keyhole surgery" is increasingly becoming the common form of surgery for gall-bladder problems. In these cases, the dosage schedule is different:

- *Arnica* (leopard's bane): one 6c dose is given just before the operation and repeated every two hours after it, for a maximum of four doses or until the bruising, if any, has settled. To be given with ...
- *Hypericum* (St John's wort): one 6c dose is given just before the operation and repeated every two hours afterwards, for a maximum of four doses or until the small incision shows signs of satisfactory healing.

# Pancreas disorders

The pancreas is essential for the control of blood sugar by secreting insulin into the blood (its endocrine function), as well as secreting enzymes into the gut (its exocrine function) to aid the absorption of food.

The pancreas can become chronically inflamed mainly from abuse of alcohol leading to an illness called *chronic pancreatitis*. An acute form of this condition can also (although rarely) result from certain viral infections such as MUMPS (*see* p. 422) and HEPATITIS (*see* p. 137).

Failure of the pancreas's endocrine function will lead to *diabetes mellitus,* which causes a high level of glucose (sugar) in the blood, extremely frequent urination, excessive thirst, weight loss and fatigue. There is a tendency for this condition to run in families, but the ultimate cause is thought to be a viral infection some years earlier. Failure of the exocrine function of the pancreas will lead to a form of *malabsorption* caused by the lack of enzymes secreted by this organ. This results in diarrhoea with greasy faeces (steatorrhoea) that are bulky and difficult to flush away in the toilet.

It is essential to obtain medical advice whenever there is disease of the pancreas. The conventional treatment for diabetes is the giving of insulin by injection, or tablets that will stimulate the pancreas to increase its production of this hormone. This treatment is given in combination with dietary advice about the intake of carbohydrates, as well as balancing calorie intake with calorie output. The conventional treatment for malabsorption is replacement of the lacking enzyme with a substitute called pancreatin, which comes in tablet and powder form.

Homeopathic treatment is best given by a specialist homeopath as disease of the pancreas is complicated. After following the advice of such a specialist, it has been shown that the insulin requirements of those who suffer from diabetes mellitus are lessened, and that the quantity of enzyme supplements needed by those with malabsorption are reduced.

If it is not possible to see a specialist homeopath, there are several remedies that have an affinity for the pancreas, and these can be used in a complementary way with conventional medical treatment. Using the 6c potency, give one dose twice a day.

Should the reason for the pancreatic disease be alcohol abuse, this must be addressed initially. As well as counselling for this addiction, the following two remedies can be used to help wean the person off alcohol:

- *Nux vomica* (poison-nut)
  This remedy picture describes sufferers who are ambitious and have a tendency to abuse alcohol, caffeine and nicotine. They are strong characters in that they want to achieve, but are weak because they damage their health by the abuse of alcohol, caffeine and nicotine. It is on this general profile of the person that this remedy will be selected for the treatment of pancreatic disease.
- *Ranunculus bulbosus* (buttercup)
  This remedy picture describes sufferers who suffer from the bad effects of alcohol. They are not as ambitious as the picture for *Nux vomica*. They can develop an irritating pain in the forehead and eyeballs, and a creeping sensation in their scalp.

Whichever of these two remedies is selected, it can be used in conjunction with the following ones.

When choosing one of these remedies, pick out a peculiar symptom that matches the remedy picture with the physical picture, or else select the remedy picture profile that suits the person as a whole. Using the 6c potency, give one dose in the middle of the day – between the morning and evening doses of one of the previous remedies if also treating alcohol abuse. If not, simply give one dose twice a day.

### *Arsenicum iodatum* (arsenic iodide)

This remedy picture describes sufferers who have severe pains in the upper part of their abdomens and are also very thirsty. Paradoxically, fluids and food are vomited quickly after they have been consumed. Sufferers also feel nauseated, which is a distressing symptom. All the symptoms are worse between midnight and 2.00 am. Sufferers easily become restless.

### *Chionanthus* (fringe tree)

This remedy picture describes sufferers who have a dull ache in the umbilical (tummy button) area that occasionally becomes a gripping pain, as if a string has been tied around the abdomen and is being gradually but progressively tightened and then suddenly loosened. The liver area is sore, the liver itself is commonly enlarged and there is jaundice. Sufferers have no appetite and are constipated. If stool is produced, it is clay-coloured and soft in texture. The tongue is heavily coated.

### *Conium* (poison hemlock)

This remedy picture describes acute inflammation of the pancreas, with pain in the liver, which is probably enlarged. There is a pressing, burning pain from the stomach through to the back and shoulders. A characteristic feature of this remedy is that the person begins to sweat on falling asleep.

### *Iodum* (iodine)

This remedy picture describes a person who has a throbbing pain in the stomach that, at times, becomes cutting in nature. Sufferers' livers and spleens are probably enlarged, and they themselves might well be jaundiced. They are also ravenously hungry and have great thirst.

### *Iris versicolor* (blue flag)

This remedy has in its picture a burning sensation of the whole of the gastrointestinal tract. There is a lack of appetite but paradoxically a profuse flow of saliva. The liver area is tender to the touch. This remedy picture also describes sufferers who have goitres (enlargement of the thyroid gland). They may also complain of headache while relaxing following a period of intense mental activity.

### *Phosphorus*

This remedy picture describes a symptom in which the whole body is consumed with a burning sensation that is particularly noticeable in the stomach and in the small intestine (this symptom will be noticed around the tummy button), and radiates through to the shoulder blades.

Generally the guiding features of this remedy will be the symptoms of the person as a whole. The remedy picture describes sufferers who possibly have an artistic temperament, as well as fine dark hair with a tint of red in it. They like salt and cold drinks. They fear being alone and tend to be socially active. They are particularly frightened by thunder, and have a perpetual feeling of someone being behind them. They gain relief from rubbing and from naps. The remedy picture also describes the presence of cutting pains and a sensation of emptiness in the entire abdominal cavity. It is common for there to be large yellow spots on the skin covering the abdominal cavity.

### *Spongia tosta* (roasted sponge)

This remedy picture describes marked effects on the pancreas. The characteristic features of this remedy are violent pains in the abdominal muscles when sufferers inhale. They feel as if their guts have been drawn upwards and are now lying just underneath the diaphragm. A woman suffering from painful periods (dysmenorrohea) will develop abdominal pains rather than uterine pains.

# Small intestine problems

The small intestine runs from the stomach and, after many metres, to the junction with the large bowel (colon). The name given to the final part of the small intestine is the "ileum" and that of the junction with the large bowel is the "ileo-caecal junction".

A very serious disease commonly affects this part of the intestine, although it can occur in any part of the gastrointestinal tract. In *Crohn's disease*, named after the physician who first described it, the intestinal wall becomes chronically inflamed and thickened, and deep ulcers may form. These changes cause abdominal pain, diarrhoea and weight loss, and in the end, can lead to blockage of the intestine.

The cause of Crohn's disease, which is much more common in women than in men, is unknown. Current thinking suggests that it might be due to an abnormal autoimmune response by the body. Several bacterial strains found in the intestines have been investigated as possible causes, particularly those associated with causing diarrhoea, but none of them has shown a convincing statistically significant result. Some people have reported that Zen meditation has helped cure Crohn's disease.

**Because this is a major illness, it is imperative that conventional medical opinion is sought.** This will involve a detailed examination and investigation (which will include a test to exclude tuberculosis, as there are certain common features between the two illnesses), followed by conventional treatment that may well include the administration of steroid therapy.

Homeopathy can be used in a complementary way with the conventional treatment, but if you decide to adopt this approach, it is essential to do so with the knowledge of your doctor and not suddenly stop any conventional treatment without mutual discussions. Using homeopathy with conventional medical treatment has been shown to increase sufferers' overall sense of well-being as well as reduce pain, the frequency of the bowels opening and the number of conventional drugs (including steroids) needed.

Homeopathic treatment differs depending on whether you are treating the acute symptomatic stage, or are giving the deeper, more fundamental treatment suitable for a recurring problem. In both of these treatments, anti-oxidant therapy and probiotic therapy are essential (*see* MYALGIC ENCEPHALOMYELITIS, p.25).

## Symptomatic treatment

Choose the remedy whose picture fits the physical symptoms most appropriately. Using the 6c potency, give one dose four times a day for as long as the symptoms are a problem.

### *Aloe* (socotrine aloes)

The remedy picture describes a person with a bloated, distended abdomen that feels full and heavy. There is general pain around the umbilicus (tummy button) that is made worse when pressure is applied. The person worries about faecal incontinence, finding that breaking wind can lead to an "accident".

### *Gambogia* (gummi gutti)

The remedy picture is similar to *Aloe* but differs in that there is a forcible ejection of stool with a strained abdominal sensation afterwards. The abdomen produces many rumbling sounds, and there is much wind after a stool is passed. The ileo-caecal area (bottom right-hand quadrant of the abdomen) is particularly tender to firm pressure. All the symptoms are worse towards sunset and at night.

### *Podophyllum* (may apple)

The remedy picture describes a gastro-enteritis with colicky abdominal pain and bilious vomiting. Stool is watery with jel-ly-like mucus; it is produced painlessly and smells very offensive. The diarrhoea is worse in the morning. Hot weather makes the whole picture worse.

## Deeper treatment

The suggested dosage schedule is to use the 30c potency and give one dose every 12 hours for a maximum of three doses. During this time, symptomatic treatment can be carried out at the same time.

The three-dose schedule of the 30c potency can be repeated according to the physical response, but a period of at least three weeks must have elapsed first.

The following bowel nosodes should be used. These are ho-meopathically prepared potencies prepared from mother tincture that has been made from bacteria from the gut. Each of these preparations has well-described and individual remedy pictures. When choosing a particular one, concentrate on the key symptom and match that with the physical presentation.

- *Dysentery co*: anticipatory worries and fears.
- *Gaertner*: malnutrition, which makes it useful in the treatment of Crohn's disease because the ileum is unable to absorb nutrients adequately.
- *Proteus*: suddenness and violence (nervous temper and mus-cular spasms).

Further remedies may be used, preferably after treatment with a bowel nosode, although they may be given in their own right.

The dosage schedule is as for the bowel nosodes: one 30c dose every 12 hours for a maximum of three doses, which may be repeated after a period of at least three weeks.

### Lycopodium (club moss)

The remedy picture describes a person who fears loneliness and has a desire for sweets. There is a feeling of constant fermentation in the abdomen, so that eating a very small amount will leave the person feeling bloated and full.

### Nux vomica (poison-nut)

The remedy picture describes an abdomen that feels bruised and sore. Intestinal gases distend it, and this is accompanied by spasmodic colic. The colic is worsened when sufferers become uncovered, and it is associated with a desire to defecate. Sufferers feel a sense of incomplete evacuation every time a stool is passed. As a whole, they are ambitious people, and tend to abuse caffeine and nicotine; they are also somewhat perfectionist.

### Phosphoricum acidum (phosphoric acid)

The remedy picture describes an abdomen that is distended and produces loud, rumbling noises. There is an aching in the umbilical (tummy button) area. The diarrhoea that occurs is painless, involuntary and accompanied by a lot of wind.

### Phosphorus

The remedy picture describes sufferers who have sharp, cutting pains in the abdomen, as well as painless and copious diarrhoea that is debilitating – it is as though the anus remains permanently open. They prefer cool liquids, as warm food and fluids cause vomiting. These people as a whole are sensitive physically and emotionally, and are fearful of thunderstorms. Sleep or just a short nap helps rejuvenate them, if only temporarily.

### *Pulsatilla* (wind flower)

The characteristic feature of this remedy is the great variability of its symptoms from hour to hour. The abdomen is painful from distension, and there are loud rumblings as though there is a stone in it. The colic is worse in the evening and is associated with chilliness. The stools vary in their consistency from watery to properly formed, no two stools being the same. Sufferers are, on the whole, mild and non-argumentative, and they yearn for physical comfort. They have little or no thirst, feel better in the fresh air and dislike warm environments as this temperature tends to weaken them.

### *Tuberculinum* (nucleo-protein from tubercular abscess)

This remedy is indicated because of the similar pathology between tuberculosis and Crohn's disease. Its remedy picture describes sudden diarrhoea, occurring early in the morning, with stools that smell offensive and are excreted explosively.

# Large intestine disorders

The large intestine, also called the colon, is much shorter than the small intestine, and is the place where the faeces are prepared and stored and where fluid is extracted from the excrement before it is evacuated from the anus. The large intestine divides into four segments – the ascending, the transverse, the descending and the sigmoid colon – before turning into the rectum and finally the anus. The appendix is a small, finger-shaped tube that projects out of the caecum, the name given to the first part of the ascending colon.

## Abdominal adhesions

These are strands of fibrous tissue that can develop inside the abdominal cavity whenever a surgical procedure is carried out in this space. They can attach previously unconnected organs, and in women, this can lead to infertility. They can also cause partial obstruction of the bowel, giving colicky pains with or without vomiting. Adhesions can be treated by further surgery, but there is a Catch 22 as any more surgery can result in more adhesion formation.

There is, however, one homeopathic remedy that can be used to resolve adhesion formation: *Thiosinaminum*, a chemical derived from mustard seed oil. Using the 6c potency, give one dose twice a day until the symptoms begin to improve.

# Appendicitis

The appendix can become inflamed, giving a condition called appendicitis. The primary symptom of this is pain in the lower right quadrant of the abdomen that is made worse on being pressed. The essential treatment is along the conventional route, with surgery an absolute necessity. If surgery is not carried out, the infected appendix will burst and spill its contents into the abdominal cavity, leading to serious infection (peritonitis) and subsequently ADHESIONS (*see above*).

Because of these serious problems, homeopathy is not considered to be a therapeutic option. However, the following remedies – which are appropriate only *after* conventional medical help has been summoned – have been used in the very early stages of acute appendicitis and have shown an ability to stop the infection from developing. Using the 6c potency, give one dose every 15 minutes.

### *Apis mellifica* (honey bee)

This remedy picture describes pains in the abdomen's right lower quadrant that the person describes as stinging. The pains develop following sleep (a symptom shared with *Lachesis*).

### *Arsenicum album* (arsenic trioxide)

This remedy picture describes abdominal pains that have a burning quality, and which are only relieved by heat. The tongue is a bluish, brown/black colour and is dry. The general profile of sufferers is that they are full of anxiety and restless and enjoy sips of fluid. Their symptoms are at their worst around midnight.

### *Belladonna* (deadly nightshade)

This remedy picture describes pain in the right lower quadrant of the abdomen that is made much worse by any jarring movement. The person cannot bear the slightest touch on the abdomen, not even the bedclothes.

### *Bryonia* (wild hops)

This remedy picture describes a person who has a dull, throbbing or sticking pain in a single spot. This pain is made easier by sufferers lying on the painful side and by drawing up their knees. They also feel better if heat is applied over the tender spot.

### *Cocculus* (Indian cockle)

This remedy picture describes a constant pain in the right lower quadrant of the abdomen that is made worse at the slightest touch, and which slowly increases in intensity. During the pain, sufferers feel as if it involves the whole of their abdomen, causing them to move their legs constantly in an unsuccessful attempt to find some relief.

### *Lachesis* (bushmaster snake venom)

This remedy picture describes pain in the right lower abdominal quadrant that is made worse at the slightest touch so that sufferers don't want to wear any clothes. This sensitivity of clothing also applies to the neck. They also feel sick, and drinking warm water makes them choke. It is typical of this remedy that the face has a purple colour to it and is puffy.

## *Lycopodium* (club moss)

This remedy picture describes colicky pains starting in the right lower quadrant of the abdomen, which radiate downwards into the bladder. This makes the person want to urinate frequently and urgently. The abdomen is sensitive to pressure and to the weight of clothes (a symptom shared with *Lachesis*).

## *Mercurius corrosivus* (corrosive sublimate of mercury)

This remedy picture describes pain in the right lower quadrant of the abdomen as well as pain across the top of it (i.e. the transverse colon). The remedy produces burning feelings in the bladder, so that hot urine is passed drop by drop, and in the lower part of the gastrointestinal tract (rectum), so that the person has a constant desire to defecate but without success.

# Constipation

People often believe that they should defecate at least once a day, but the normal range is far wider: 3–14 times a week. However, the stool should be soft and easily expelled. If the frequency of defecation is decreased or the stool becomes hard, lumpy and difficult to expel, the person is said to be constipated. Abdominal pain may or may not be a symptom.

> If the stool frequency or consistency begins to change, and particularly if the person is over the age of 40 and blood is present in the stool, it is extremely important to obtain a medical opinion as these symptoms may mark the beginning of a serious problem such as cancer of the colon.

The treatment of constipation involves a number of factors. A proper diet is very important, and changing this should be the first step in treating the condition. It should include as much fibre (roughage) as possible as well as an adequate amount of fluid so that the stools become bulky and soft.

Exercise is also essential in restoring normal bowel activity. If the person is sluggish, the bowels also become sluggish. This is most noticeable in those who have to have long periods of bed rest.

There are a number of "natural" laxatives: syrup of figs; dried fruits, particularly apricots and prunes; linseed soaked in boiled water and drunk as a herbal tea two or three times a day (linseed can also be sprinkled on cereals or into soup); and molasses (black treacle), 10–15 ml (2–3 teaspoons) to be taken three times a day, as it comes or spread on food. However, it is far preferable to deal with constipation through diet and exercise, rather than resorting to these substances, however "natural". It is probably a good idea to take probiotic supplements (*see* MYALGIC ENCEPHALOMYELI-TIS, p. 25), as they help restore the micro-flora of the gastrointestinal tract and therefore normal bowel activity.

Constipation occurs in all ages, apart from the breast-fed baby, but the symptoms vary between the different age groups. In the older person, it may cause colicky abdominal pain, a feeling of not being right, tension headaches and ultimately the formation of HAEMORRHOIDS. In the younger person, the symptoms include a poor appetite. Depressed persons may have a reduced energy level, and children experience increased stress and anxiety, which almost certainly spills over on to the parents.

For the homeopathic remedies for babies, see p. 406, and for children, p. 442. Those for adults follow, with their remedy pictures. Select the remedy by matching its picture with the physical symptoms. Using the 6c potency, give one dose twice a day for as long as necessary. Remember that, when taking a homeopathic remedy, the broad guidelines about diet and pro-biotic therapy still apply.

### *Aesculus hippocastanum* (horse chestnut)

This remedy describes sufferers who have dry, hard stools and difficulty in defecation. They feel as though their rectums are dry and hot, and also have a sensation that their rectums are "full of small sticks". These symptoms cause them to feel a knife-like pain shooting upwards, giving them severe backache in the lower back. Whenever a stool is passed, there is a spasmodic and constrictive pain in the anus, which can last for many hours (a symptom shared with *Nitric acidum*).

### *Alumen* (potash of aluminium)

This remedy picture describes sufferers whose bowels are inactive and also their bladders. They cannot defecate for days on end. It is as though the rectum is paralysed, and sufferers don't feel anything in it. They also find that, in order to urinate, they need to strain to pass a stool. They feel worse in cold environments, except for a headache that is improved by exposure to the cold. If this remedy picture matches the physical symptoms of the person, check that the cooking utensils are not made of aluminium as this will aggravate the symptoms.

### *Bryonia* (wild hops)

This remedy picture describes the person who has to strain repeatedly in order to defecate. This considerable straining causes a rush of blood to the head, giving a headache and a possible nose bleed. The stools are hard, dry and dark as if burned (a symptom shared with *Sulphur*). Sufferers probably have distended abdomens with much rumbling and colicky pains, as though there is about to be an easy defecation. However, there is still an obstinate constipation. When a stool is finally passed, sufferers are left with a long-standing burning pain in the rectum. The sort of person that this remedy suits is irritable (like *Nux vomica*), feels worse with movement, very probably has a white-coloured tongue and is extremely thirsty.

### *Conium* (poison hemlock)

This remedy picture describes sufferers who have an ineffectual urge to defecate and produce hard stools. They cannot strain to produce these stools because of a seemingly paralytic weakness of the muscles used for evacuation. Every time they go to defecate, they develop a tremulous weakness associated with palpitations. The picture of *Conium* has a peculiar symptom: copious sweating that occurs when sufferers fall asleep or merely close their eyes.

## *Natrum muriaticum* (sodium chloride)

This remedy picture describes sufferers who tend to be shy and irritable and hate fuss of any sort. They have an aversion to fatty food (unlike *Sulphur*) and also to bread, but crave salt. They have an irregular bowel action, commonly defecating on alternate days, and cannot be sure whether a stool has been passed or not.

## *Magnesia muriaticum* (magnesium chloride)

This remedy picture describes a person whose symptoms are worse from salt, including salty food, salt baths and sea air. It is the remedy to be considered for constipation that may occur at the seaside. The stools are dry and crumble at the anus.

## *Nitric acidum* (nitric acid)

This remedy picture describes a person who notices a pricking pain in the rectum whenever a stool is being passed, as though something is being torn. This pain can last for many hours after a stool has been passed (a symptom shared with *Aesculus*). Its quality is described as a burning in the anus and an itching in the rectum. The person as a whole is similar to a *Sepia* person, but craves fatty food and salt.

## *Nux vomica* (poison-nut)

This remedy picture describes sedentary people who are probably workaholic, and are generally irritable and perfectionist. They have a sensation of continually wanting to defecate, but little or no stool appears. If it does, they are left feeling that there are more faeces that still need to come out. They also experience a tearing, sticking and contracting pain in the rectum as if from

HAEMORRHOIDS. These sensations come on particularly after a meal and when the brain has been overextended through work or study. Bowel activity is abnormal, causing an irregular peristalsis (the muscular movement of food through the gastrointestinal tract) that drives the intestinal contents backwards and then forwards, giving rise to spasmodic contractions.

### *Opium* (dried latex of the poppy)

This remedy picture describes totally obstinate constipation that is almost unconquerable. This state can last for many weeks at a time and is associated with a loss of appetite. Any stool that does appear is a hard, small ball that has a tendency to retreat backwards into the rectum (a symptom shared with *Silicea*).

### *Platina* (platinum)

This remedy picture describes sufferers who travel around a great deal and are constantly changing the food they eat and the water they drink. This remedy shares with *Plumbum metallicum* the symptom of feeling as though the abdominal wall is being drawn into the back by a string, a feeling that extends into the pelvis. The stool is sticky and sticks to the rectum and anus like putty. Like *Alumen,* this remedy picture has the symptom of a frequent urge to defecate but with an inability to strain to complete an evacuation. A peculiar symptom of this remedy is that sufferers feel tall and everything looks small to them. Mentally they feel proud and look down on others around them.

### *Plumbum metallicum* (lead)

This remedy picture describes people who experience a lot of intestinal colic, the pain radiating to all parts of their bodies. They have a peculiar symptom: a sensation that the abdominal wall is being drawn into the back by a string. They have a paralysis of the intestines and are unable to strain at stool and so are totally unable to defecate. Any stool that does appear is like a conglomerate of small hard balls, reminiscent of sheep dung.

Sufferers experience considerable urges to defecate, with terrible pains from the constriction and spasm of the anus.

### Sepia (inky juice of cuttlefish)

This remedy picture describes a woman who is constipated during pregnancy. She has an ineffectual urge to defecate, causing such discomfort that it is as if she is in labour. This straining is accompanied by much sweating. The woman has the sensation of "a ball in the rectum". The woman as a whole tends to have low self-esteem, is indifferent to those around her, tends to feel that she has a vaginal prolapse and, for this reason, prefers to sit with her legs crossed. She also loves high winds and craves vinegar.

### Silicea (pure flint)

This remedy picture describes sufferers who have great difficulty in expelling stools because no sooner does one appear than it recedes back into the rectum. This is known as the "bashful stool"! Sufferers' straining is so strong because the anal sphincter goes into an intermittent contractile spasm, and their heads and particularly their feet break out in a sweat. They generally lack confidence and tend to feel cold. Pains similar to gallstone colic (see p. 141) are felt under the left lower ribs (although the gall-bladder is sited under the right ribs), and they are made worse by anything hot and by being touched. Sufferers aren't thirsty.

### Sulphur

This remedy picture describes people who have intermittent constipation, passing a stool every three to four days. The stools themselves are hard as if burned (a symptom shared with *Bryonia*), and they tend to be large and are held back because of the pain they cause on defecation. After passing a stool, sufferers always have the feeling as if "something has been left behind"(a symptom shared with *Nux vomica*). They are generally warm-blooded people who tend to kick off the bedclothes at night in order to put their feet outside. They become hungry at 11.00 am and enjoy all types of foods, particularly fatty ones.

# Diverticulosis and diverticulitis

Diverticula are small pouches that protrude from the wall of the colon into the abdominal cavity. The term "diverticulosis" simply means the presence of these pouches. You can be born with these, but more usually they are the result of ageing. They seem to arise where pressure in the colon forces its lining through areas of weaknesses in the intestinal wall. A lack of fibre in the diet is thought to be the primary cause.

If you have diverticula, it is important to eat a high-fibre diet and avoid becoming constipated. It is also a good idea to use probiotics (*see* MYALGIC ENCEPHALOMYELITIS, p. 25) as these will help to regulate the microflora of the small intestine, which in turn will enhance the mobility of the large intestine, making food move through more quickly and relieving any constipation.

Diverticula can become infected, causing pain that is localized and constant and which is usually associated with fever and vomiting. This illness is known as *diverticulitis*. It is important to seek conventional medical advice to establish this as a diagnosis for two reasons: diverticulitis shares many symptoms with the early stages of colonic cancer; and antibiotic therapy will probably be necessary. As well as a physical examination, there will also be a detailed investigation including X-ray, sigmoidoscopy (examination of the rectum and the sigmoid colon through a rigid or flexible fibreoptic tube) or colonoscopy (examination of the length of the colon through a flexible fibreoptic tube).

Homeopathic remedies can also be given in a truly complementary way with the conventional approach. Select the remedy picture that matches the physical symptoms most accurately, employing the principle of "like cures like". Using the 6c potency, give one dose every hour when the pain is at its worse, for a maximum of ten doses. Then reduce to one dose every two hours for one day, and further reduce the schedule to one dose every six hours until the person recovers.

### *Aconitum napellus* (monk's-hood)

This remedy picture describes an abdomen that is hot, tense and sensitive to the touch. There is also colic that no change in position makes better. Unusually, the abdominal symptoms are relieved after the drinking of warm soup.

### *Belladonna* (deadly nightshade)

This remedy picture describes a situation where the transverse colon is prominent and the person is aware of it, it is tender to the touch and feels as if it is being clutched by a hand. The pain is made worse by the least jarring movement and the least pressure.

### *Colocynthis* (bitter cucumber)

The characteristic feature of this remedy picture is a colicky pain that is made easier by the person bending over double thereby creating pressure on the pain which is the primary relieving action. The person is generally irritable and this mood makes the pains seem even worse.

### *Magnesium phosphoricum* (magnesium phosphate)

The characteristic feature of this remedy picture is that the colicky pains are alleviated more by warmth than by pressure.

# Enterocolitis

This terms includes the infective causes of diarrhoea – from gastroenteritis to cholera and salmonella – as well as "holiday diarrhoea", which may not necessarily result from an infection.

The primary treatment of any type of diarrhoea is the adequate replacement of fluids and minerals, particularly sodium (as found in salt). Dehydration is the most physically important factor to avoid. It is essential to seek medical help as stool culture for bacterial growth may be necessary to identify the bug causing the diarrhoea, which will help to determine which (if any) anti-biotic should be prescribed.

To prevent diarrhoea, observing stringent personal hygiene measures is vital, as well as – especially when travelling to those parts of the world where there is a high risk – avoiding non-bottled water, ice in drinks and particular foods that are known to be potential sources of the bacteria that cause diarrhoea: shellfish, unpeeled raw fruit and vegetables, foods containing raw eggs, reheated packaged meals. For information on diarrhoea in infants, *see* GASTROENTERITIS on p.414.

# Gastroenteritis

This illness, in which the stomach and intestines become in-flamed, is characterized by the sudden onset of diarrhoea with or without vomiting. The cause is usually a virus, but it can occur in travellers who eat and drink things that unsettle the microflora of the gastrointestinal tract. Acute diarrhoea can also occur when an infant starts teething. (For information on gastroenteritis in newborn babies, *see* p. 396, in infants generally, p. 414, and in teething infants, p. 435.)

The main concern with this illness is dehydration, and so fluid intake must be increased to match the fluid that is lost. It is also important to replace lost minerals (primarily sugar and salt). There are especially prepared packets of minerals – known as "rehydration salts" – that can be dissolved in water to give to sufferers. Dehydration is a particular problem of the very young and also the elderly. Medical opinion must be sought if there is any cause for concern.

Homeopathic treatment can either be used independently (while dealing with any dehydration) or in a complementary way with conventional medication. When selecting the homeopathic reme-dy, identify the most prominent symptom that the person is show-ing and match this with the appropriate remedy picture. Using the 6c potency, give one dose every four hours until the symptoms improve, when the frequency of medication can be slowly reduced.

### *Aethusa cynapium* (fool's parsley)

This remedy picture describes a situation of violence: violent diarrhoea, violent vomiting and violent abdominal colic. It applies particularly to children, who collapse very easily and will probably need medical attention. Sufferers have an intolerance of milk and their faces show much anxiety and pain.

### *Arsenicum album* (arsenic trioxide)

In this remedy picture, sufferers have simultaneous vomiting and diarrhoea. They are restless and anxious and feel very cold, and need sips, rather than gulps, of cold water. The symptoms are at their worst between midnight and 2.00 am.

### *Belladonna* (deadly nightshade)

The typical remedy picture is of diarrhoea in people who are twitchy and start at every noise. They are drowsy, and their faces are flushed, with widely dilated pupils. They usually have colic before the passage of diarrhoea.

### *Carbo vegetabilis* (vegetable charcoal)

The characteristic feature of this remedy picture is weakness to the point of collapse, associated with burning sensations. The anus is reddened (like *Sulphur*) and raw, and itches and bleeds easily. The diarrhoea is of a watery consistency and contains blood. Because the person is so weak, medical attention is obviously needed. It is useful to note that the remedy picture describes sufferers who feel better if air can be fanned directly over their faces.

### *Cinchona officinalis (China)* (Peruvian bark)

The diarrhoea in this remedy picture consists of undigested food particles, is painless and is worse at night and in hot weather. The picture describes a very weakened person who has much wind as well as diarrhoea.

### Croton tiglium (croton oil seed)

This remedy picture describes copious and watery diarrhoea associated with a lot of anal urging. The motions are shot out in a forcible manner; any food or drink (including a breast feed) will initiate this explosive evacuation. The symptoms are generally worse in the summer and are made worse by the slightest touch.

### Cuprum metallicum (copper)

The characteristic feature of this remedy picture is the intense cramping of all body muscles, associated with diarrhoea. The abdominal colic is relieved by firm pressure, and the muscle cramps are alleviated by the person doing appropriate body-stretching movements.

### Ignatia (St Ignatius' bean)

This remedy picture describes an upset gastrointestinal tract with colic and diarrhoea, particularly in the breastfed infant whose mother is undergoing a grief reaction.

### Ipecacuanha (ipecac root)

In this remedy picture, the characteristic feature is a continuous feeling of nausea. The diarrhoea smells offensive and contains a lot of undigested food.

### Nux vomica (poison-nut)

This remedy picture has a characteristic feature that, when a stool is passed, it eases the abdominal pain. The diarrhoea may have been caused by over-indulgence of alcohol or caffeine, and it may, in turn, worsen HAEMORRHOIDS.

### Phosphorus

This remedy picture describes diarrhoea that causes a burning sensation as the stools are being passed. The person vomits a lot and craves ice-cold water and ice cream, which is promptly vomited as it heats up in the stomach.

### Pulsatilla (wind flower)

This remedy picture describes diarrhoea that is made worse by the eating of fatty food. The person is of a tearful nature and feels more comfortable when given physical and emotional support. All the symptoms are worse at night and improve whenever the person gets out into the fresh air.

### Sulphur

In this remedy picture, the diarrhoea is much worse in the early morning, and can force sufferers out of bed. The whole remedy picture is full of burning sensations, so that the anus becomes red and itches a great deal. It is common for sufferers to develop haemorrhoids. They easily become hot and prefer their feet to stick out of the bedclothes in order to cool down.

## Cholera

This is a bacterial infection of the gastrointestinal tract caused by drinking contaminated water or eating vegetables and fruit washed in it. It causes severe abdominal pain, continuous diarrhoea with vomiting and a great thirst, but with no fever.

Conventional treatment consists of antibiotic therapy and correction of dehydration by intravenous fluid replacement. The illness lasts for about two weeks.

It was in the treatment of this disease that Samuel Hahnemann made a considerable reputation for himself when cholera epidemics swept through Europe in the early 1800s. The three remedies that he used were *Camphor* (for the feverish state; give a single dose of the 30c potency), *Cuprum* (for the spasmodic stage; give a single dose of the 30c potency) and *Veratrum album* (for a state of total collapse; give a single dose of the 30c potency). Nowadays, with improved water supplies, cholera epidemics are a rare occurrence.

The most recent one was in Peru, where Hahnemann's original three remedies were used to good effect.

# Salmonella poisoning

This is caused by infection with any one of the *Salmonella* group of bacteria. One type causes typhoid fever, but far more common is food poisoning by some of the other types. The source of the poisoning is very often found to be contaminated poultry and eggs, and strict food hygiene practices are necessary to avoid it. The symptoms of salmonella food poisoning are the same as for gastroenteritis, and it can be treated by the homeopathic remedies given in that section. In addition, one remedy – *Baptisia*, given below – is specifically useful in treating this condition.

It is important to obtain medical assessment as conventional treatment with antibiotics and intravenous fluid replacement (if necessary) may be required in severe cases.

## *Baptisia* (wild indigo)

This remedy is of particular use in the treatment of salmonella. The diarrhoea is profuse and bloody and smells offensive. The illness starts very suddenly, and the person quickly becomes very weak, as though drugged. The tongue is swollen, dry and coloured yellow in the centre.

# Haemorrhoids

Haemorrhoids – commonly called "piles" – are swollen veins in the anal lining. They can cause irritation around the anus as well as bleeding, with or without defecation. If a clot forms inside a haemorrhoid (thrombosed haemorrhoid), this can be very painful. It is important to get a medical opinion to establish the precise diagnosis, as haemorrhoids can be a precursor of other, more serious problems. The examination that the doctor will perform is simple and painless.

The broad guidelines about diet in relation to treating CON-STIPATION (*see above*) also apply to the treatment of haemorrhoids. In addition, the conventional medical approach includes analgesics for pain relief, surgery to remove the haemorrhoids (haemorrhoidectomy) and an anal stretch to relieve spasm of the anal sphincter – i.e. the muscles controlling its opening and closing. Conventional ointments are available for relief of anal irritation, as are homeopathic ointments and remedies for treating haemorrhoids: using the 30c potency, give one dose daily for one week, reducing to the 6c potency twice a day for two weeks. With all treatments, it is important to keep the stool soft so that it can be evacuated without any strain.

### *Aesculus hippocastanum* (horse chestnut)

This remedy picture describes engorged haemorrhoidal veins associated with lower backache. The anal margin feels as if small sticks are attached to it, causing a raw and sore feeling. The passage of a stool is obviously very painful and may or may not be accompanied by blood.

### *Aloe* (socotrine aloes)

This remedy picture describes haemorrhoids that protrude like grapes from the anus, and are very sore and tender. These symptoms are improved by the application of cold water (from a bidet spray, for example). The person is aware of a burning sensation in the rectum and anus.

### *Ammonium carbonicum* (ammonium carbonate)

This remedy picture describes haemorrhoids found in a woman, which bleed a great deal and are particularly worse during menstruation. The bleeding is also worse after the evacuation of a stool, but is improved when the woman lies down.

### Collinsonia canadensis (stone-root)

This remedy picture suits women in particular. There is a sensation that the rectum is constricted, together with a feeling of sharp sticks there. The haemorrhoids are painful and bleed, and are associated with itching around the anus. The person has alternating constipation and diarrhoea, both of which are associated with a lot of wind.

### Hamamelis virginica (witch hazel)

This remedy picture describes an anus that feels raw and sore, with haemorrhoids that bleed profusely. The person is aware of a pulsating feeling in the rectum.

### Nitricum acidum (nitric acid)

This remedy picture describes a person who feels a sensation of splinters around the anal margin. This causes violent cutting pain after the passage of a stool, and the pain persists for a long time afterwards. The haemorrhoids bleed easily. The person may also notice a colicky pain that is eased by tightening their clothes.

### Nux vomica (poison-nut)

This remedy picture describes a person who has an ineffectual urge to defecate and believes that the effort is not worthwhile since, even after a stool has been passed, there remains a feeling that the bowel still needs evacuating. The overall characteristics of the person can also influence the choice of this remedy: a hardworking, high achiever who probably overindulges with alcohol, caffeine and tobacco.

### *Paeonia* (peony)

This remedy picture describes irritation around the anus. The remedy is used as an ointment that is applied topically as often as the haemorrhoidal irritation requires. It can also be used with other homeopathic remedies when treating haemorrhoids.

### *Pulsatilla* (wind flower)

This remedy picture describes painful haemorrhoids, and the pain is increased when the person lies down. He or she is characteristically not at all thirsty and has a malleable personality.

### *Ratanhia* (krameria and mapato)

This remedy picture describes a person who feels as if the rectum is filled with broken glass, and it takes extreme pain and effort to pass any stool. This pain lasts for hours. This remedy is also useful for the homeopathic treatment of a condition called anal fissure (fissure-in-ano), in which there is a tear in the anal sphincter (the ring of muscle surrounding the opening of the anus) that can ulcerate and cause pain and bleeding.

### *Sulphur*

This remedy picture describes sufferers who notice a burning and pinching sensation around the anus, and are aware of prolapsed haemorrhoids – that is, they protrude outside the anus. The overall picture of these people is an important influence on the choice of this remedy: rather laid-back individuals who are jovial and good fun to be with, enjoy beer and a joke and have a definite point of view, as well as a violent temper from which they are able to recover very quickly and forget all about.

# Irritable bowel syndrome (IBS)

In irritable bowel syndrome – formerly known as spastic colon – sufferers notice a variety of symptoms, including colicky pains and a change in bowel habits, all of which need detailed medical assessment, as these symptoms could be a precursor of more serious illnesses. It is by exclusion of these that the diagnosis of irritable bowel syndrome can be confidently made.

Bowel activity is closely linked with diet, exercise and the mind. It is important to eat a high-fibre diet and to take plenty of exercise. Probiotic therapy (*see* MYALGIC ENCEPHALOMYELITIS, p. 25) will help settle the intestinal tract. The emotions and the mental state should not be ignored. This can be quite a upsetting condition and stress may make it worse (it has also been implicated in its cause). Therefore, psychotherapy or counselling is an important option to clarify any effects that the mind may be having on the overall illness.

In the conventional medical approach, antispasmodic drugs are used, as well as tranquillizers and antidepressants.

Homeopathic treatment is best obtained by consulting a specialist homeopath. If this is not possible, the following homeopathic remedies can be used. Using the 6c potency, give one dose four times a day until the symptoms diminish.

### *Argentum nitricum* (silver nitrate)

This remedy picture describes sufferers who feel very nervy, and this is associated with a rumbling, fluttery abdomen. They notice a lot of wind, as well as diarrhoea that alternates with constipation. The colicky pains appear mainly on the left side of the abdomen. The person as a whole prefers refined sugar and has a fear of heights and of crowded places.

### *Cantharis* (Spanish fly)

This remedy picture describes sufferers who notice burning all over the abdomen. They have a dislike of food and drink, and particularly of tobacco. Their thirst is unquenchable, although drinking coffee causes a serious deterioration of symptoms. After passing a stool, they shudder.

### *Colocynthis* (bitter cucumber)

This remedy picture describes sufferers who develop serious colicky abdominal pains that are eased when they bend double, or by applying firm pressure to the site of the pain. The colic is more easily stimulated if they have just become irritated or angry about something.

### *Magnesium phosphoricum* (magnesium phosphate)

This remedy picture describes sufferers who notice that their colicky abdominal pain is eased more by warmth than by firm pressure.

# Ulcerative colitis

In this condition, the lining of the colon becomes ulcerated, giving symptoms of pain and a disturbance of defecation: painless diarrhoea with or without blood and mucus. It is essential to have conventional treatment as this form of colitis, if it affects the entire colon and is present for more than ten years, can lead to cancer of the colon in a small percentage of cases. The investigations will include sigmoidoscopy (examination of the rectum and sigmoid colon through a rigid or flexible fibreoptic tube), bowel biopsy and X-ray examination.

In most cases, treatment is medical, with the steroid drug prednisolone being given by mouth or enema, or one of the derivatives of the antibacterial drug sulphasalazine. In severe cases, surgery may be necessary, with the removal of the colon. The person will be required to attend a clinic regularly as an outpatient for follow-up appointments.

The illness can also be treated in a complementary way with one of the homeopathic remedies listed below. When the condition is acute, with much pain, bleeding and inflammation, use the 6c potency and give one dose every hour, for a maximum of 12 doses or until medical advice can be obtained.

In the chronic phase, it is best to consult a specialist

homeopath, but if this is not possible, a homeopathic remedy may be used. Select the remedy by matching its picture closely with the physical symptoms. Using the 30c potency, give one dose twice a week. In this chronic phase, it is also important to take nutritional supplements: vitamin C, multi-mineral tablets and probiotics (*see* MYALGIC ENCEPHALOMYE-LITIS, p. 25).

## *Aloe* (socotrine aloes)

This remedy picture describes sufferers with a constant bearing-down feeling in their rectums. There is a feeling of insecurity when they pass wind because of a fear of defecation. The stool itself, jelly-like and covered with much mucus, is passed without effort, almost unnoticed. However, it leaves a residual pain in the rectum.

## *Antimonium crudum* (black sulphide of antimony)

This remedy picture describes a person who is excessively irritable and fretful and has a thickly coated white tongue. Diarrhoea alternates with constipation (like *Podophyllum*), but when there is diarrhoea, the stool consists entirely of mucus. In fact, there is usually a continual loss of anal mucus.

## *Magnesium phosphoricum* (magnesium phosphate)

This remedy picture describes an abdomen that feels very sore and swollen, and the person dislikes any tight clothing around it. The pains in it are relieved when warm pressure is applied to it, such as a hot-water bottle applied with minimal pressure. There is much intestinal gas and wind.

## *Mercurius corrosivus* (corrosive sublimate of mercury)

The person has a continuous straining sensation in the rectum, which is not relieved by the passage of a stool. The stool itself is hot, bloody, slimy and offensive. The passage of this stool is accompanied with cutting pains and associated with the appearance of shreds of mucous membrane.

### *Podophyllum* (may apple)

This remedy picture describes constipation alternating with diarrhoea, and a rumbling and shifting of wind within the ascending colon. Sufferers' abdomens are distended, and they have a sensation of weakness or just a sinking feeling. They find comfort in lying on their stomachs.

# Eating disorders

The eating disorders considered here – *anorexia nervosa, binge eating* and *bulimia nervosa* – all stem from a person's changed attitude to his or her (but most often her) own body shape. They are essentially psychological in nature, and therefore psychotherapy is a cornerstone of treatment.

In anorexia nervosa, sufferers refuse to maintain a normal body weight to the point of starvation. This they do by the abuse of laxatives or diuretics and/or by excessive self-induced vomiting.

Binge eating is characterized by eating a great deal of food much more rapidly than normal and when not physically hungry, until the sufferers feel uncomfortably full. They eat alone through embarrassment, and afterwards feel very guilty, depressed and/or disgusted with themselves for the amount of food consumed.

Bulimia nervosa is a condition of repeated episodes of binge eating with a lack of control over the amount of food actually eaten. However, unlike binge eaters, sufferers of bulimia nervosa develop compensatory behaviour to maintain their body weight by self-induced vomiting and the abuse of laxatives and diuretics.

Sufferers of all these conditions require dietary advice, medical supervision and intensive counselling. In addition, there are certain homeopathic remedies that can be used in a complementary manner with the conventional treatment. Select the remedy picture that most suits the person's physical picture. Using the 6c potency, give one dose four times a day.

## *Abrotanum* (southernwood)

This remedy picture describes sufferers who are underweight and have particularly thin lower limbs, yet have good appetites. They develop a gnawing pain in their stomachs and tend to vomit large quantities of offensive-smelling fluid.

## *Argentum nitricum* (silver nitrate)

This remedy picture describes people who show a progressive and steady weight loss. Their faces are old-looking and pale with a bluish tinge, and the skin generally has a dried-up appearance like that of a "mummy". They crave sweets, although sweet food can disagree with them, and also crave salt. They feel more comfortable in cold air and prefer drinking cold drinks. Their abdomens are distended almost to the point of bursting. They experience a lot of wind, and there is an emotionally based diarrhoea (with the emotion identified as an anticipatory anxiety). They also have a fear of heights and of crowded places.

## *Arsenicum album* (arsenic trioxide)

This remedy picture describes anxiety, coldness, restlessness, prostration and diarrhoea with vomiting. Sufferers are, on the whole, very neat and tidy. Like *Argentum nitricum*, their faces are pale and anxious-looking and are "dried up like a mummy". The diarrhoea begins as soon as they eat anything. The stools contain a lot of undigested food, and they smell very offensive. The weight loss is rapid, and sufferers find the least effort exhausting.

## *Baryta carbonicum* (barium carbonate)

The general feature of this remedy picture is a feeling of dwarfishness both in mind and body. The limbs and organs of the body become emaciated, and the person feels as if he or she has become a dwarf.

### *Calcarea carbonica* (calcium carbonate)

This remedy picture describes younger people who have large heads, distended abdomens and thin, emaciated lower limbs. They are generally cold, and sweat profusely from the scalp particularly at night. They find that milk disagrees with them. On the whole, they are obstinate and easily frightened and have a tendency to develop constipation. In their past medical history, they usually show a delay in the eruption of their teeth, and there is generally a fault in the development of their bones. When they stopped growing, the emaciation began.

### *Iodum* (iodine)

This remedy picture shares with *Abrotanum* the loss of weight despite a ravenous hunger. However, this remedy picture includes a great thirst, too. The person feels anxious and becomes very worried if food is not consumed.

### *Lycopodium* (club moss)

This remedy picture describes sufferers who become thin from the top down, so that the lower limbs are fairly well nourished. Their abdomens are distended like drums (a symptom shared with *Argentum nitricum*), so much so that they can hardly breathe and feel so full that no food can be eaten. They crave sweets (a symptom shared with *Argentum nitricum*) and feel worse between 4.00 and 8.00 pm. They suffer an anticipatory anxiety (a symptom shared with both *Argentum nitricum* and *Arsenicum album*) and lack self-confidence. They feel better in a cold room and worse in a warm one (a symptom shared with *Iodum*), and characteristically one part of their body is warm while the other is cold. Their faces are dry and wrinkled, and they usually have a frown on their forehead.

### *Medorhinum* (gonorrhoeal bacteria)

This remedy picture describes a coppery taste in the mouth and a ravenous hunger soon after eating. The person is very thirsty for warm drinks and has a craving for alcohol, salty foods and sweets. In this remedy picture, vomiting is a prominent feature.

### Natrum muriaticum (sodium chloride)

Like the two previous remedies, this one's picture includes a hungry person who still loses weight. He or she has an unquenchable thirst, sweats while eating, craves salt and has an aversion to bread and to anything that is slimy (such as oysters and fatty food).

### Nux vomica (poison-nut)

This remedy picture describes people who have a characteristic habit of always meticulously selecting their food but digest almost nothing. They are very sensitive to the cold and cannot bear to be uncovered in bed. They have a problem with their bowel action: they are primarily constipated with unproductive urging to defecate, but this can alternate with diarrhoea. They tend to be over-sensitive and never satisfied and can have uncontrollable tempers. The symptoms are aggravated by the overuse of alcohol, nicotine and caffeine.

### Pulsatilla (wind flower)

This remedy describes sufferers who dislike fatty food and warm food and drink. They aren't thirsty, and they tend to vomit food that has been eaten some time ago. They notice pain in their stomachs about one hour after eating food. The general characteristic of these people is a yielding personality that is very apt to cry. They respond well to emotional and physical comforting.

### Petroleum (crude rock oil)

This remedy picture describes emaciation that is associated with diarrhoea that occurs only during the day. Sufferers are constantly hungry and yet cannot eat because eating causes abdominal pain.

Paradoxically they feel hungry after a bowel action. They have an aversion to fatty food, meat and the open air. Their skin is fragile and has deep cracks in it. They may have had a problem with travel sickness, and can sweat offensively from their feet and armpits while generally feeling cold.

### Phosphorus

This remedy picture describes young people who have grown up rapidly and quickly become emaciated. They bleed and bruise easily and are very sensitive to the cold. They are very sociable, enjoying other people's company very much. They are frightened by thunderstorms and the dark and of being left alone. They tire quickly but can be rejuvenated by a short nap.

### Sanicula (water from the Sanicula Springs, Ottawa)

This remedy picture describes a progressive weight loss in a person who kicks off the bedclothes even in the coldest weather (a symptom shared with *Sulphur*), and craves meat, fatty food and salt. When defecating, the stool protrudes, only to recede back into the rectum (a symptom shared with *Silicea*). The person's feet sweat and smell foul (a symptom shared with *Silicea*).

### Silicea (pure flint)

This remedy picture describes sufferers who become increasingly debilitated because of a defective assimilation of food. They have large heads but small, emaciated bodies, apart from their abdomens, which are plump. They feel cold and, during sleep, sweat easily from the head and feet. As a whole, they lack confidence and are shy by nature but, when disturbed, can lose their temper quite suddenly.

# Heart and Circulatory Disorders

The heart has four chambers. The right atrium collects all the blood that has travelled through the veins. This blood is then pumped into the right ventricle, from where it is pumped into the lungs in order to be oxygenated. This oxygenated blood then flows into the left atrium, which in turn pumps the blood into the left ventricle. This is the principal muscular pump that forces the blood into the arteries of the whole body.

## Atherosclerosis

The single most common factor underlying all heart and circulatory conditions is atherosclerosis, the build-up of cholesterol in the arteries, in the form of atherosclerotic plaques. If this happens in the heart (coronary) arteries, it results in a progressive reduction in the blood supply to the heart (cardiac) muscle as the inner diameters of the coronary arteries slowly become smaller. This causes an equally progressive weakening of the cardiac muscle as they are starved of properly oxygenated blood.

Because of the serious implications of all of these illnesses, conventional medical attention is essential.

Self-help is also extremely important, preferably at an early stage so that these illnesses can be prevented or, if already present, their progress minimized. The following steps are the ideal:

- Maintenance of an ideal body weight.
- A restriction in alcohol consumption to one unit a day – that is, half a pint of beer, a glass of wine or one pub measure each of sherry or spirits.
- A dietary restriction of fatty foods (particularly saturated fats from animal foods) to keep the blood cholesterol low.
- Stopping smoking, as it increases atherosclerotic formation.

A daily dose of the herbal supplement ginkgo has been shown to decrease the formation of atherosclerotic plaques. It can also be taken as a preventative measure. Garlic also appears to have a cholesterol-lowering effect, and therefore should be used in the management of atherosclerosis. A single clove of garlic should be eaten every day, but if you are worried about the bad breath this can cause, you can instead take garlic in capsule form, two capsules a day to be taken as divided doses.

There are a number of conventional drugs available for lowering a persistently elevated level of cholesterol in the blood.

In addition, there is one homeopathic remedy that can be used either as a complementary remedy with conventional therapy or on its own.

### *Crataegus* (hawthorn berries)

This remedy acts as a heart tonic, and its remedy picture also describes a weak and irregular heart rate, fluid retention in the lower limbs and in the lungs. It acts on atherosclerosis directly as a solvent. Using the mother tincture, put 5 to 15 drops in 20 ml (4 teaspoons) of pure water. This is swallowed three times a day. This schedule should be considered a long-term measure.

## Angina

This comprises isolated attacks of central, constricting chest pains that result from the fact that the cardiac muscle is getting an insufficient blood supply and therefore is suffering a lack of oxygen. There can also be repeated attacks of angina at short intervals, a condition known as crescendo angina. This is potentially serious as it can be signalling an impending HEART ATTACK. For both of these conditions, medical advice is essential.

There are certain homeopathic remedies that can be used either on their own or in a complementary way with any conventional drugs that may be prescribed. After reading the remedy pictures, select the remedy that matches the physical symptoms. Using the

6c potency, give one dose every two minutes until the attack subsides, for a maximum of ten doses. If there is no improvement, immediate medical help is required.

### *Aconitum napellus* (monk's-hood)

This remedy picture describes a rapid heart rate with a feeling of pressure on the heart, giving a pain in the left shoulder. The characteristic feature of this remedy is the suddenness of an attack associated with a shock or fright. The person is restless and is full of fears, particularly of dying.

### *Apis mellifica* (honey bee)

This remedy picture describes characteristically stinging and burning pains in any part of the body, including the heart. There is a sudden swelling of the lower limbs (oedema) associated with shortness of breath whenever the person lies down (orthoponea) – see HEART FAILURE. The picture also describes a person who is generally thirstless and feels better from cold applications, the reverse of *Arsenicum album*.

### *Arnica* (leopard's bane)

This remedy picture describes pains as if the heart is being squeezed (a symptom shared with *Cactus grandiflorus* and *Lilium tigrinum*) or stitching pains that are referred into the left elbow. The heartbeat is irregular. Sufferers have a horror of instant death and feel worn out from physical or mental strain. They are restless in bed because they feel that it is too hard. They usually do not want to be touched.

### *Arsenicum album* (arsenic trioxide)

This remedy picture describes a sudden tightness above the heart with agonising pains in the organ itself, which extend into the neck and the back of the head and into the left arm and hand. The least motion makes sufferers breathless, and they feel most comfortable sitting bent forward with their head thrown back. They feel at their worst at night, particularly between 1.00 and 5.00 am. The characteristic features of this remedy are usually present: extreme restlessness, symptoms that are worsened by cold applications relieved by heat, and a desire for small quantities of fluid at frequent intervals. All these symptoms are worse late at night (towards midnight).

### *Aurum metallicum* (gold)

This remedy picture describes frequent concern about the heart, associated with a peculiar symptom of feeling as though the heart is loose within the body and seems to shake when the person goes for a walk. The mental state of the person is characteristic: he or she is very depressed, has a disgust for life and has suicidal thoughts.

### *Cactus grandiflorus* (night-blooming cereus)

This remedy picture describes a constricting chest pain, as though an ever-present iron band is around the chest. The pain radiates down the left arm, and is made worse by lying on the left side. The person feels suffocated and is usually in a cold sweat. The heart beats rapidly (palpitations), giving a dizzy feeling (vertigo) and shortness of breath (dyspnoea).

### *Glonoine* (nitroglycerine)

The remedy picture is of blood rushing into the heart, causing palpitations and shortness of breath, which stops the person from walking uphill or anything else that causes over-exertion. The symptoms are worse in the heat of the sun and from any stimulants consumed.

### *Haematoxylon* (logwood)

This remedy picture describes a feeling of a constrictive pain that extends into the stomach area (epigastrium). The person also feels as though a bar lies across the chest. This is commonly associated with heart palpitations.

### *Kalmia latifolia* (mountain laurel)

This remedy picture describes pains in the heart that are so sharp that they take the breath away. They shoot through the chest and into the shoulder blades. There is an association between the heart disease of the person with their rheumatic complaints (e.g. arthritis): if one of them is bad, the other is better.

### *Lachesis* (bushmaster snake venom)

This remedy picture describes cramp-like pain in the heart causing palpitations and anxiety. Sufferers feel as though their hearts are too large for their bodies. It is common for their lips to go blue (cyanosis), and they are intolerant of anything touching their throats. The symptoms are worse following sleep.

### *Latrodectus mactans* (spider)

The remedy picture describes a violent chest pain that radiates into the left armpit and down the left arm and into the fingers, making the arm feel as though it is paralysed. The pulse rate is rapid and difficult to feel because it is so weak.

### *Lilium tigrinum* (tiger lily)

This remedy picture describes a symptom as though the heart is gripped in a vice (a symptom shared with *Cactus grandiflorus*). Sufferers feel as if all the blood has gone from their hearts and that they must bend double (the reverse of *Spigelia*). This is the only remedy picture in which the pain radiates down the *right* arm. The heart beats rapidly, and these palpitations extend through the whole body. Sufferers feel as if their hearts will burst, and they feel worse in crowded rooms, especially if it is warm.

### Naja tripudians (cobra venom)

This remedy picture describes chest pains extending into the throat, nape of the neck and forehead. Sufferers' pulses are irregular, and they are full of anxiety and have a real sense of dying. Their symptoms are made worse by the use of any stimulants.

### Oxalicum acidum (sorrel acid)

The remedy picture describes a sharp, lancing pain in the left lung that comes on suddenly and causes the person to be short of breath. Alternatively, the chest pains dart to the left shoulder. In both situations, the pains are worsened by the person thinking about him or herself.

### Spigelia (pinkroot)

This remedy picture describes stitching pains in the chest. Sufferers have a craving for drinks of hot water, which relieves the pain. They are short of breath, which is relieved if they lie on their right sides with their heads held high (the reverse of Lilium tigrinum).

### Syphilinum (bacteria of syphilis)

This remedy picture describes the characteristic pains and pressures that occur behind the breastbone. The symptoms are much worse at night.

### Tuberculinum (nucleo-protein from tubercular abscess)

This remedy is particularly indicated when there is a personal or family history of tuberculosis. The symptoms are palpitations and heaviness over the heart. The person is irritable about everything, and nothing seems to satisfy; he or she also has a desire to travel.

### Nosode therapy for angina

Nosodes – Hahnemann's miasms, see p. 95 – are useful in the treatment of angina when other homeopathic treatment has not been as successful as hoped. However, this treatment should be continued, with one of the following nosodes being used as an additional form of therapy. Using the 30c potency, give one dose every 12 hours, for a maximum of three doses. Repeat this schedule every month. Select the appropriate nosode from the following remedy pictures.

### Medorhinum (gonorrhoea bacteria)

This remedy picture describes painful symptoms that are worse during daylight. The pains extend into the left arm and into the throat. Sufferers are anxious, find difficulty in concentrating and are always anticipating that something bad is going to happen (as if someone is always following them). They also feel that time moves too slowly and everything seems unreal, as if a dream.

## Heart attacks

A heart attack – medically called a *myocardial infarction* – is the sudden death of part of the heart muscle, usually caused by a complete blockage of one or more of the coronary arteries by atherosclerosis (*see above*) and a blood clot. **This is an emergency requiring immediate medical attention.** Heart attack victims may complain of severe chest pains with or without shortness of breath, and if they do not receive help within minutes, they will collapse and require immediate mouth-to-mouth resuscitation (the kiss of life) and chest compressions.

Conventional medical treatment is the recommended approach. It begins with immediate pain relief (with diamorphine) and soluble aspirin (which will help dissolve the blood clot obstructing the coronary artery). Urgent hospital admission is arranged where the drug streptokinase is given; this also helps to dissolve clots. On discharge from hospital, the person will take a daily dose of aspirin.

The homeopathic treatment for such a medical emergency is very much the second choice. While waiting for emergency medical attention, the following homeopathic remedies can be given.

- *Aconitum napellus* (monk's-hood)
  This is the first remedy to be given, as one dose using the 30c potency. It will help alleviate the anxiety and fear of dying.

This can be immediately followed by one of the two following remedies, matching its picture with the physical symptoms. Using the 30c potency, give one dose every 30 minutes.

- *Cactus grandiflorus* (night-blooming cereus)
  This remedy picture describes a person who develops a sudden crushing chest pain that radiates down the left arm. The person is in a cold sweat.
- *Carbo vegetabilis* (vegetable charcoal)
  This remedy picture describes a person who suddenly collapses and whose body becomes blue and icy cold. He or she feels terrible but is helped when the face is fanned with fresh air.

The following is given to help dissolve the clot in the coronary artery.

- *Lachesis* (bushmaster snake venom)
  This remedy picture describes an ability to dissolve blood clots. Using the 30c potency, give one dose with one of the preceding two remedies. When the person is discharged from hospital, this remedy can be given on a monthly basis.

# Heart failure

When there is heart failure, it can be either right-sided or left-sided. Right-sided failure – also known as congestive heart failure – causes a venous congestion, leading to a build-up of fluid in the lower limbs (oedema) and in the lungs (pulmonary congestion). This causes shortness of breath that is worse when the person lies down (orthopnoea) and a feeling of general weakness. Left-sided failure is due to a failure of the left ventricle to pump the blood from the lungs around to the rest of the body, usually because of a

HEART ATTACK or sustained HIGH BLOOD PRESSURE. It causes a build-up of fluid in the lungs, which results in a condition similar to ASTHMA and it is called cardiac asthma.

Heart failure, whether right or left, requires urgent medical attention and treatment, probably with drugs such as digoxin (to stimulate the heart), diuretics (to cause the kidneys to pass more urine) and drugs to control raised blood pressure.

There are homeopathic remedies that can be used in a complementary way with the conventional treatments, or individually on their own but under medical supervision (ideally from a medically qualified homeopath). Caffeine-containing tea and coffee should be avoided; herbal teas are a suitable alternative. In congestive heart failure, a herbal tea containing fennel is ideal as this herb is a natural diuretic.

*Remedies for right-sided heart failure (congestive heart failure)*

### *Adonis vernalis* (pheasant's eye)

This remedy is a heart tonic that is of particular use after influenza or any other viral condition where there has been a fatty degeneration of the heart muscle, or where there is heart valve disease from any cause (but especially following rheumatic fever). The main cardiac symptom is an irregular, rapid heartbeat. The person has a frequent desire to take deep breaths and has a feeling of a weight on the chest. There is marked pulmonary congestion with swelling of the lower limbs (oedema). Using the mother tincture, place 1–10 drops in 20 ml (4 teaspoons) of pure water and swallow this once a day. The number of drops depends on the severity of symptoms.

### *Convallaria majalis* (lily of the valley)

This remedy increases the energy of the heart muscle and makes the heart rate more regular and forceful. The remedy picture shows marked venous stasis (pooling of the blood in the veins), causing oedema (swelling of the lower limbs), as well as shortness of breath due to pulmonary congestion, which is worse when lying down (orthopnoea). Using the mother tincture, place 1–15 drops in 20 ml (4 teaspoons) of pure water and swallow this once a day. The number of drops depends on the severity of the oedema and pulmonary congestion.

### *Crataegus* (hawthorn berries)

A homeopathic heart tonic that should be used as previously discussed in the section on ATHEROSCLEROSIS.

### *Digitalis* (foxglove)

This remedy is made up in the homeopathic way and is not the same as the conventional drug, although its actions are similar. This remedy picture describes weakness of the heart and a heart rate that is irregular, weak or abnormally slow. This remedy is the mainstay of treatment where there is pulmonary congestion and oedema. Using the mother tincture, place 5–20 drops in 20 ml (4 teaspoons) of pure water and swallow this once a day.

### *Remedies for left-sided heart failure (cardiac asthma)*

There are several homeopathic remedies that can be used while awaiting the medical attention. Using the 6c potency (apart from *Aurum metallicum,* when the 30c potency should be used), give one dose every ten minutes.

### *Aconitum napellus* (monk's-hood)

This remedy is the first choice in treating this condition. Its remedy picture shows sufferers who are fearful of death. Their breathing is difficult, with shortness of breath and a hoarse, dry cough. Their hearts beat rapidly and have a crushing pain that can radiate into the left shoulder area. They usually feel faint and are in a cold sweat. Their fingers are commonly tingly.

The following homeopathic remedies may also be given following the use of *Aconitum napellus*.

### *Arsenicum iodatum* (arsenic iodide)

This remedy picture is seen in a person with serious heart problems due to atherosclerosis, where the extreme shortness of breath is associated with a heart that is weakening – i.e. a senile heart. These symptoms occur towards midnight. The person is restless and anxious, and needs sips of water.

### *Aurum metallicum* (gold)

This remedy picture describes pulmonary congestion, particularly associated with disease of the heart valves. The heart stops beating for a few seconds and the person falls down unconscious. This remedy is also associated with deep depression, with the person feeling hopeless and suicidal. Using the 30c strength, give one dose twice a day for two days, reducing to one a day for a further week.

### *Cactus grandiflorus* (night-blooming cereus)

This remedy picture describes suffocative breathing associated with a feeling that the chest is bound up tight, thereby hindering respiration. The heart beats rapidly, giving violent palpitations that are worse when lying down, particularly on the left side, and, in women, at the approach of menstruation.

### *Iberis* (bitter candytuft)

This remedy picture describes a person who commonly wakes up at 2.00 am with heart palpitations, and whose windpipe (trachea) fills up with mucus, causing shortness of breath with a cough that makes the person go red in the face.

### *Lachesis* (bushmaster snake venom)

This remedy picture describes a suffocating cough that comes on when sufferers are asleep, falling asleep or waking. They feel better leaning forward and when breathing cool, fresh air. They feel much worse if anything touches their throats, and so feel much better when clothing is removed from their necks.

### *Laurocerasus* (cherry laurel)

This remedy picture describes a person who is very short of breath and, while gasping, clutches at the heart. Unusually he or she feels worse when sitting up.

### *Naja tripudians* (cobra venom)

This remedy picture is characterized by a sense of choking. Sufferers are frequently seen grasping at their throats while coping with their pulmonary congestion.

### *Spongia tosta* (roasted sponge)

The remedy picture describes sufferers with wheezing asthmatic coughs that are worse in the cold air and when they are lying with their heads low. Their chests feel hot, and as a whole, they feel very weak. Their heart rates are rapid, and they are commonly woken from sleep at midnight with chest pains and a feeling of suffocation. They feel very frightened (similar to *Aconitum napellus*), and because of this, they develop a cold sweat.

### *Sumbul-perula* (musk root)

This remedy picture shows a person with cardiac asthma, and who, on the whole, has many hysterical and nervous symptoms. The heart suffers from a nervous palpitation, and the person is aware of a nagging pain around the left breast.

# High blood pressure

**High blood pressure is a serious condition, requiring expert medical advice.** This will include medical investigations and probably drug therapy.

Self-help includes weight and stress reduction. Meditation, massage, yoga, aromatherapy and creative activities are all useful for reducing stress. Dietary adjustments are important, too, particularly a reduction in salt, caffeine and excess alcohol. Smoking should be stopped or at least reduced.

Garlic has been shown to have an effect on lowering blood pressure. One clove of garlic should be eaten every day. If you are worried about bad breath, you can take garlic capsules instead, two a day.

There are two specific homeopathic remedies, either of which can help reduce blood pressure, and one or the other should be used in conjunction with a general, holistic remedy prescribed by a consultant homeopath. If the blood pressure does not respond in a satisfactory way, the two remedies can be taken together, three times a day using the 6c potency.

### *Lycopus virginicus* (bugle-weed)

This remedy has a specific effect on the heart, reducing its rate and lowering the blood pressure. It is associated with coughing up blood (haemoptysis) where the person has heart valve disease. Using 6c potency, give one dose three times a day. It is important to measure the blood pressure at regular intervals.

### *Spartium scoparium* (broom)

This remedy also has a specific action on the heart, reducing the heart rate and the blood pressure. It is thought that this effect is caused by the remedy stimulating the vagus nerve. The person notices that the volume of urine passed increases. This remedy therefore has a diuretic action as well which is useful where there is swelling of the ankles (oedema). The dosage schedule is 6c potency, one dose to be taken three times each day. It is important to measure the blood pressure at regular intervals.

The following remedies also have a specific action in lowering blood pressure and can be used if the above treatment does not work. Select the remedy according to the remedy picture, matching it with the physical symptoms. Using the 6c potency, give one dose three times a day until the blood pressure is under control, at which point reduce the dose to a minimum, starting with one 6c potency a day and reducing it further according to the blood pressure readings.

### Aurum metallicum (gold)

This remedy picture describes high blood pressure associated with angina and palpitations. The person is seriously depressed.

### Baryta carbonicum (barium carbonate)

This remedy picture describes high blood pressure, angina and palpitations in people who are growing old before their time. They tend to be continually tired.

### Baryta muriaticum (barium chloride)

This remedy picture describes high blood pressure with a high systolic pressure but a low diastolic pressure (the systolic and diastolic pressures are the two measurements made when the blood pressure is taken). The person has characteristic movements, tossing about periodically as if having convulsions.

### Coffea cruda (unroasted coffee)

This remedy picture describes a person who is nervous and probably has palpitations and trembling limbs, and who develops sudden rises in blood pressure.

### Strontium carbonicum (strontium carbonate)

This remedy picture describes high blood pressure in a person who develops widespread pains that are localized in the bone marrow.

### *Sumbul-perula* (musk root)

This remedy picture describes high blood pressure in a nervous person who suffers from nervous palpitations and whose blood pressure rises by just thinking about it.

# Low blood pressure

Apart from medical emergencies, this condition is not recognized as a medical problem in the United Kingdom but is recognized as such in continental Europe.

The symptoms are lethargy and muscular fatigue. The homeopathic treatment includes the following nutritional supplements: vitamin C (at least 1 gram a day), multi-mineral tablets (to include magnesium and zinc, both of which will improve neuromuscular activity), and lecithin and ginkgo capsules, both of which will improve brain function.

The following homeopathic remedies will help restore the body to its normal vitality. Using the 6c potency, give one dose twice a day for one month, reducing thereafter to one a day.

### *Cactus grandiflorus* (night-blooming cereus)

This remedy picture describes low blood pressure in a person who has a weak pulse, is exhausted from the least effort and tends to be melancholy and ill-humoured.

### *Radium* (radium bromide)

This describes low blood pressure in a person showing great weakness. He or she also tends to wake up panting, with palpitations.

### *Theidion* (orange spider)

This remedy picture describes low blood pressure in people who are anxious about their hearts. They develop pain in their hearts that radiates to the left arm and shoulder; their pulse rates are usually slow; and they suffer from attacks of giddiness (vertigo).

### *Veratrum viride* (white American hellebore)

This remedy picture describes a particular sort of person who has a red, livid face and a quarrelsome personality. The heart is liable to have an irregular rate (atrial fibrillation; *see* ARRHYTHMIAS), and there is also a reduction in blood pressure (in both the systolic and diastolic pressures).

### *Viscum album* (mistletoe)

This remedy picture describes blood pressure that is low and the heart rate slowed. The person that this remedy will match will also probably have gouty and rheumatic complaints and, especially, SCIATICA.

# Arrhythmias

A cardiac arrhythmia is an abnormality of the rhythm or rate of the heartbeat. This is caused by a disturbance in the electrical impulses produced by the heart to regulate its beating rhythm and rate. There are two main types of arrhythmias. Tachycardias are heartbeats that are faster than normal (more than 100 beats per minute); bradycardias are heartbeats that are slower than normal (fewer than 60 beats per minute).

The diagnosis of a cardiac arrhythmia needs accurate medical assessment, which will almost certainly include an electrocardiogram. In this way, the electrical problem of the heart can be accurately diagnosed and appropriate treatment given. Conventional medical treatment can include drugs and a heart pacemaker.

There are several homeopathic remedies that are applicable to the treatment of cardiac arrhythmias, but these must always take second place to conventional treatment. They can be used in a complementary way if the conventional therapy is not working and while waiting for medical attention.

## Atrial fibrillation

This arrhythmia of the heart occurs through an electrical disharmony so that both the left and right atria beat much faster than both ventricles. This can produce such symptoms as breathlessness, chest pains (similar to ANGINA) and faintness. This is not normally life-threatening; however, blood clots can form in the atria, which can become dislodged and will cause problems wherever they finally end up, but especially in the lungs or the brain. For this reason, conventional medical therapy may well include an anticoagulant drug to break down any clots. Sometimes, medical practitioners recommend that the arrhythmia be corrected by defribrillation, in which case anticoagulant therapy will almost certainly be advised.

The following homeopathic remedy should only be used while awaiting expert medical attention. Using the 6c potency, give one dose every 15 minutes until the medical practitioner is available.

## *Veratrum viride* (white American hellebore)

This remedy has a marked effect on atrial fibrillation. Sufferers will probably notice, or will have been told about, a fall in blood pressure. This remedy suits full-blooded people who will also probably feel the irregular pulse beating throughout their entire body. This sensation is most marked in the right thigh.

## Supraventricular tachycardia (SVT)

In this arrhythmia – also known as paroxysmal tachycardia – the heart rate is doubled and causes the person to feel breathless and faint. **These symptoms must be reported immediately to a medical practitioner for accurate diagnosis.**

Once this has been established and treatment commenced (usually with anti-arrhythmic drugs), it is still possible for the arrhythmia to return. If it does, there are several simple things that can be done to correct the heart rhythm: massaging the carotid arteries (the large blood vessels just underneath the jaw, extending from the chest); forcibly breathing out while holding the mouth closed and pinching the nostrils together; and even just drinking some cold water.

The following homeopathic remedies can be used while awaiting medical attention. Using the 6c potency, give one dose every 15 minutes.

### *Arsenicum album* (arsenic trioxide)

This remedy describes a person who has SVT and is chilly, restless and very anxious, and craves sips of cold water. All the symptoms tend to be worse between midnight and 2.00 am.

### *Cactus grandiflorus* (night-blooming cereus)

This remedy picture describes violent palpitations that are worse when the person lies on his or her left side and, if a woman, before her menstrual period.

### *Iberis* (bitter candytuft)

This remedy picture describes violent palpitations that can have been induced by the slightest exertion, such as laughing or coughing. They can cause extreme shortness of breath and stitching pains in the heart. The person feels worse when lying down and particularly when lying down on the left side.

### *Lilium tigrinum* (tiger lily)

This remedy picture describes rapid palpitations that can also give an irregular pulse, which can be felt throughout the entire body. If these individuals already suffer from ANGINA, they will almost certainly develop an anginal attack, with the result that they will feel as if their hearts are gripped in a vice.

### *Spigelia* (pinkroot)

This remedy picture describes violent palpitations, with shortness of breath (dyspnoea). Sufferers must lie on their right sides with their heads held high. They develop neuralgic pains that extend into one or both arms. If they also suffer from angina, they find that drinking hot water relieves the symptoms.

# Palpitations

If a person has palpitations, he or she either is abnormally aware of the heartbeat (which normally would not be noticed) or feels that it is beating unusually forcefully or rapidly.

It is quite normal to experience palpitations after hard exercise or a severe fright. However, they can also be caused by ATRIAL FIBRILLATION or SUPRAVENTRICULAR TACHYCARDIA (*see above*).

In addition, palpitations that occur when an individual is at rest may be a cause for concern. However, these "ectopic heartbeats" are simply the result of a premature heartbeat followed by comparatively long pauses. They are usually not a serious problem, often occurring during periods of mental stress and/or following an overdose of caffeine, alcohol and/or nicotine. They are also common during the MENOPAUSE. They are diagnosed from an electrocardiogram. The only time that these ectopic heartbeats are a serious medical condition and require immediate medical attention is when the person has an already diagnosed major heart problem such as serious ischaemic heart disease, when the coronary arteries have become very blocked and the heart is being starved of oxygenated blood. The palpitations could then be a prelude to a serious cardiac arrhythmia known as ventricular fibrillation, which unless immediately treated can be life-threatening.

Simple adjustments to lifestyle will usually help stop palpitations: reducing the consumption of caffeine, stopping smoking, reducing alcohol consumption and avoiding stress (and dealing with what can't be avoided). If a woman is going through the menopause, consider treatments that may help during this time (*see* p. 488).

The following homeopathic remedies can also be used. Select the remedy by matching its picture with the physical symptoms. Using the 6c potency, give one dose twice a day.

## *Aurum metallicum* (gold)

This remedy picture describes an abnormal heart rhythm: the heart stops beating for two or three seconds, and this is immediately followed by a tumultuous rebound thump, associated with a sinking feeling in the stomach.

## *Cactus grandiflorus* (night-blooming cereus)

This remedy picture describes sufferers who develop violent palpitations that are worse when they lie on their left sides. In women, these palpitations are worse premenstrually, and they are common in heavy cigarette smokers.

## *Lachesis* (bushmaster snake venom)

This remedy picture describes palpitations associated with fainting spells, which may be brought on by a feeling of constriction around the throat and a feeling of anxiety. This remedy suits women who are going through the menopause.

## *Moschus* (musk)

This remedy picture describes a highly nervous person who may show bouts of uncontrollable laughter that may be precipitated by anxiety. This hysteria initiates palpitations. These feelings may also be associated with trembling around the heart that itself can lead to fainting episodes.

## *Natrum muriaticum* (sodium chloride)

This remedy picture describes a person with palpitations that make the whole body shake, giving a constricting sensation in the chest. This feeling is made worse by heat in any form, and by other people making a fuss.

### *Nux vomica* (poison-nut)

This remedy picture describes people who overuse alcohol, nicotine and caffeine, or have been subjected to an unusual amount of stress. On the whole, they are generally feeling irritated and are ambitious and workaholics. They are sensitive to the cold.

### *Pulsatilla* (wind flower)

The remedy picture describes palpitations brought on by the eating of fatty food, or when sufferers become overheated or engage in an argument. They cry easily and often and respond well to physical and emotional support.

### *Spigelia* (pinkroot)

The remedy picture describes violent and repeated attacks of palpitations associated with foul-smelling breath. If these palpitations give an attack of ANGINA, sufferers commonly crave hot liquids that, they find, relieve the symptoms. If there is also shortness of breath, they alleviate this by lying on their right sides with their heads held high.

## Rheumatic heart disease

This condition arises from RHEUMATIC FEVER (*see* p. 424). The illness can cause infection of the heart muscle (endocarditis), thickening of the heart valves leading to HEART FAILURE, and the loss of a regular heart rhythm (this ARRHYTHMIA is usually atrial fibrillation). The homeopathic and conventional treatments for these complications have already been covered.

In addition to these, the following homeopathic remedies can be used as a baseline of therapy for a heart that has become infected from the streptococcal toxin. To select the remedy, match its picture with the physical features. Using the 30c potency, give one dose twice a week.

### *Aurum metallicum* (gold)

This remedy picture describes inflammation that moves quickly from joint to joint, finally settling in the heart. Sufferers find it difficult to lie flat, fighting for their breath and then leaning forwards. When they are fighting for breath, their faces become blue (cyanosis), they can only speak in a whisper, their feet and legs begin to swell (oedema) and the main blood vessels in the neck are seen to bulge and throb irregularly from atrial fibrillation. The principal picture of this remedy is its extreme depression and despondency that can lead to suicide attempts.

### *Kalmia latifolia* (mountain laurel)

This remedy picture describes rheumatic fever where the joint pains shift from joint to joint suddenly, and the pain in any particular joint comes and goes suddenly. This remedy picture particularly describes thickening of the heart valves. The heart can be seen to beat violently, but paradoxically it can also be seen to beat very slowly.

### *Naja tripudians* (cobra venom)

This remedy is the most useful in treating rheumatic heart disease. The picture describes disease of the heart valves. Sufferers wake up choking with a feeling of suffocation, and they commonly complain of a pain between their shoulder blades.

### *Spigelia* (pinkroot)

This remedy picture describes rheumatic heart disease that affects the heart muscle (endocarditis) and also the lining of the heart (pericarditis). The heart beats so violently that the whole body shakes. The heart rhythm is usually irregular with this remedy. Sufferers feel a violent shooting pain in their hearts, as though a hot needle was being passed through their bodies. They feel better lying on their right sides with their heads held high. They are sensitive to the cold and to loud noises, and become worse when moved. They have a peculiar symptom: a fear of pointed objects such as pins.

# Deep vein thrombosis

In this condition, a clot of blood (thrombus) forms in a vein, obstructing the flow of blood from the vein back to the heart. These clots form most commonly in the lower legs, giving symptoms of localized pain, redness and swelling (oedema) of the affected limb.

This is a serious condition requiring medical attention. The thrombus can become dislodged (when it becomes known as an embolus) and travel through the vein back to the heart and finally the lungs. This can be life-threatening.

The conventional treatment is to prescribe anticoagulant drugs that will break up the clot.

Certain conventional drugs predispose people to form these clots, notably the oestrogen component of the oral contraceptive pill and certain hormone replacement therapy pills used in treating the MENOPAUSE. Thrombus formation is more likely to occur in people who are overweight, and after periods of inactivity, such as a long air flight and convalescence following an operation. On long air flights, it is important to walk about to keep the circulation moving, and similarly after an operation; if walking is impossible, the advice is: keep wiggling the toes!

There are several homeopathic remedies that can be used while awaiting medical assessment. Using the 6c potency, give one dose every hour until the medical practitioner has made an accurate diagnosis. If the diagnosis of a deep vein thrombosis is established, a homeopathic remedy can be used to prevent the blood from clotting in a complementary way with the conventional anticoagulants.

However, the decision to use homeopathic remedies for this condition must be discussed with the medical practitioner. Some people are unsuitable for conventional anticoagulant therapy, and so, for them, a homeopathic remedy for treating deep vein thrombosis is a real option.

### Bothrops lanciolatus (yellow viper)

This remedy picture describes symptoms that are mainly right-sided, and shares with *Lachesis* an ability to dissolve clots. It is of particular use in those who have suddenly become paralysed down one side from a stroke (hemiplegia) and in those who are badly bruised. Using the 6c potency, give one dose twice a day for six months.

### Lachesis (bushmaster snake venom)

This snake venom has in its remedy picture the characteristics of the snake venom itself, in that it dissolves blood clots. For this reason and in certain cases, it can be used as a preventative instead of conventional anticoagulant therapy. However, to use *Lachesis* in this way requires the agreement of the medical practitioner. Using the 6c potency, give one dose twice a day for the rest of the person's lifetime. If using the remedy for an acute episode of deep vein thrombosis, use the 6c potency and give one dose four times a day for six months.

### Vipera (German viper)

The remedy picture describes an inflammation of the veins that causes a bursting sensation that is relieved by elevating the affected limb and is correspondingly made worse when the limb is allowed to hang downwards. As well as suffering this bursting pain, the limb also becomes swollen. Using the 6c potency, give one dose twice a day for six months.

## Thrombophlebitis

This is an inflammation of a vein wall. It usually follows an injury in someone who probably already suffers from VARICOSE VEINS. He or she may also develop a fever with this condition.

Conventional treatment will include pain relief, antibiotic therapy and supportive bandaging. Homeopathic treatment involves the use of one of the following remedies. Using the 6c potency, give one dose twice a day until the condition improves.

### Arnica (leopard's bane)

This remedy is indicated where the thrombophlebitis has followed an injury involving the affected vein.

If there is no improvement after ten days' treatment with *Arnica*, proceed to using one of the following:

### Hamamelis virginica (witch hazel)

This remedy picture describes a person who has varicose veins in which thrombophlebitis is a common occurrence.

### Lachesis (bushmaster snake venom)

This remedy picture describes thrombophlebitis where the surrounding skin has a purple colour despite no previous damage to it.

### Pulsatilla (wind flower)

This remedy picture also describes a person who suffers from varicose veins in which thrombophlebitis is a common occurrence. However, in this remedy picture, the condition is made worse whenever the person gets hot or allows the limbs to hang down.

## Varicose veins

These enlarged, twisted veins just below the skin occur as a result of excess pressure building up in the main drainage system of veins. Varicose veins are usually found in the lower limbs and particularly in women following pregnancy. They can also occur around the anal orifice, when they are called HAEMORRHOIDS (piles).

Conventional treatment of varicose veins in the lower limbs is to strip out the section of the affected veins, or to inject them with an irritant substance and then tightly bandage the leg, to effect a closure of the veins' walls.

As a general measure, support stockings are often prescribed, with the advice to keep the legs well elevated to help the blood drain upwards.

There are also several homeopathic remedies that can be used to help this condition. Using the 6c potency, give one dose twice a day until an improvement is noted.

### Carbo vegetabilis (vegetable charcoal)

This remedy picture describes a person with varicose veins who has a peculiar marbling coloration of the skin. The skin also feels very cold. It is a common feature of pregnancy and is therefore a good remedy to use for women who are pregnant.

### Hamamelis virginica (witch hazel)

This remedy picture describes a person with varicose veins who also probably has haemorrhoids. He or she notices a bruised soreness in the affected parts.

### Pulsatilla (wind flower)

This remedy picture describes a person whose varicose veins become more prominent in heat. The symptoms of tiredness and discomfort in the veins become worse when the limb is allowed to hang down.

## Raynaud's disease/phenomenon

This is a condition caused by impaired circulation, resulting in the fingers and possibly the toes becoming white/bluish, stiff and numb. As the circulation slowly returns to normal, the digits are affected by pins and needles.

In Raynaud's *disease*, these symptoms can occur spontaneously, whereas in Raynaud's *phenomenon*, they are brought on by certain factors – cold weather, use of a pneumatic drill or chain saw, an abnormal reaction to certain drugs such as beta-blockers – and in association with certain medical conditions.

It is important to seek medical advice to obtain an accurate diagnosis. The conventional treatment is with drugs that dilate the small blood vessels in the digits as well as advice on keeping hands and feet as warm as possible.

A daily dose of a herbal ginkgo supplement will also help, not only as a therapeutic measure (with both conventional and homeopathic treatments) but also as a preventative.

In addition, there are certain specific homeopathic remedies available. Select the remedy picture that most closely matches the physical symptoms. Using the 6c potency, give one dose every 30 minutes, for a maximum of 12 doses or until the circulation in the affected digit(s) improves.

### Arsenicum album (arsenic trioxide)

This remedy picture shows a very anxious person who feels generally cold, and whose hands and feet become swollen with a sensation of burning and itching. The symptoms deteriorate with the application of anything cold, and are worse towards midnight.

### Cactus grandiflorus (night-blooming cereus)

This remedy picture describes a person with hands and feet swollen through oedema (fluid retention). The hands feel icy cold, and the person has restless legs.

### Carbo vegetabilis (vegetable charcoal)

This remedy picture describes skin that is icy cold and mottled in colour. The remedy is particularly suitable for the older person: the skin responds well, returning to a normal colour after it is fanned.

### *Pulsatilla* (wind flower)

In this remedy picture, the symptoms of the cold hands and feet are made worse by letting the feet hang down from the side of the bed or by the application of anything hot.

### *Secale* (ergot)

This remedy picture describes sufferers whose digits are cold and painful yet are made worse from heat and improved by cold. They develop violent cramps in the digits, violent pain in their finger-tips and a tingling sensation in their toes. Their bodies are generally cold yet feel hot. They are ravenously hungry and unquenchably thirsty.

## Spleen disorders

The spleen is sited underneath the lower left ribs and usually cannot be felt on physical examination (except in the newborn child). Its function is to mop up damaged red blood cells and to produce various constituents of the blood that fight infection.

The spleen may have to be removed if it becomes ruptured in an accident or as a preventative measure when treating a form of cancer called Hodgkin's disease. When the spleen is removed, the person becomes more susceptible to infection by *Pneumococcus* bacteria, for which there is a specific vaccine available.

The spleen can become enlarged in certain conditions that cause red blood cell production to be dramatically increased: polycythaemia, certain types of anaemia, leukaemia, GLANDULAR FEVER, TUBERCULOSIS and liver diseases causing cirrhosis. Apart from the symptoms of the particular illness causing the enlarged spleen, the only symptom from the spleen will be a feeling of heaviness under the left lower ribs. Any case of an enlarged spleen should immediately be referred to a medical practitioner for full investigation.

While this is taking place, there are several homeopathic remedies that will not only help the spleen but will also work as a truly complementary method of therapy with whatever conventional drug therapy is prescribed. Using the 6c potency, give one dose twice a day.

### *Arsenicum album* (arsenic trioxide)

This remedy picture describes a swollen liver and spleen. The spleen area – the left upper quadrant of the abdomen – is tender to the touch, and stitching pains in this area precede the vomiting of blood.

### *Ceanothus* (New Jersey tea)

This remedy picture only describes problems with the spleen – that is, pains in the left upper quadrant of the abdomen, with the person unable to lie on his or her left side. Physical examination reveals a considerably enlarged spleen.

### *Cinchona officinalis (China)* (Peruvian bark)

This remedy picture describes pains in the area of the spleen that are made worse when sufferers walk slowly. On the whole, they feel worse from the slightest touch and from any draught of air, and they feel better when firm pressure has been applied to their bodies. Associated with this remedy, but not necessarily in connection with the spleen, is painless, debilitating diarrhoea that contains undigested food.

### *Helianthus* (sunflower)

This remedy picture describes pain in the spleen area where the symptoms are made worse from heat and improved by vomiting.

### *Ignatia* (St Ignatius' bean)

This remedy picture describes enlargement of the spleen where the person prefers to lie on the left side, although this is the side of discomfort (mainly in the left upper quadrant).

## *Iodum* (iodine)

This remedy picture describes pains in the left upper outer quadrant of the abdomen, which is also very tender to the touch. The liver may also be enlarged, and there may be a disorder of the pancreas. The person is usually very nervous and very hungry and yet loses weight quickly and easily.

## *Quercus glandium spiritus* (spirit from acorn kernels)

This remedy has a specific action on the spleen. The remedy picture also describes a person who has cirrhosis of the liver following alcohol abuse, and whose feet are usually swollen.

# Disorders of the Urinary System

The body's two kidneys are the principal organs that excrete waste products and maintain fluid balance. They also adjust the acidity and alkalinity of the blood. It is on all these fine and correct balances that the chemical reactions of the body depend.

The liquid produced by the kidneys is called urine. It flows from them into the ureters and collects in the bladder. From the age of about four, we have voluntary control over when the bladder is emptied of urine. The prostate gland, only found in males, is located around the neck of the bladder. The final passage of urine is through the urethra to the outside.

The urethra is much longer in males than in females, as a result of which the female urethra is much closer to the anus and therefore to possible faecal contamination. This is one of the reasons why bladder infections are more common in women.

Urine is sterile and usually straw-coloured. If it is dark, this indicates that the person is probably dehydrated. Cloudy urine may also indicate dehydration, the cloudiness resulting from a chemical released by the kidney in an attempt to adjust the fluid balance. However, if cloudiness persists after the urine has been heated, this probably means that the urine is infected and medical advice is needed. If the urine is extremely dark, this may indicate that bile is present and that the person is jaundiced (*see* p. 398) and needs immediate medical attention. A distinguishing feature of urine that contains bile is that, when the urine sample is shaken, a froth appears on its surface that takes a long time to disperse. It may also contain blood, another indication of infection that certainly requires medical investigation.

Infection can occur at all levels of the urinary tract:

- in the urethra, causing *urethritis*.
- in the bladder, causing *cystitis*.

- in the upper part of the ureter where it is immediately attached to the kidney, causing *pyelonephritis*.
- in the body of the kidney, causing *nephritis*.

The minerals that the kidney extracts from the blood can accumulate in the urine and form a stone. When this stone passes from the kidney down the ureter, it causes such severe pain – called renal colic – that it calls for medical attention to alleviate it. There are homeopathic remedies that can be used to good effect as an immediate treatment for this condition while awaiting medical attention.

Stones can also form in the bladder. These do not cause nearly as much pain as kidney stones, but urine infections are common. The conventional treatment is to remove the stone surgically, as well as checking to see if there is any metabolic reason for the stone formation. There are several homeopathic remedies available for treating bladder stones, but it is still important to check on the metabolic status of the person and treat any condition that may be revealed in the conventional way.

Select the appropriate homeopathic remedy and, using the 30c potency, give one dose daily for two weeks, reducing to one dose on alternate days for two weeks, finally reducing to one dose weekly as long-term therapy.

# Urethritis

In this condition, pus is seen to emerge from the end of the urethra: the end of the penis in the male and just behind the clitoris in the female. There may be pain, itchiness and an alteration in bladder activity, and there may or may not be a fever. It is very important to seek medical advice if this condition ever occurs as conventional treatment (which will be antibiotic therapy) is usually indicated as the first choice of treatment.

There are several homeopathic remedies for the treatment of urethritis, and these can be used in a complementary way with the conventional therapy, as they will help alleviate some of the symptoms. Select the remedy by matching its picture with the physical symptoms. Using the 6c potency, give one dose every hour for a maximum of six doses while medical attention is being obtained.

### Apis mellifica (honey bee)

This remedy picture classically describes a stinging quality in the pains in the urethra, which are particularly prominent when urinating. It is the last few drops of urine that particularly burn and smart. There is a frequent desire to urinate and there may well be incontinence of urine.

### Argentum nitricum (silver nitrate)

This remedy picture describes pain as if from a splinter, and the person also feels a burning and itching discomfort. There is a dribble of urine after the act of urination has apparently finished. In a man, he may notice a divided stream of urine and in both sexes the urine may contain blood. There is a profuse discharge from the urethra. The general profile of the person that this remedy would particularly suit is someone who has a specific fear of heights and of crowded places. The person likes refined sugar and salty food.

### Barosma crenata (buchu)

This remedy picture describes an irritable bladder and a discharge of mucus and pus from the urethra. There may be gravel in the urine, and males may well have prostate troubles.

### Cantharis (Spanish fly)

This remedy picture describes not only pain in the urethra, such that urine has to be passed drop by drop because it scalds so much. There is a constant desire to urinate with cutting pains before, during, and after urinating. Blood is a common occurrence in the urine.

### Clematis erecta (virgin's bower)

This remedy picture describes a person who has a tingling sensation in the urethra that lasts for a long time after the act of urination has finished. The urethra feels constricted, and the urine flow is interrupted and incomplete; dribbling at the end of urination is common. The person feels a burning sensation at the end of the urethra, a sensation that is worse at night.

### Doryphora (Colorado potato bug)

This remedy picture describes urethritis particularly in children. There is an excruciating pain in the urethra whenever the child urinates, which extends into the back and the loins. The child's lower limbs tremble markedly.

### Ferrum picricum (iron pictrate)

This remedy picture describes pain along the whole course of the urethra, associated with frequent urination at night. The person is aware of a sensation of fullness in the bladder and pressure in the rectum. There is a smarting sensation at the neck of the bladder, and in males, this travels along the penis. The person may retain urine.

### Mercurius corrosivus (corrosive sublimate of mercury)

This remedy picture describes an intense burning sensation in the urethra, making the urine feel hot and scalding. The urine is commonly bloodstained, and there is usually a greenish discharge from the end of the urethra. The sensation in the urethra extends into the bladder, giving a tremendous urge to urinate. The person commonly sweats after urinating.

### Thuja occidentalis (arbor vitae)

This remedy picture describes a swollen, inflamed urethra. Characteristically the urine stream is split and weak. There is pain at the end of urination. The desire to urinate is urgent and frequent, and the person suffers from urine incontinence (trickling urine).

# Bladder dysfunction

## Cystitis

In this condition, inflammation of the bladder results in an urgent and frequent need to urinate and then painful urination, with or without fever. Blood in the urine is also a common feature. The cause of this inflammation is usually bacterial, for which antibiotic therapy is generally prescribed. The management of cystitis depends on the age and, in later life, the sex of the sufferer (*see later*).

---

## General measures for avoiding cystitis

Double urination is important to practise. This means urinating as completely as possible, then waiting for a few minutes and attempting to urinate again. In this way, any residual urine does not stagnate but is expelled from the bladder.

- Drinking a lot of liquid helps to "wash out" the infection. If cystitis occurs as a single episode, a suitable fluid to drink is barley water, to be taken as often as possible, at least 100 ml (3.5 fl. oz) an hour.
- It is important to maintain an adequate fluid intake so that the urine remains a light straw colour and does not darken, which shows that the person is becoming dehydrated. Caffeine and alcohol consumption should be reduced as both of these can encourage dehydration. In this state of relative urine stagnation, bacteria can easily grow in the bladder.
- Drink 250 ml (9 fl. oz) of cranberry juice four times a day as a herbal therapy to discourage bacterial growth in the bladder and prevent recurrent bouts of cystitis.

---

### General homeopathic treatment

The homeopathic approach would be to ensure an adequate fluid intake (*see box*) and to consult a specialist homeopath who will be able to give specific advice about any local symptoms as well as a remedy that will suit the general profile of the individual. If this is not possible, choose one of the following remedies, which can be selected by matching its picture with the physical symptoms. Using the 6c potency, for the acute attack of cystitis give one dose four times a day until the symptoms improve. For repeated attacks of cystitis, give one dose twice a day as a long-term strategy.

### *Aconitum napellus* (monk's-hood)

This remedy picture describes people who are full of anxiety and fears, particularly of dying. They have cystitis and become very agitated and anxious at the prospect of urination because of the pain that this will cause. The pain is a violent burning and the urine feels hot. It may also contain blood. Sufferers are thirsty, which differs from *Apis mellifica,* which is a thirstless remedy. All symptoms can be brought on and are made worse by dry cold weather (as compared with *Dulcamara,* whose symptom picture is brought on and made worse by damp cold conditions).

### *Apis mellifica* (honey bee)

This remedy picture describes sharp, stinging pains in the lower abdomen, with a frequent desire to urinate. The pain is of such intensity that the person shrieks with anticipatory fear of the pain to come (a symptom shared with *Aconitum napellus*). The urine is passed in small volumes and may contain blood, and it is the last few drops that particularly burn and smart. There may be incontinence of urine. Heat makes all the symptoms worse, and they are improved by the cold. The person is not particularly thirsty, as compared with *Aconitum napellus* which is a thirsty remedy.

### *Arnica* (leopard's bane)

This remedy picture describes symptoms of cystitis following a traumatic injury. With this remedy, the whole body feels so sore and bruised that the bed feels too hard. *Arnica* has a peculiar symptom: sufferers say that they feel well when, in fact, they are quite ill.

### *Belladonna* (deadly nightshade)

This remedy picture describes a symptom as if there was a worm in the bladder. There is usually a lot of blood in the urine, the person may be incontinent of urine or may have such difficulty in urinating that the person goes into retention of urine. The urge to try to urinate continues even after urine has been passed.

### *Cantharis* (Spanish fly)

This remedy picture describes sufferers who have an unbearable urgency to urinate, with spasm in the urethra and bladder when urinating. They have a cutting pain before, during and after urinating. The urine usually contains blood.

### *Causticum* (Hahnemann's mixture of quicklime {calcium oxide} with potassium bisulphate)

This remedy is the most common one used for treating cystitis. Its remedy picture shows sufferers with a great feeling of urgency to urinate, who then find themselves unable to do so. Later, while sitting or coughing or on exertion, there is urine incontinence that occurs without warning. When they are unable to urinate properly, they develop a shooting pain in the rectum. Retention of urine can occur after surgical operations, particularly gynaecological ones, and this remedy, given as a single 30c dose, often prevents unnecessary catheterization (when a narrow tube is inserted into the urethra to drain urine). Sufferers are very sensitive to the cold.

### *Chamomilla* (camomile)

This remedy picture describes a sticking pain in the neck of the bladder that becomes a burning pain during urination. Sufferers have an ineffectual urging to urinate, which causes them much anguish. Any urine that is passed is hot, red in colour and scanty in volume. The mental picture of the person is significant. Children have a contrary attitude; nothing seems to please them. Adults are irritable and impatient. Both adults and children are oversensitive to pain – they cannot bear it.

### Chimaphila umbellata (pipsisewa)

This remedy picture describes cystitis where the urine contains great quantities of ropy, bloody mucus, and produces a peculiar symptom: the sensation of a ball between the legs, in the region known as the perineum. Sufferers must stand with their feet wide apart and their bodies leaning forwards in order to be able to pass urine.

### Clematis erecta (virgin's bower)

This remedy picture describes a burning sensation at the beginning of urination, which remains in the urethra for a long time afterwards. The feeling is as if the urethra will close up – a feeling of constriction. The flow of urine is very slow, and the bladder is seldom properly emptied.

### Dulcamara (bittersweet)

This remedy picture describes the development of cystitis after the person has become hot either from the weather or from exertion and then has suddenly become cold either from the weather or from paddling in cold water. When chilled in this way, he or she feels an urge to urinate.

### Epigea repens (trailing arbutus)

This remedy picture describes a pain in the neck of the bladder during urination, with a straining sensation of wanting to urinate even after urination has finished. The urine is brown and contains a fine sand of uric acid crystals, and there is occasional urine incontinence. The infection in the bladder commonly ascends into the kidneys, causing pyelonephritis (*see below*).

### *Equisetum* (scouring-rush)

This remedy picture describes a dull pain in the bladder as though it were distended. Sufferers have a constant desire to urinate, and pass large quantities of pale-coloured urine without this easing the symptom of discomfort. They also have a severe pain at the end of urination (a symptom shared with *Sarsaparilla*). Children often wet their beds while dreaming of passing urine. In older people, there is often incontinence not only of urine but also of faeces.

### *Lachesis* (bushmaster snake venom)

This remedy picture describes a cystitis that results in the passing of offensive-smelling urine. Sufferers' abdomens are so sensitive to the touch that any clothing they are wearing cannot be fastened too tightly. They also have a feeling as though a ball is rolling around their bladder or lower abdomen. They always have to urinate after lying down and especially after a period of sleep.

### *Lycopodium* (club moss)

This remedy picture describes a heavy feeling in the bladder that is made better when sufferers hold their abdomens (a symptom shared with *Sepia*). Although having an urge to urinate, they have to wait a long time before any urine begins to flow. It is common for the urine to contain a red sediment. Sufferers may find that they pass large volumes of urine during the night, while during the day, only normal amounts of urine are passed. They also may find that urine is passed at night involuntarily. The mental symptoms are important with this remedy. The symptoms are at their worst between 4.00 and 8.00 pm, and the person has a desire for sweet foods and hot drinks.

### Pareira brava (virgin vine)

This remedy picture describes a constant urge to urinate, and severe pains radiating down both thighs during urination. In order to urinate, sufferers have to bend over so that their hands and knees are touching the floor and their foreheads are almost touching the floor.

### Petroselinum (parsley)

This remedy picture describes sudden, agonizing urges to urinate. These urges are associated with such severe pains that sufferers have to shiver and dance around the room in order to reduce the agony.

### Populace tremuloides (American aspen)

This remedy picture describes symptoms that suggest that this remedy is particularly useful in treating cystitis in older people and pregnant women and following a surgical operation. Sufferers have pain behind their pubic bones at the end of urination, and their urine contains blood and pus. They experience a strong urge to urinate and may become incontinent when they sit down. In men, it is common to find that the prostate gland is enlarged.

### Pulsatilla (wind flower)

This remedy describes cystitis in which urine cannot be retained in the bladder (a symptom shared with Cantharis). Sufferers are unable to lie on their backs without having the desire to urinate. They have to concentrate on the necks of their bladders in order to remain continent of urine. The slightest movement in coughing or sneezing will cause urine to dribble out (a symptom shared with Causticum). They are also so sensitive to noise that they can become incontinent of urine when a door is slammed shut (a symptom shared with Sepia). The general profile of the person that this remedy will particularly suit is someone who feels worse in hot environments and after eating fatty foods, and feels much better in the fresh air.

## Sepia (inky juice of cuttlefish)

This describes symptoms of cystitis that are similar to those of *Pulsatilla*. It is the mental symptoms that distinguish the two remedies. The *Sepia* person wants to retreat into a private space, whereas the *Pulsatilla* person craves company.

## Tarentula hispania (Spanish spider)

The characteristic feature of this remedy picture is one of intense restlessness. Sufferers are hurried, fidgety and roll from side to side. With cystitis, they can develop a high body temperature and also have gastrointestinal tract disturbances.

## Staphysagria (stavesacre)

For this remedy picture, see the description on p.223.

## Terebinthina (turpentine)

This remedy picture has a peculiar symptom in that the urine smells of violets. There are violent sensations of burning and cutting pains in the bladder, the urine is bloodstained and the person has a constant desire to urinate. Apart from the burning sensation in the bladder – the characteristic feature of this remedy – there are three other important features: drowsiness even when in pain; a humming sensation in the ears, like having sea shells placed over them; and a dry, red, sore and shiny tongue with a burning pain on the tip.

### Children and cystitis

In children, a full medical assessment is imperative as the infection may indicate an abnormality of the urinary tract that causes urine to stagnate and which may need surgical correction. This assessment will include an ultrasound investigation.

### Cystitis in adults

Between the ages of 20 and 50, cystitis is more common in women than in men. This is because, in women, the urethra's opening is comparatively closer to the anus, making it easier for bacteria from the anus to enter the urethra. Therefore, personal hygiene is particularly important in stopping recurrent urine infections. Women should wash daily the vulval area with non-irritant soaps and, following defecation, should wipe the anus from the front towards the back. Wearing cotton underwear will also help, but bathing in bubble baths for long periods should be avoided.

During sexual intercourse, a woman's urethra can become injured and bacterial infection can occur leading to cystitis. To avoid this, the vagina should be as lubricated as possible before intercourse takes place, either by natural processes or by applying a lubricant. It is also important for the woman to empty her bladder before intercourse, and to empty it again as soon as is conveniently possible afterwards. Similar injuries to the urethra can also happen as a result of catheterization (in which a tube is placed in the urethra to collect urine), which may occur during childbirth or an operation. There is a specific homeopathic remedy that is applicable in these cases:

### *Staphysagria* (stavesacre)

This remedy picture describes frequency of urination with pain in the bladder or loin (the kidney area in the back) or along the track of the urethra. The person has a sensation as if a drop of urine is rolling continuously along the urethra. The symptoms occur particularly with sexual intercourse excesses. Using the 30c potency, take one dose immediately after sexual intercourse or if the infection has become apparent only after the event has taken place, then a 6c potency four times a day for three to four days.

If the person has a neurological condition so that complete emptying of the bladder is not possible, the urine stagnates in the bladder, creating the ideal environment in which bacteria can grow. In this situation, medical advice is important because long-term antibiotic therapy may have to be considered. An alternative strategy would be to consume about 1 litre (2 pints) of cranberry juice a day in four equal amounts, and to apply pressure to the bladder to help empty it as much as possible.

### Cystitis and older people

In older men, the prostate gland can slowly enlarge, causing an obstruction at the neck of the bladder, leading to stagnation of urine in the bladder and providing an ideal environment for the growth of bacteria and the development of cystitis.

In older people of both sexes, the power of urinating decreases due to weakening of the muscle that expels urine from the bladder. This results in an enlarged bladder and urine stagnation. As well as conventional drug therapy for improving the bladder muscle power, there are two homeopathic remedies that can be considered. These can be used either as a complementary method of treatment with the conventional drug therapy or on their own. Using the 6c potency, give one dose twice a day as a long-term policy.

### Alumina metallicum (aluminium)

This remedy picture describes people whose bladder muscles are so weak that they have to strain to defecate in order to urinate. Although they have a frequent desire to urinate, they have difficulty in initiating a flow.

### Plumbum metallicum (lead)

This remedy picture describes frequent but ineffectual urges to urinate, and when there is urination, it only comes drop by drop.

## Bladder stones

A stone can form in the bladder. This does not cause the same amount of pain as a KIDNEY STONE and it is more likely to cause symptoms of CYSTITIS. The diagnosis of a stone in the bladder is made by either a special type of X-ray called an intravenous pyelogram (IVP) or by a cystoscopy, a procedure whereby a thin telescope is inserted through the urethra.

Bladder stones are usually removed surgically, or crushed by lithotripsy (shock waves). However, a medical workup must be carried out to find the reason why the stones have formed in the first place. They can occur if the diet is low in phosphate and protein (as it often is in developing countries), or if there is an obstruction to the flow of urine from the bladder and/or a long-standing urinary tract infection. Whatever is the cause, it must be treated to avoid further bladder stones forming.

There are several homeopathic remedies that can treat bladder stones. These can be used in a complementary way with conventional therapy or as a separate form of therapy. Using the 30c potency, give one dose daily for two weeks, reducing the 30c potency to one dose on alternate days for two weeks, and finally changing to a 6c potency and giving one dose of this twice a day for as long as necessary.

### Calcarea carbonica (calcium carbonate)

This remedy picture describes the presence of gravel in the urine. This can not only cause stone formation in the ureters but also within the bladder. The general features of the person will point to this remedy: sweating, particularly of the head and feet; physical chilliness; a tendency towards obesity; and a craving for eggs.

### Sarsaparilla (similax)

This remedy picture describes either a white sediment in a scanty, slimy or flaky urine or a red sediment in clear urine. This remedy has a peculiar symptom: urine only flows freely when the person is standing upright.

### Sepia (inky juice of cuttlefish)

This remedy picture describes urine containing gravel that leaves an adhesive sediment in the toilet. The general features of the individuals as a whole will give added pointers to using this remedy: they prefer their own space; they may have a saddle-shaped rash across their noses and cheeks; they feel tired and have a downward dragging feeling in their genitals and bowels so that they prefer to sit with their legs crossed.

### *Silicea* (pure flint)

This remedy picture describes the presence of bladder stones. Sufferers may have an involuntary discharge of urine after urination has apparently finished. They have a constant urge to urinate, and they may be urine incontinent at night. The general features of this remedy picture as applied to the person as a whole may provide added pointers to the use of this remedy: such individuals have sweaty feet and tend to be weak in mind and body, although they can occasionally be stirred into action.

### *Uva ursi* (bearberry)

This remedy picture describes the stopping of urine flow as if a stone has rolled over in the bladder, blocking the opening of the urethra. The urine that is passed is ropey from a thick mucous sediment, and it burns and scalds the person.

# Enuresis (bedwetting)

Babies normally develop bladder control during the day between the ages of two and three, while they might be five or even seven years old before they develop control at night during sleep.

*Primary enuresis* describes a condition where children have never developed bladder control. This needs medical assessment. If no abnormality is found, the children can be "trained" to control their bladder sphincter through such techniques as using a "star chart" (where dry nights are rewarded with stars in a diary), by a rearrangement of fluid intake before going to bed and by "lifting" the children from their beds and sitting them on a toilet to urinate.

*Secondary enuresis* describes a condition where, although they have acquired bladder control, individuals subsequently become incontinent of urine at night. This is usually associated with a stress reaction, but it can also be due to a urine infection or mark the beginning of a neurological illness. It is always advisable to seek medical advice about the cause of secondary enuresis.

There are several homeopathic remedies that are useful in treating secondary enuresis. Having selected a remedy from the following remedy pictures, use the 6c potency and give one dose four times a day until the enuresis has improved.

### Apis mellifica (honey bee)

This remedy picture describes enuresis in a person who is without any joy, is apathetic, is easily made jealous and hides in indifference. The enuresis occurs with a burning and stinging pain and may be associated with faecal incontinence as well. Generally the person that this remedy will suit will be intolerant of heat and will be thirstless (symptoms shared with *Pulsatilla*).

### Argentum nitricum (silver nitrate)

This remedy picture describes enuresis with daytime incontinence as well. However, the features that distinguish this remedy will be the general and the mental. The person will crave salt and sugar, will be very anxious, will have a fear of high places and crowded places, and will prefer cooler environments and the fresh air.

### Arsenicum album (arsenic trioxide)

This remedy picture describes enuresis, and its use will be determined by the basic characteristics of sufferers. They will be nervous, anxious, restless and fastidious (to the point where they will get out of bed to put one of their hairs straight), and they feel the cold intensely. Their worst hour is approximately between 1.00 and 2.00 am.

### Belladonna (deadly nightshade)

This remedy picture describes individuals with the sensation of a continual motion in the bladder, as if a worm were present. There can be blood in the urine even though no cause can be found for its appearance. Sufferers dream of passing urine and then do so (a symptom shared with *Equisetum* and *Kreosotum*). The general profile of such individuals is that of redness in the face, widely dilated pupils, a rapid heart rate and a probable fever.

### *Benzoicum acidum* (benzoic acid)

This remedy picture describes urine that has a characteristic repulsive odour and a changeable and highly coloured nature. The person may well be asthmatic and/or have a uric acid problem.

### *Causticum* (Hahnemann's mixture of quicklime [calcium oxide] with potassium bisulphate)

This remedy picture is of sufferers who are enuretic during the first sleep at night (a symptom shared with *Kreosotum* and *Pulsatilla*) and from the slightest emotional excitement. The person has no awareness of passing urine.

### *Cina* (worm seed)

This remedy picture describes copious and involuntary urination associated with symptoms of threadworm infestation (anal irritation) and a ravenous appetite. The characteristic feature of this remedy is that the person is cross and doesn't want to be touched or looked at.

### *Equisetum* (scouring-rush)

This remedy picture describes enuresis that occurs when the person is actually dreaming of passing urine. In older people, enuresis is associated with the involuntary passing of faeces.

### *Hepar sulphuris* (Hahnemann's calcium sulphide)

This remedy picture has a specific indication: the urine flow is very slow, being voided without any force so that the urine drops vertically. It is in this situation that the person becomes enuretic.

### Kreosotum (beechwood kreosote)

The remedy picture describes a sudden urging to urinate during the very deep sleep at the beginning of sleep. Either sufferers cannot get out of bed quick enough or they dream of urinating. Either way they become enuretic.

### Lycopodium (club moss)

This remedy picture describes involuntary urination during sleep. A marked feature of this remedy is that a large quantity of clear urine is passed at night, while during the day, a normal quantity is passed. With this remedy, there is also incontinence of urine between 4.00 and 8.00 pm. The urine commonly contains a red-coloured sediment. Adults may show a peculiar symptom: they may cry when being thanked.

### Natrum muriaticum (sodium chloride)

This remedy picture describes the involuntary escape of urine when walking, coughing or sneezing (a symptom shared with *Causticum*). Sufferers have an urgency to urinate but an inability to retain the urine (a symptom shared with *Sulphur*). When other people are around, they have to wait a long time for urine to appear. The general symptoms that indicate that this remedy will suit the person as a whole are a craving for salt, a deep crack in the middle of the lower lip, a dislike of sympathy and throbbing headaches.

### Phosphorus

This remedy picture applies to children who are enuretic and who are going through a growth spurt. The other general features that point to this remedy are that sufferers have a preference for salt, cold drinks and ice cream, and they fear the dark, being left alone, ghosts and thunderstorms.

### Rhus aromatica (fragrant sumach)

This remedy picture is of enuresis in a person who has bladder muscle weakness. He or she has severe pain at the beginning or even before urination begins. The enuresis is associated with DIABETES MELLITUS.

### Sepia (inky juice of cuttlefish)

This remedy picture describes enuresis that occurs during the first part of sleep (a symptom shared with *Causticum* and *Kreosotum*). The indications for using this remedy depend on the general features of sufferers. They are indifferent to loved ones, want their own space and dislike sympathy (all of which are similar to *Natrum muriaticum*, but *Sepia* does not crave salt and has a preference for vinegar and windy weather).

### Sulphur

This remedy picture describes untidy individuals who urinate frequently, especially at night when enuresis occurs. They may also complain of a burning sensation in the urethra during urination, which lasts for a long time afterwards.

### Uranium nitricum (uranium nitrate)

The keynote of this remedy picture is great emaciation and debility with the presence of ascites (fluid in the abdominal cavity) and swelling of the lower limbs (oedema). In this physical condition, sufferers pass a copious amount of urine, being unable to retain urine without pain in the bladder. Enuresis is a common feature. They have an excessive thirst and may well have DIABETES MELLITUS.

## Stress incontinence

This type of incontinence is caused by physical forces that override the sphincter at the bladder outlet or by muscle weakness resulting from illness, a surgical operation or childbirth.

If the stress incontinence occurs following childbirth, pelvic floor exercises are important to increase the tone of the muscles in this part of the woman's body. This is done by squeezing the cheeks of the buttocks together for at least 10 to 15 minutes, as many times as possible throughout the day.

The existence of CONSTIPATION (*see* p. 158) is an important finding as this condition can cause stress incontinence. The urine should be tested for infection, and a detailed neurological examination should be made by a medical practitioner to exclude any treatable condition.

There are several homeopathic remedies to be considered. Using the 6c potency, give one dose twice a day as a long-term strategy.

### *Causticum* (Hahnemann's mixture of quicklime [calcium oxide] with potassium bisulphate)

This remedy picture describes sufferers who are incontinent of urine whenever they cough or sneeze and whenever they get excited.

### *Ferrum phosphoricum* (iron phosphate)

This remedy picture describes an irritation at the neck of the bladder (the outlet into the urethra). This results in a lack of control over urine function so that urine spurts out with every cough.

### *Gelsemium* (yellow jasmine)

This remedy picture describes sufferers who show a lack of muscle co-ordination, muscular weakness (their eyelids droop) and even paralysis of certain muscles. This also applies to sphincters, particularly the bladder sphincter, which allows urine to come out involuntarily. The general profile of such individuals will help select this remedy: they are nervous with a feeling in their stomach as if they are going into an examination.

### Nux vomica (poison-nut)

This remedy picture describes irritable individuals with irritable bladders and an unstable sphincter. This results in the involuntary dribbling of urine. The general profile of these people is of ambitious individuals who are also perfectionists and workaholics, and who overindulge in alcohol, coffee and cigarettes.

### Pulsatilla (wind flower)

This remedy picture describes involuntary urination, particularly at night and also when coughing or passing wind through the anus. The general profile of such individuals, which will help in the selection of this remedy, is that they dislike hot environments and fatty foods, and feel at their best in the fresh air.

# Retention of urine

There are occasions when a person is unable to pass any urine at all, not because of kidney failure but because the bladder sphincter is unable to relax and let the urine in the bladder out. This causes considerable pain and requires urgent medical help. It can result from an injury to the urethra, after abdominal surgery and from an enlarged or infected PROSTATE GLAND.

A first step to overcome urine retention is to sit in a warm bath. If this does not help, urgent medical help is needed, which involves putting a catheter (narrow tube) through the urethra and into the bladder, to let the urine drain out.

While waiting for this help, the following homeopathic remedies can be taken every 15 minutes, using the 6c potency.

### Aconitum napellus (monk's-hood)

This remedy picture describes retention of urine after becoming cold, from a fright or injury and following a surgical operation. The retention is characterized by the person tossing about in agony and experiencing extreme anxiety. This last symptom is shared with *Arsenicum album*. The person also has a fear of dying.

### *Apis mellifica* (honey bee)

This remedy describes retention of urine associated with stinging pains. The person has no thirst and is intolerant of heat.

### *Arnica* (leopard's bane)

This remedy picture describes retention of urine where there has been an injury to the lower abdomen, and also when the person has over-exerted. As such, it is useful to treat retention of urine that may occur just after a woman has given birth. Sufferers feel bruised on the whole, and they complain that their beds feel too hard.

### *Arsenicum album* (arsenic trioxide)

This remedy picture describes urine retention in the older person who has probably lost the desire to urinate and who now has no power to do so. The other pointers to using this remedy are sufferers' coldness, restlessness and anxiety, with an associated degree of perfectionism – for example, they may get out of bed just to check that their hair is in place.

### *Belladonna* (deadly nightshade)

This remedy picture describes violent twitching movements (compared with the tossing movements of *Aconitum napellus*) as soon as urine starts to collect in the bladder and sufferers feel the need to urinate. Typically those that this remedy will match will have reddened faces that do not sweat, widely dilated pupils, a throbbing heartbeat, a thirst for cold drinks and jerking movements during sleep.

## *Cantharis* (Spanish fly)

This remedy picture describes intense pains when sufferers try to urinate. The urge to pass urine is a constant feature, but they sit on the toilet straining to urinate without any success.

## *Causticum* (Hahnemann's mixture of quicklime [calcium oxide] and potassium bisulphate)

This remedy picture describes retention of urine that follows abdominal surgery, and when the urine has been retained in the bladder for too long and the person subsequently is unable to pass any.

## *Ignatia* (St Ignatius' bean)

This remedy picture describes retention of urine that follows a grief reaction.

## *Lycopodium* (club moss)

This remedy picture describes a urine flow that stops and starts. There is a characteristic backache in the area of the kidneys, which disappears as soon as the urine begins to flow. Children cry out in pain whenever they attempt to pass urine, and they grasp their abdomens for support. In both adults and children, the urine may contain a sediment of red sand. This remedy picture describes individuals whose symptoms are worse between 4.00 and 8.00 pm and who prefer warm food and drink. They also prefer someone else to be around in their house.

## *Natrum muriaticum* (sodium chloride)

This remedy picture describes individuals who retain urine because they were being watched while urinating. They find it difficult to accept any fuss being made about them, and they will also probably have a desire for salt.

## Nux vomica (poison-nut)

This remedy picture describes retention of urine following the overuse of alcohol. Sufferers have painful and ineffective urges to urinate. The general profile of these individuals is of ambitious people who are perfectionists and workaholics and prefer the outdoor life.

## Opium (dried latex of the poppy)

This picture describes retention of urine that occurs following a fright. The other characteristic feature is that the retention is unusually painless except that sufferers have a feeling as though their bladders are going to burst (a symptom shared with *Pereira brava*).

## Pareira brava (virgin vine)

This remedy picture describes those who, in order to urinate, have to get on to their knees and press their foreheads to the floor. In this situation, and while they sweat profusely, urine may or may not appear. They also feel as if their bladders will burst (a symptom shared with *Opium*).

## Stramonium (thorn apple)

This remedy describes retention of urine that is eased by drinking vinegar. When attempting to urinate, sufferers may experience vigorous shaking. They have violent thoughts and carry out violent physical actions.

## Tarentula cubensis (Cuban spider)

This remedy picture describes an overactive person who is unable to relax their bladder sphincter and so is unable to let their urine out. It is common with this remedy to have an unsettled gastro-intestinal tract.

*Terebinthina* (turpentine)

This remedy picture describes muscle spasms whenever the person tries to urinate, which causes the retention of urine. In turn, this may be due to a sexually transmitted disease. The retention is associated with a burning and cutting feeling in the bladder.

# Prostate problems

The prostate is a gland situated in males around the urethra at the neck of the bladder. For remedies to deal with enlarged prostate and prostitis (inflamed prostate), *see* p. 475.

# Kidney disorders

## Kidney stones

The kidney acts as a filter for the blood, and minerals such as calcium and substances such as uric acid can precipitate out to form stones. Those with calcium in them are radio-opaque and will show up on X-rays, whereas uric acid and oxalic acid stones are radio-translucent. These will only show up on an X-ray if a contrast medium is injected into the bloodstream; when this is filtered out in the kidneys, it will show up any stone. This investigation is called an intravenous pyelogram (IVP).

The cause of kidney stone formation is an abnormality in the metabolism of certain body functions. A high urine level of oxalate, a waste product, can lead to stones; this high level may result from a diet with a high oxalic acid content: spinach, rhubarb, leafy vegetables, coffee. Too much calcium in the urine, due to overactivity of the parathyroid glands, can also result in stones. Finally, stones can occur as a result of chronic urinary tract infection and, less importantly, gout, cancer and chronic dehydration.

A kidney stone can cause excruciating pain as the stone passes down the ureter, and immediate medical attention is needed to alleviate it. The follow-up from this consultation will be an assessment to find the cause of the stone formation, which will then be treated.

There are homeopathic remedies that can be used either in their own right or in a complementary way with conventional therapy. If it is necessary to remove a stone surgically, a course of the following remedy should be taken:

### *Staphysagria* (stavesacre)

This remedy picture describes the remedy's use in any surgery of the urinary tract. Using the 30c potency, take one dose every day for five days. Follow this remedy with the appropriate remedy from those described below.

There are several homeopathic remedies that can be used to good effect to help alleviate the pain from a kidney stone while awaiting medical attention. Choose the remedy whose picture most closely fits the symptoms. Using the 6c potency, give one dose every 15 minutes for a maximum of ten doses – but medical attention will undoubtedly have been received well before a decision has to be made on the maximum dose.

### *Argentum nitricum* (silver nitrate)

This remedy picture describes the passage of stones from the kidney that causes a dull ache in the small of sufferers' backs and over their bladders. The urine has a burning quality while being passed (a symptom shared with *Cantharis*) and the urethra feels swollen. The type of person that this remedy will suit craves sweet foods, has an anticipatory anxiety and suffers from a disturbed gastrointestinal tract.

### *Belladonna* (deadly nightshade)

This describes typically colicky pains. The person will be red faced, hot but not sweating and hypersensitive to any sudden body movement (a symptom with *Berberis*).

### *Benzoicum acidum* (benzoic acid)

This remedy picture describes severe colicky pains associated with very offensive-smelling urine that is as thick in consistency as pea soup.

### *Berberis vulgaris* (burberry)

This remedy picture describes stitching pains that shoot out from a single point, usually in the region of the kidneys, and extend into the bladder and down the legs. It also describes pains extending into the loins and thighs, which are worse when the person is urinating. In fact, he or she is made worse by any motion and prefers to sit quietly on the painful side for relief. The desire for urination is increased and the urethra burns even when not urinating.

### *Cantharis* (Spanish fly)

This remedy picture describes a person who has a great thirst and yet, paradoxically, has an aversion to all liquids and food. There is a specific problem in attempting to drink any fluid that contains caffeine: it can cause violent vomiting and make the pain in the bladder much worse. The person has bouts of pain in the kidney area, which are cutting and burning. The person has a continuous desire to urinate, but the action is painful before, during and afterwards.

### *Calcarea carbonica* (calcium carbonate)

This remedy picture describes pain in one of the ureters as the stone leaves the kidney and travels down it (ureter colic). However, the remedy will be prescribed because of the type of person as a whole. The general symptoms from a homeopathic point of view are obesity and weakness. Sufferers sweat easily from their heads and feet. They prefer eating eggs and tend to be constipated.

### *Chimaphila umbellata* (pipsisewa)

This remedy picture describes, as well as a constant pain in one of the kidneys, also a fluttering sensation in the person's kidneys with smarting pains going from the neck of the bladder into the end of the urethra. There is also a peculiar symptom: a sensation as though the person is sitting on a ball.

### *Lachesis* (bushmaster snake venom)

This remedy picture describes symptoms that are mainly left-sided, sufferers noticing stitching pains in the kidney area and a dull pain in the left back. They are aware of tenderness on the left side of the abdomen, which is made worse from any contact and therefore clothing is removed from that area. The symptoms are made worse from sleep and particularly on waking up.

### *Lithium carbonicum* (lithium carbonate)

This remedy picture has a peculiar but characteristic symptom: pains in the heart area while the person is urinating or bending over. The colicky pains are generally in the right kidney, with a feeling of soreness and sharp, sticking pains on the right side of the bladder.

### *Lycopodium* (club moss)

This remedy picture describes symptoms that are worse on the right side and between the hours of 4.00 and 8.00 pm. Sufferers have a low backache that eases as soon as the urine flows from the bladder. They must strain in order to urinate, and it is common for them to develop an acute retention of urine. They tend to produce a lot of urine at night, and it is common for it to contain a red sediment. Those whom this remedy suits are worriers with frowns on their foreheads, prefer warm food and drinks and like sweet foods. They enjoy their own private space, provided that somebody is present in the house.

### Nitric acidum (nitric acid)

This remedy picture specifically describes renal colic (pain in the kidneys) in those who have a proven raised oxalic acid level or a past history of passing an oxalic acid stone. The urine has a distinctive, intolerable smell of horse's urine. Sufferers may feel cold while the stone is being passed. The pain is described as if a splinter is being passed, and this pain is made easier by firm pressure being applied over the area where it is felt.

### Nux vomica (poison-nut)

This remedy picture describes irritable and cold individuals with colicky pains extending from the kidney into the genital area and down into the legs. They often feel nauseated and may vomit whenever the pains are present. This remedy is especially suited for colic pain in the right kidney. The urine stream is weak and dribbles out even though the bladder is full. Sufferers have to strain in order to urinate, and when the urine stream starts, the dribbling stops. While they urinate, there is an itching sensation in the urethra and pain in the neck of the bladder. These pains can extend into the rectum, giving an urge to defecate.

### Ocimum canum (Brazilian alfavaca)

This remedy picture suits a person who has a medical history of gout (and therefore a raised blood uric acid level). The kidney colic tends to be on the right side and is associated with considerable bleeding into the urine and with violent vomiting (every 15 minutes). The urine has a characteristic smell of musk.

### Pareira brava (virgin vine)

This remedy picture describes excruciating pain radiating from the left kidney, following the course of the left ureter and into the groin, with particular pain at the end of the urethra. This is associated with much urging to urinate, such that sufferers have to go down on all fours, almost touching the floor with their foreheads in order to be able to pass urine. They may be nauseated and may vomit bile.

### *Tabacum* (tobacco)

This remedy picture describes pain that shoots downwards from the kidneys along the course of the ureters to the bladder. When experiencing pain, the person is in a cold sweat and feels nauseated. There is a feeling of a burning heat in the abdomen, the rest of the body being cold. Despite feeling cold, the person persists in uncovering the abdomen.

# Nephritis

Nephritis – also known as glomerulonephritis and Bright's disease – is an inflammatory illness of the *glomeruli*, the very small filter units of the kidneys. It tends to occur in children and causes red blood cells and protein (albumin) to leak into the urine through the damaged glomeruli. This is a serious illness needing expert medical advice.

If the protein loss is severe, sufferers will develop swelling of their limbs (oedema) that may become generalized to include the whole body, a condition called *anasarca*. Together, these symptoms make up the "nephrotic syndrome" and it requires careful assessment of kidney function and blood pressure measurements. The conventional treatment will probably include steroids as a primary option, as kidney failure and long-term raised blood pressure must be avoided.

Homeopathic treatment for this disease is available but should be regarded as the second choice. However, one of the following remedies can be given while waiting for medical assessment: using the 6c potency, give one dose every hour. If one of the remedies is given as a complementary method of therapy with the conventional treatment, use the 30c potency and give one dose a day for one week reducing to one dose twice a week for as long as the illness lasts.

### *Aconitum napellus* (monk's-hood)

This remedy is the first remedy to use when the diagnosis of nephritis has been made. The remedy picture describes a sensitive kidney region in which there are shooting and stinging pains. The urine contains albumin and fragments that look like tissue (these are called "casts"). The picture has much fear in it, particularly fear of the night-time and of dying.

### *Apis mellifica* (honey bee)

The remedy picture describes pains in both kidneys, with pressure felt in the left kidney on stooping. The person feels burning and soreness when urinating, which occurs frequently and often involuntarily. It is the last drop of urine that particularly burns and smarts. The urine is scanty in volume and dark in colour and contains many deposits. The limbs show signs of oedema, and the person typically is thirstless and is intolerant of heat.

### *Arnica* (leopard's bane)

This remedy picture describes nephritis with a bruised feeling all over the body. The person does not want to be touched and is fearful of the night (a symptom shared with *Aconitum napellus*). The inflammation is associated with a pain that feels as though a knife is being plunged into the kidney. The person is inclined to vomit.

### *Arsenicum album* (arsenic trioxide)

This remedy picture describes stitching pains in the kidney area on breathing or sneezing. Sufferers are nauseated and feel faint at the sight and smell of cooking. The urine is like thick beer and has a rotten smell. Sufferers are extremely restless, very anxious and quite weakened by the illness. They prefer drinking sips of cold water.

### *Belladonna* (deadly nightshade)

This remedy picture describes stinging, burning pains that come and go quickly and are felt from the kidney region down into the bladder. Characteristically the person that this remedy will suit is red in colour and hot to the touch and has widely dilated pupils.

### *Cantharis* (Spanish fly)

The main symptom picture of this remedy is irritation and inflammation in the whole urinary tract. There is a discharge of bloody urine that burns like fire, and a dull pressing or a cutting and burning pain in both kidneys that comes and goes. The person is very sensitive to the slightest touch, and has a great urge to urinate, which is painful before, during and afterwards.

### *Colchicum* (meadow saffron)

This remedy picture shows a person with urine that is like ink. This remedy is particularly useful when nephritis is caused by an illness called SCARLATINA, a mild form of scarlet fever, or by scarlet fever itself.

### *Helleborus* (Christmas rose)

This remedy is useful in treating nephritis following an attack of SCARLATINA or scarlet fever. The person has swollen lower limbs (oedema) and also has free fluid in their abdomen (ascites). The person finds difficulty in breathing, but breathes easier when lying down. The urine is scanty, dark with decomposed blood that looks like coffee grounds.

### *Ocimum canum* (Brazilian alfavaca)

This remedy picture suits people with a uric acid problem. The urine contains spiky crystals of uric acid and a brick dust red or yellow sediment, and it also has the odour of musk. The kidneys are afflicted by cramp-like pains, more commonly on the right side.

*Streptococcin* (streptococcal bacteria)

This remedy is to be used in those people who develop nephritis following acute TONSILLITIS from streptococcal bacteria.

*Terebinthina* (turpentine)

This remedy picture describes burning in the kidney region that is worse when the person is sitting and improves when he or she begins to move about. Characteristically the urine smells of violets. The tongue is smooth, glossy and red.

# Pyelonephritis

Pyelonephritis is another inflammatory condition of the kidney, but this is caused by bacterial infection in the part where the ureter emerges. It usually occurs as a result of an infection lower down in the urinary tract. The symptoms are back pain over the site of the affected kidney and very high fevers associated with shivering attacks (called rigors). Medical advice is essential; the conventional treatment will include antibiotic therapy, bed rest and intravenous fluid replacement.

Homeopathic treatment for this disease is available but should be regarded as the second choice. However, one of the following remedies can be given while waiting for medical assessment: using the 6c potency, give one dose every hour. If one of the remedies is given as a complementary method of therapy with the conventional treatment, use the 30c potency and give one dose a day for one week; then change to the 30c potency and give one dose twice a week for as long as the illness lasts.

*Aconitum napellus* (monk's-hood)

This remedy picture describes a sudden onset of the illness, associated with much anxiety and fears, particularly of dying. The feeling of anxiousness is worse when the person is beginning to urinate. The kidney area is very sensitive to the touch, and there is a lot of perspiration associated with diarrhoea. The urine may be passed in large quantities, or if it is hot and painful to pass, it may be scanty.

### *Cantharis* (Spanish fly)

This remedy picture is of a furious disturbance in the entire urinary tract. In particular, there are violent cutting and burning pains in the kidney area. These are associated with painful and continual urges to urinate, as well as cutting pains in the bladder and urethra before, during and after urination.

### *Cuprum arsenitum* (copper arsenite)

This remedy picture describes a remedy that suits a person with kidney illness in pregnancy and while also suffering from DIABETES MELLITUS. The main urinary symptom is that the urine smells of garlic, which may be associated with abdominal symptoms of colicky pains and diarrhoea.

### *Epigea repens* (trailing arbutus)

This remedy picture describes sufferers who have a uric acid problem. They also have a continuing problem with CYSTITIS and a burning feeling in the neck of their bladder while urinating, which is followed by a straining feeling to urinate again afterwards. Finally, they have a peculiar symptom: a croaking noise with rumbling in their bowels.

### *Juniperus communis* (juniper berries)

This remedy picture is of an older person who suffers from repeated attacks of pyelonephritis. The kidneys feel heavy in the body, and the urine has a violet odour (a symptom with *Terebinthina* – see sections on CYSTITIS and NEPHRITIS).

## *Natrum muriaticum* (sodium chloride)

This remedy must be considered where there has been exposure to malaria and quinine. The person has a strong desire to urinate but can only do so when alone.

## *Uva ursi* (bearberry)

This remedy picture is of painful urination with much spasm in the bladder. The urine contains blood, pus and much mucus that collects into large clumps.

# *Disorders of the Skin, Hair and Nails*

T he skin is the largest organ of the body. It is able to regulate body temperature by constricting or dilating the blood vessels lying within the skin – when they are constricted, heat is conserved, and when they are dilated, heat is lost – and by raising the hairs on the skin thereby increasing the area of insulation over the skin. The skin is also able to regulate the blood chemistry through the loss of sweat containing salt (sodium chloride). It is through the nerve endings in the skin that we are mainly able to detect pain and changes in temperature and feel pleasure.

The health of the skin, nails and hair acts as a barometer to individuals' general health. It can reflect the diet that they are eating – in general, excess refined sugar, alcohol and fats all have an adverse effect, as does a state of CONSTIPATION. The amount of exercise that they take also has an effect on their skin, nails and hair.

Homeopathically, a deep-seated illness can be reflected as a skin disorder. The obvious example is the association between ASTHMA and ECZEMA. The disorders of the skin that follow will be described with this implication in mind. The homeopathic dosage schedules will be discussed separately with each individual remedy.

## Abscess

When the skin is cut, bacteria that naturally cover the whole skin penetrate into the deeper parts, where they multiply to form a abscess – a collection of pus – which builds up until it bursts. Until then, it causes pain and a hot swelling.

Conventionally the abscess can be treated with antibiotics or by surgically lancing it to let the pus drain away. The medical danger of not letting the pus be properly dealt with is that the bacteria may enter the bloodstream, causing the much more serious infection *septicaemia*, which will certainly mean hospitalisation.

Abscess formation can be due to poor skin hygiene, a poor diet that impairs the immune system or stress, or a combination of all these factors. Certain medical illnesses predispose to skin infections, notably DIABETES MELLITUS. If there are recurrent attacks of skin infection, it is important to seek medical advice so that an underlying physical condition can be treated.

The following homeopathic remedies are known to treat early abscess formation successfully.

## *Anthracinum* (anthrax poison)

This remedy is a nosode (*see* p. 95) and has been shown to be useful in treating septic conditions of the skin, particularly when the infection collects in a single focus such as an abscess. It locally creates a terrible burning sensation. The surrounding skin becomes swollen and there is a risk of the localized infection spreading into the bloodstream (septicaemia). Using the 30c potency, give one dose twice a day for one week, reducing to one dose daily for the second week, and finally one dose twice a week until the infection subsides.

## *Belladonna* (deadly nightshade)

This remedy describes an early abscess. It is a hot, angry swelling, tender to the touch and about to burst. The person that this remedy suits will have a red face with widely dilated pupils and a fast heart rate, as well as probably a fever. This remedy should be taken in the first place, using the 6c potency and giving one dose every two hours for a maximum of 12 doses.

## *Hepar sulphuris* (Hahnemann's calcium sulphide)

This remedy picture describes an abscess that has burst. The skin around it is usually tender to the touch, and the person may sweat profusely day and night. Using the 6c potency, give one dose every four hours for two days, and then decrease the dose to one every eight hours until the abscess improves.

### Silicea (pure flint)

This remedy picture describes a more deeply sited abscess giving pain not only over the area of the abscess but also in the lymph glands draining it. The remedy encourages the abscess to come out from the deeper parts and thereby is more easily treated. It is also helpful in resolving any residual infection in an abscess that has been lanced. Using the 6c potency, give one dose every six hours for a maximum of 12 doses.

## Acne rosacea

This is a condition that produces similar spots to those seen in ACNE VULGARIS, but it occurs in middle life. It affects women more than men, and is made worse by stimulants such as hot spicy foods, anything containing caffeine and alcohol, as well as by stress, and long-term steroid applications on the face.

The conventional treatment is antibiotic therapy with possible vitamin supplements – vitamin $B_2$ (riboflavin) deficiency may be a cause – and avoidance of any of the above-mentioned causative factors.

The following homeopathic remedies are also useful in treating this condition. Select the remedy picture that most closely matches the physical symptoms. Using the 6c potency, give one dose twice a day until the condition begins to improve.

### Arsenicum album (arsenic trioxide)

This remedy picture describes a dry, rough and scaly skin with eruptions of papules (small, slightly raised areas). These are itchy and are made worse from cold applications and by scratching. The person is probably restless and anxious and feels very cold.

### Belladonna (deadly nightshade)

This remedy picture describes skin that is dry and hot. Its redness can alternate with pallor very quickly as can the burning sensation. Pustules (pus-filled blisters) can form and may leave permanent scars.

### Lachesis (bushmaster snake venom)

This remedy picture describes skin that is always covered in hot perspiration and has a bluish-purplish appearance. The pustules are surrounded by bluish-purple skin. The rash is worse after a period of sleep, from heat (including hot drinks) and pressure and in the spring. It improves with warm applications.

### Nux vomica (poison-nut)

This remedy picture describes faces that are burning hot yet sufferers cannot move or uncover them without feeling cold. The skin has a blotchy appearance that is made worse from alcohol, spicy food, mental exertion, scratching and dry, cold weather.

### Rhus toxicodendron (poison ivy)

This remedy picture describes an intensely itching blister-type rash that has a tendency to scale. The face is swollen, and the condition is made worse in cold and wet weather.

### Sanguinaria (blood root)

This remedy picture describes a blotchy rash around the bridge of the nose, which has a seasonal variation, being worse in spring. It burns and itches and is made worse from heat. This remedy particularly suits women who are going through the MENO-PAUSE.

*Sulphur iodatum* (sulphur iodide)

This remedy picture describes a particularly resistant pustular eruption on the face. Sufferers feel as if their hair stands erect and that their faces are always red.

# Alopecia (hair loss)

Most hair loss – alopecia – is hereditary and is the normal loss that occurs as a result of ageing. It is called "male-pattern baldness", but it can affect women as well. A new (and expensive) conventional treatment for treating this type of premature hair loss is now available without a prescription. Minoxidil (brand name Regaine) is recommended for adults aged between 18 and 65. One millilitre of the liquid is applied to the bald scalp twice a day; if no improvement is seen after one year, it should be discontinued.

Although it is relatively rare, alopecia can also be the outcome of a stressful situation such as childbirth, a long illness or an emotional shock. In these cases, natural recovery will usually take place and will lead to restoration of normal hair growth. To hasten this recovery, certain specific homeopathic remedies can be used.

Some medical conditions – low thyroid activity, anaemia – can also cause thinning of the hair. For this reason, it is reasonable to seek a medical opinion so that the correct treatment of the underlying condition can be given.

Occasionally no obvious cause can be found, and in these cases, hypnotherapy can be helpful in finding out whether there is any hidden reason.

The following remedies – given with the relevant predisposing factors – are the most usual homeopathic treatments:

- **Severe emotional shock**: *Aconitum napellus* (monk's-hood) – give a weekly dose using the 30c potency.
- **Grief**: *Ignatia* (St Ignatius' bean) – give a weekly dose using the 30c potency.

- **Break-up of a relationship**: *Natrum muriaticum* (sodium chloride) – give a weekly dose using the 30c potency.
- **Hormonal (following childbirth, during the menopause)**: *Sepia* (inky juice of cuttlefish) – give a weekly dose using the 30c potency.
- **Severe accident**: *Arnica* (leopard's bane) – give one dose twice a day for two weeks, using the 6c potency.

If none of these causes are applicable, consider using one of the following homeopathic remedies, matching the remedy picture with the profile of the individual person. Using the 6c potency, give one dose twice a day as a long-term policy.

### *Alumina metallicum* (aluminium)

This remedy picture describes alopecia in those whose skin is dry and wrinkled, making them look older than they really are. They are constipated, having no desire nor the power to defecate.

### *Baryta carbonicum* (barium carbonate)

This remedy picture describes an older person who is physically and mentally slowing down and whose hair is beginning to fall out.

### *Fluoricum acidum* (hydrofluoric acid)

This remedy describes alopecia in people who may have had a long illness. Their teeth may show early signs of decay. Mentally they are inclined to be indifferent to their loved ones and show a lack of responsibility. They are prone to ear infections that discharge profusely after a long illness with a fever or following a particularly stressful situation leading to depression. They may also notice that their hair falls out easily.

### *Kali carbonicum* (potassium carbonate)

This remedy picture describes very dry hair that falls out easily.

### *Lycopodium* (club moss)

This remedy picture describes a person whose hair begins to go grey at an early age and it subsequently begins to fall out.

### *Pix liquida* (pine tar)

This remedy picture describes alopecia in a person who may have an irritating cough and itchy skin that cracks easily and bleeds on scratching.

### *Phosphoricum acidum* (phosphoric acid)

This remedy describes a person who is mentally depressed and whose hair has become grey early in life and falls out easily.

### *Phosphorus*

This remedy picture describes a person with dandruff and an itchy scalp, whose hair falls out in large bunches.

### *Selenium*

This remedy picture describes a person who can easily develop a headache, particularly over the left eye and after drinking tea. The hair falls out easily.

### *Thuja occidentalis* (arbor vitae)

This remedy picture describes a person with dry hair that has a tendency to fall out. The person that this remedy will suit will probably have left-sided headaches, as if a nail is piercing the head.

# Blushing

When a person blushes, the blood vessels in the face, neck and upper chest dilate to cause redness and embarrassment. It usually occurs in moments of emotional stress and because of fear of losing control in a particular situation. In the menopausal woman, hot flushes are common as a result of a falling oestrogen level, causing an instability of the circulatory system. The homeopathic approach for this is discussed on p. 493.

For all other situations, the following homeopathic remedies can be used. Using the 6c potency, give one dose as an immediate therapy, and possibly one dose before an event where blushing is a possibility.

### *Ferrum phosphoricum* (iron phosphate)

This remedy picture describes individuals who are not robust but are nervous, sensitive and pale because of anaemia. However, they have a tendency to blush easily, giving them a false appearance of well-being. If this remedy picture matches, it is important also to have the blood checked as anaemia is a real possibility and needs conventional therapy.

### *Lycopodium* (club moss)

This remedy picture describes an unstable circulatory system and blushing is a common occurrence. One ear or one foot can be red while the other is pale, and the person's nose is usually red.

### *Phosphorus*

This remedy picture describes people who are usually tall, extrovert and fearful of thunderstorms and of being alone in the dark. They can become easily and quickly excited and, in this state, blush easily.

### *Pulsatilla* (wind flower)

This remedy particularly suits fair-haired persons who dislike the heat and fatty foods and who feel better in the fresh air. They tend to cry easily and dislike disagreements, and when they become involved in an argument, they blush easily.

# Boils and carbuncles

A boil is an infection in one of the hair follicles, usually by specific bacteria (*Staphylococcus aureus*). If a boil becomes particularly large or if several boils become united, this is known as a carbuncle.

The conventional treatment is antibiotic therapy, and the boil or carbuncle is surgically lanced. Homeopathically, at the first sign of infection make a mixture of the mother tinctures of *Calendula oficinalis* (marigold) and *Hypericum* (St John's wort) and bathe the affected area three times a day.

If the boil or carbuncle does not resolve, use the remedy pictures for abscesses (*see* pp. 248–9) and select a remedy that matches the physical picture of the boil or carbuncle. The same potency and dosage schedules apply.

# Burning feet

In this condition, the person has a continuous feeling of burning in the feet. It can be due to a vitamin deficiency or to MULTIPLE SCLEROSIS, but usually no cause can be found. There is no conventional treatment available, but encouraging the person to walk barefoot can help, together with a multi-vitamin supplement.

Homeopathic treatment is to use one of the following remedies, matching the picture of the remedy with the physical symptoms. Using the 6c potency, give one dose three times a day for two weeks. If there is no improvement, select a different remedy, using the same dosage schedule. If there is an improvement, slowly reduce the dosage to one 6c potency dose daily for as long as necessary.

### *Apis mellifica* (honey bee)

The characteristic feature of this remedy is a stinging, burning discomfort that is made worse from heat and touch. The feet tend to be swollen.

### *Chamomilla* (camomile)

This remedy picture describes angry individuals who have a burning sensation in the soles of their feet, which is particularly bad at night and during a fit of anger. They may also have severe rheumatic pains that make them get out of bed at night in order to walk about, which eases the pains.

### *Graphites* (black lead)

This remedy picture describes a burning sensation in the feet that is improved by firmly wrapping up the feet.

### *Pulsatilla* (wind flower)

This remedy picture describes burning feet that are made worse in heat and when the legs are allowed to hang down. However, the sensations are improved when the feet are placed in a bowl of cold water and when the person lies down.

### *Silicea* (pure flint)

This remedy picture describes burning feet that are also sweaty although they feel cold. The sweat becomes offensive to the smell.

### *Sulphur*

This remedy picture describes hot burning feet such that sufferers have to put their feet out of the bed clothes at night to cool them down. Most of the time, they feel generally hot all over, wearing seemingly inappropriate clothes on cold days.

# Burns and sunburn

**Emergency procedure for burns**
- Remove the person from the source of the burn, making sure that you do not become injured as well.
- Immerse the burned part in water as fast as you can. Place it under a running tap or, if the affected part is too large, put the person in the bath and fill it.
- If the person who has been burned is a baby or young child, the water should be room temperature. If the person is an older child or adult, it should be cold.
- Gently remove any jewellery, watches or constricting clothing.
- Do *not* remove any clothing or debris that may have become stuck to the burned part.
- Keep the burned part in the water for about ten minutes. Then cover it with a clean, non-fluffy cloth.
- If the burn is a bad one or very extensive, or if the injury involves the mouth, dial the emergency services.

Burns are classified into three degrees:

1 **First degree burns** involve only the outer layer of the skin, which remains intact and may form a blister.
2 **Second degree burns** involve the deeper layers of the skin, which means that the outer layer is broken.
3 **Third degree burns** involve all the layers of the skin, down to the muscles.

Anything but the first degree burns need medical assessment as fluid loss is an important factor, as is adequately protecting the skin from infection.

For all burns, follow the instructions in the emergency procedure box. Then, for first degree burns where the skin is not broken, bathe the skin with a mixture of *Calendula* and *Hyper-*

*icum* mother tinctures, adding 20 drops of each tincture to 2 litres of water. Continue for as long as the burn hurts. If a blister forms over the skin, do not burst it as the sealed skin protects against infection. In addition, do not apply any creams, but protect the burn with a non-fluffy dressing.

The following homeopathic remedies can be given:

*For immediate use:*
**Arnica** (leopard's bane): using the 30c potency, give one dose every 15 minutes for a maximum of three doses.

*Follow this with:*
**Cantharis** (Spanish fly): using the 30c potency, give a further three doses every 15 minutes.

*If the skin is still stinging use:*
**Urtica urens** (stinging nettle): using the 6c potency, give one dose every 30 minutes for a maximum of 12 doses.

*If the skin ulcerates, it needs careful dressing with a non-sticking dressing. Then use:*
**Kali bichromium** (potassium bichromate): using the 6c potency, give one dose every four hours for two days, reducing to one dose every six hours until the skin begins to heal.

*If this ulcer becomes infected, the conventional treatment is to use antibiotic therapy. The homeopathic therapy is to use:*
**Hepar sulphuris** (Hahnemann's calcium sulphide): This remedy picture describes skin ulcers that have become infected and have a discharge of pus with possible blood. Using the 6c potency give one dose every four hours for two days, reducing to one dose every six hours until the infection is under control.

*Sunburn*
This causes initial reddening of the skin, which becomes sore and painful to touch; it may later cause blister formation. Because of the risk of skin cancer (melanoma), it is important to take preventive measures by using an adequate sun screen.

Should the skin become burned, it is important to cool down the skin and to moisturize it adequately. This can be done with *Calendula* (marigold) or *Urtica urens* (stinging nettle) ointment or *Aloe vera* gel.

For conditions that are brought on by sitting in the sun (but not necessarily developing sunburn), the following homeopathic remedy can be used:

**Natrum carbonicum (sodium carbonate)**

This remedy picture describes the ill effects of sunstroke. Give the 6c potency twice a day.

# Cellulitis

This is an infection of the skin caused by a bacterium, either *Staphylococcus* or *streptococcus*.

Conventional treatment is with antibiotics. See the sections on ABSCESSES and ERYSIPELAS for homeopathic remedies that can be used.

# Chilblains

This condition affects both the fingers and the toes and occurs with repeated cold and damp weather. Initially the fingers and/or toes become pale and numb and then reddened, swollen and itchy. Eventually the skin breaks and can become infected. To prevent chilblains, it is advisable to keep the fingers and toes as warm and as dry as possible during cold, damp weather.

Conventional treatment is with a drug that opens the capillaries (the smallest blood vessels), which helps to keep the fingers and toes warm.

If the skin becomes dry and breaks appear in it, using a homeopathic ointment called *Calendula* (marigold) will help to soothe it. A herbal supplement of ginkgo will also be beneficial, not only as a therapeutic measure but also as a preventative. Take one capsule or tablet every day as a long-term therapy.

There are several other homeopathic remedies that can be used in the treatment of chilblains. Using the 6c potency, give one dose every 30 minutes for a maximum of ten doses.

### Agaricus muscarius (toadstool)

The remedy picture describes skin that burns and itches, and then becomes red and swollen as if suffering from frostbite.

### Calcarea carbonica (calcium carbonate)

This remedy picture describes individuals who are probably over-weight, notice the cold a lot and are prone to a lot of head sweats. They suffer from chilblains that are worse in cold weather.

### Petroleum (crude rock oil)

This remedy picture describes skin that itches and burns, and then goes on to weep with a watery discharge. The person is prone to rough skin that can easily become infected from the slightest of scratches.

### Pulsatilla (wind flower)

In this remedy picture, the skin problems become worse when the limbs hang downwards, making the veins swollen. This remedy is unusual in that warmth makes the symptoms worse.

## Corns, bunions and callosities

With repeated pressure on bones in the feet and hands, the skin becomes thickened to form a callus. The cause of this is usually a problem of the skeletal system that produces prominent joints of the hands or feet. This can result from illness or it may be a congenital abnormality (i.e. the way the person was born). Ill-fitting shoes can aggravate this situation in the feet, causing a corn to develop from the initial callus. And a corn can go on to become a bunion.

Corns and bunions can become infected, giving a lot of pain. Individuals with certain illnesses (e.g. DIABETES MELLITUS and ARTHRITIS) are particularly prone to these problems, and therefore the treatment of the underlying disease is the priority in treating a corn or bunion. Attention to footwear is important, and advice and treatment from a chiropodist is essential. As a final method of therapy, surgery – to correct a bony abnormality or remove a bunion – can be considered.

Alternatively, the skin can be softened with *Calendula* (marigold) ointment and the following two homeopathic remedies used:

### *Antimonium crudum* (black sulphide of antimony)

This remedy picture describes very tender feet, with particular pain in the heels. Corns and bunions are a feature. Using the 6c potency, give one dose twice a day in conjunction with ...

### *Calendula officinalis* (marigold)

Mother tincture to be applied on lint and placed over the bunion as a daily dressing.

# Cracks in the skin

Some people suffer from cracked skin, possibly due to insufficient moisturization or a diet deficient in vitamin C, but more usually this is simply the way the person was made. The treatment is to use either *Petroleum* (crude rock oil) or *Calendula* (marigold) creams in order to moisturize the skin, and to take supplements of vitamin C.

The following homeopathic remedies are also useful when the remedy picture matches the physical condition. Using the 6c potency, give one dose three times a day until the condition improves.

### *Calcarea carbonica* (calcium carbonate)

This remedy picture describes people who are overweight, sweat easily and are sensitive to the cold. They develop cracks in their skin, which become deeper in the winter.

### *Graphites* (black lead)

This remedy picture describes cracks around the nostrils, behind the ears, around the nipples of the breast and on the fingertips. It is common for these cracks to ooze a honey-like discharge.

### *Petroleum* (crude rock oil)

This remedy picture describes skin that is dry and rough with a leathery feeling to it, and in which cracks commonly appear. These cracks have a tendency to bleed.

### *Silicea* (pure flint)

This remedy picture describes a person who has sweaty hands and feet and in whom cracks in the skin, particularly in the fingertips, are a common occurrence. These become deeper in colder weather, and if they become infected, they are slow to heal.

### *Sulphur*

This remedy picture describes dirty-looking skin that is itchy and has a tendency to crack. Washing the skin makes the cracks worse. The skin is generally hot and moist, and the cracks easily become infected.


# Dandruff (including seborrhoeaic dermatitis)

When a person has dandruff, skin flakes from the superficial layer of the scalp, which is shed in the normal way, stay visibly within the hair and descend on to clothing, generally causing embarrassment.

There are some skin conditions in which dandruff is a prominent feature, notably ECZEMA (*see* p. 267), and these need to be treated initially.

It is important to brush the hair regularly in order to stimulate the scalp and to get rid of the superficial layer of scalp skin naturally. Restricting the amounts of refined sugar and animal fats in the diet will help to reduce the stickiness of the flaking scalp skin, thereby reducing dandruff.

There are numerous dandruff shampoos on the market, and finding one that may work for you is a matter of trial and error. You may find that those containing coal tar or those containing selenium are more effective than the more commercial types.

The following homeopathic remedies can be used to good effect. Using the 6c potency, give one dose twice a day for at least four weeks.

### *Arsenicum album* (arsenic trioxide)

This remedy picture describes an itchy scalp that is so sensitive that sufferers find it difficult to brush their hair. The scalp feels as if it is burning, particularly at night, and parting the hair reveals bare patches and a skin surface consisting of dry scales from which dandruff is produced.

### *Badiaga* (freshwater sponge)

This remedy picture describes a sore scalp that has dry flaky skin, and the person feels fuzzy headed.

### *Fluoricum acidum* (hydrofluoric acid)

This remedy picture describes sufferers who have lost their hair probably quite suddenly (ALOPECIA) and whose skin becomes flaky.

### *Graphites* (black lead)

This remedy picture describes an itchy scalp that has crusts on it, which extend to behind the ears. The scalp has a nasty odour of faeces and a burning feeling right on the top.

### *Kali muriaticum* (potassium chloride)

This remedy picture simply describes dandruff, and therefore this remedy can be used if the pictures of the other remedies do not fit the symptoms.

### *Kali sulphuricum* (potassium sulphate)

This remedy picture describes generalized flaking of the skin of the entire body including the scalp, which shows profuse dandruff.

### *Mezereum* (spurge olive)

This remedy picture describes a scalp whose skin is thick and leathery and has crusts that flake. Underneath the crusts, pus collects, and when this is discharged, white scabs form.

### *Natrum muriaticum* (sodium chloride)

This remedy picture describes greasy hair that has a tendency to flake around the hairline on the forehead. The person that this remedy will suit has a food preference for salt.

### *Oleander* (rose laurel)

This remedy picture describes intense itchiness of the entire scalp, which is made worse from heat. There are moist spots behind the ears that have an offensive odour.

### *Sepia* (inky juice of cuttlefish)

This remedy picture describes greasy hair that has a tendency to fall out. The roots of the hair are particularly sensitive. The skin is flaky along the hairline on the forehead, which causes dandruff. This area can also develop pimples.

## Sulphur

This remedy picture describes an itchy scalp and scratching it causes a burning sensation. The skin of the scalp is dry and flaky. The hair, which is dry and brittle, falls out easily. All of these symptoms are made worse by washing the hair.

# Erysipelas

This is a highly infectious skin disease that affects the young and the elderly more than other people. It is caused by streptococcal bacteria. It is characterized by the formation of blisters mainly around the mouth and nose (although they can be present on any part of the body). When the infection spreads into the lymphatic system, red lines are seen to emerge from the blisters and there are enlarged lymph glands and a fever. Rarely, the infection spreads into the bloodstream, causing kidney damage in the form of GLOMERULONEPHRITIS.

The conventional treatment is with antibiotic therapy.

Homeopathic treatment is with one of the following remedies. Select the remedy by matching its picture with the physical symptoms. Using the 6c potency, give one dose twice a day for five days.

## Apis mellifica (honey bee)

This remedy picture describes infected skin that is swollen and has a burning, stinging pain that is made worse by anything hot and from being touched.

## Belladonna (deadly nightshade)

This remedy picture describes a skin infection that is bright red, throbs with pain and is made worse by anything cold. The person has a dry mouth, yet is not thirsty.

### Borax (sodium borate)

This remedy picture describes erysipelas causing swelling of the face. The person may also suffer from CHILBLAINS, which – unusually – are better when in the open air. As a whole, the person has a fear of downward movement and of any sudden noise.

### Cantharis (Spanish fly)

This remedy picture describes a blister-type rash that is intensely itchy, causing the person to become very restless.

### Croton tiglium (croton oil seed)

This remedy picture describes a pustular blister-type eruption that itches intensely. This itchiness is followed by a feeling of painful burning. This skin symptom may also be associated with diarrhoea.

### Graphites (black lead)

This remedy is useful for recurrent attacks of erysipelas. The remedy picture also describes blisters that, when they break, exude a honey-coloured exudate.

### Lachesis (bushmaster snake venom)

The characteristic feature of this remedy picture is a bluish-purple coloration around the site of the infection. The person easily sweats. This remedy is of particular use for older people.

### Mercurius (quicksilver)

This remedy picture describes a blister-type rash that becomes pustular. The rash is itchy, and the skin is moist with sweat that has an offensive odour.

### Rhus toxicodendron (poison ivy)

This remedy picture describes a blister-type rash that is intensely itchy and feels more comfortable for warm applications. The person tends to be very restless.

### Sulphur

This remedy picture describes erysipelas that creeps along the skin. The person's skin is generally dry.

### Taxus baccata (yew)

This remedy picture describes pustular blister formation on the skin associated with bad-smelling night sweats.

# Eczema and dermatitis

Eczema is a complicated inflammatory condition of the skin that can occur at any age, although it is especially common in babies and young children. It causes itchiness, cracking of the skin, blisters, discharges, and dryness leading to the scaling and flaking of the skin. Some types of eczema are better known as dermatitis – e.g. seborrhoeic dermatitis, contact dermatitis and photodermatitis.

The conventional treatment is to use steroid creams, antihistamines to control the itchiness and antibiotics to control any infection.

The homeopath regards eczema as an important disease representing a deep-seated problem that is expressing itself in a superficial manner as a skin problem. Since there can be a family history of eczema, ASTHMA, HAYFEVER, ALLERGIC RHINITIS, VASOMOTOR RHINITIS and allergies, it is very important to discuss the ailments of close relatives when the medical history is taken.

It is best to consult a specialist homeopath for this condition in order to assess accurately all the relevant indicators for this skin problem. If this is not possible, use the following approach.

First, dietary management must be tackled. Supplements of evening primrose oil should be taken, at least 1,500 milligrams each day. A careful dietary history, particularly of a young child, will show whether the person has an allergy or intolerance to cow dairy products. If this is the case, it is important to exclude these dairy products from the diet. Goat or sheep dairy products or soya preparations can be consumed instead. It is also important to exclude any products containing caffeine (cola drinks, chocolate, coffee) as these can aggravate the eczema.

To moisturize dry, flaking skin, use *Calendula* (marigold) ointment as often as necessary. *Graphites* (black lead) ointment can be used to treat active, inflamed eczema, usually once a day. This is the homeopathic equivalent to conventional steroid ointment.

If the person has a strong family history of these problems, use **Psorinum** (scabies vesicle) as a nosode (*see* p. 95). Using the 30c potency, give one dose every 12 hours for a maximum of three doses every month.

This nosode can be used with the following homeopathic remedies, which are selected by matching the remedy picture with the physical state of the eczema. Using the 6c potency, give one dose three times a day. As the eczema improves, the nosode and the specific remedy can be slowly withdrawn.

### *Anacardium* (marking nut)

This remedy picture describes intensely itching eczema that is made worse by mental stress and by applying warm water. The eczema may form blisters, particularly on the forearms where they can then turn into ulcers.

### *Arbutus andrachne* (strawberry tree)

This remedy picture describes eczema in a person who also suffers from GOUT and OSTEOARTHRITIS. The intensity of symptoms shifts between the skin and the joints.

### Arsenicum album (arsenic trioxide)

This remedy picture describes a dry, burning eczema that is made worse from cold applications. This remedy should be used when the skin picture fits sufferers as a whole. They are very anxious, feel the cold, are very restless and are extremely neat and tidy. Their physical symptoms are worse between midnight and 1.00 am. Those whom this remedy will suit are thirsty for sips of fluid rather than gulps.

### Bovista (puff ball)

This remedy picture describes eczema in a person who also has such a sensitive skin that any excitement brings on a nervous rash. It is a remedy that particularly suits children who have a stammer and older people who suffer from PALPITATIONS.

### Clematis erecta (virgin's bower)

This remedy picture describes eczema that is worse on the hands, face and scalp, particularly at the back of the head. It is red, burning and scaly with a tendency to form blisters. The itchiness is made worse by washing in cold water. This remedy has a peculiar symptom: the eczema has a monthly aggravation coinciding with the new moon.

### Kali arsenicum (Fowler's solution)

This remedy picture describes itchy eczema that is made worse by the act of undressing and from warmth and walking. The skin in the bends of the elbow and knees has a tendency to develop cracks.

### Oleander (rose laurel)

This remedy picture describes an intensely itching eczema. The itchiness is particularly marked on the scalp, and is made worse by the person undressing. In an attempt to ease the itchiness the person scratches the skin until it bleeds.

### Petroleum (crude rock oil)

This remedy picture describes a dry skin that develops eczema that causes the skin to crack easily.

### Sulphur

This remedy picture describes a hot, dry skin that develops an itchy eczema that is made worse from heat, washing and the process of undressing.

### Viola tricolor (pansy)

This remedy picture describes eczema of the scalp and so is useful in treating "cradle cap" in babies and young children.


## Greasy skin and hair

Greasiness of the skin and hair is due to overactivity of the sebaceous glands that naturally moisturize the skin and hair. It can run in families and is made worse by the eating of animal fats and by over-vigorous use of certain shampoos (particularly the anti-dandruff varieties) and soaps. It is advisable, therefore, to eat a diet low in animal fats, to use simple, unscented soaps on the skin and simple, unscented shampoos, and not to wash the hair too frequently.

An ideal wash for the skin and the hair is a solution of the mother tincture of *Hamamelis virginica* (witch hazel). Put ten drops of the tincture into 250 millilitres of pure water. This solution can be applied daily.

If these measures are not completely effective, the following homeopathic remedies can be used. Match the remedy picture with the physical profile of the person. Using the 6c potency, give one dose twice a day for one month, then one dose daily for two weeks, finally reducing to single doses as required.

### *Bryonia* (wild hops)

This is the first choice of remedy for greasy hair. The remedy picture describes excessive production of sebum (from the sebaceous glands), giving greasy skin and particularly greasy hair.

### *Mercurius* (quicksilver)

This describes a person with a consistently greasy skin due to the production of a sticky sweat that has an offensive odour and is made worse by heat. The person may produce a lot of saliva.

### *Natrum muriaticum* (sodium chloride)

This remedy picture describes someone with a greasy skin and hair who also probably suffers from seborrhoeic dermatitis (a form of dandruff). The person that this remedy suits will also have a liking for salt.

### *Phosphoricum acidum* (phosphoric acid)

This remedy picture describes a person with generalized greasiness of their skin. The person's mood is depressed, particularly when they have had an emotional loss.

# Greying hair

As part of the ageing process, both men and women lose the pigment in their hair. This is quite normal, but if it occurs at an earlier age, other explanations can be explored. It may be associated with severe stress, vitamin deficiencies (particularly the B vitamins) and mineral deficiencies (particularly zinc).

The first line of treatment, therefore, is to correct these problems. If, after a few weeks, there is no improvement, the following homeopathic remedies can be used. Select the remedy by matching the remedy picture with the physical symptoms. Using the 6c potency, give one dose twice a day as a long-term policy.

### *Arsenicum album* (arsenic trioxide)

This remedy picture describes a very sensitive scalp such that sufferers find it difficult to brush their hair, which turns grey and falls out easily. The scalp is itchy and slightly burning and there is dandruff. A dry, scaly eczema may be present, too. The general profile of such people is that they feel at their worst towards midnight, they are excessively neat and tidy, and they are anxious and restless.

### *Lycopodium* (club moss)

This remedy picture describes grey hair associated with early balding. Sufferers may have moist eczema behind their ears and in the deep folds of their foreheads. The general profile of such individuals is that they feel at their worst between 4.00 and 8.00 pm, they show an anticipatory anxiety and they have a liking for warm food and drink.

### *Natrum muriaticum* (sodium chloride)

This remedy picture describes a person with greying hair, associated with seborrhoeic dermatitis (a form of dandruff). He or she may show a preference for salt and have a central crack in the lower lip.

### *Phosphoricum acidum* (phosphoric acid)

This remedy picture describes the appearance of grey hair at an early age in a person who also goes bald early. It is common for these to occur in someone who has suffered a severe shock, is convalescing from a serious illness or has just experienced a grief reaction.

### *Silicea* (pure flint)

This remedy picture describes a person with greying hair, who may have headaches that are relieved by wearing a hat. The feet tend to sweat easily and smell.

*Sulphuricum acidum* (sulphuric acid)

This remedy picture describes greying hair associated with septic spots like boils. The person may also complain of "writer's cramp".

# Icthyosis

In this inherited condition, the skin is very dry and flakes easily. Treatment involves the liberal use of moisturizing creams: *Petroleum* (crude rock oil) is ideal or aqueous cream.

The following homeopathic remedies can also be used. Select the remedy by matching the remedy picture with the physical symptoms. Using the 6c potency, give one dose four times a day for three weeks, reducing to one dose twice a day for one month and finally to one dose a day for as long as necessary.

*Arsenicum album* (arsenic trioxide)

This remedy picture describes rough, dry scaly skin that is made worse from anything cold and by scratching. The general profile of sufferers is that they are anxious, fearful and restless, and feel at their worst towards midnight.

*Arsenicum iodatum* (arsenic iodide)

This remedy picture describes dry, scaly, itchy skin, large areas of which come off, revealing a raw, exuding surface underneath.

*Kali sulphuricum* (potassium sulphate)

This remedy picture describes skin that is dry, burning and itchy. It is associated with profuse desquamation (the flaking off of the surface of the skin).

### *Plumbum metallicum* (lead)

This remedy picture describes a rough, itchy skin covered with yellow-to-dark brown patches. The veins of the forearms and legs tend to stand out as if they are dilated.

### *Thuja occidentalis* (arbor vitae)

This remedy picture describes skin that is particularly sensitive to the touch, is very dry and has a tendency to develop warts. The skin of the hands and forearms is usually covered with freckles and brown spots. The person will also usually have brittle, deformed nails.

# Impetigo

This is a very infectious disease mainly affecting children. It is caused by bacteria, giving blister-type rashes mainly around the nose and mouth.

Affected children should be kept away from school. The infection is spread by direct contact with the rash, and therefore it is imperative that affected individuals and anyone who comes into contact with them should wash their hands. The infection is more serious in babies and very young children as it can spread to the kidneys causing GLOMERULONEPHRITIS.

The conventional treatment is with antibiotic tablets and ointments.

The following homeopathic remedies can be used. Select the remedy from the remedy picture that most closely matches the symptoms. Using the 6c potency, give one dose four times a day for 12 doses. If there is no improvement, consult a medical practitioner for conventional treatment.

---

Babies and young children should be given one dose of the selected remedy, using the 6c potency, and then taken to see a medical practitioner. In this situation, it is reasonable to use homeopathy in conjunction with conventional therapy.

---

### *Antimonium crudum* (black sulphide of antimony)

This remedy picture describes pimples on the face, particularly around the nose and mouth, which leave yellow crusted scabs on the skin, which are sensitive to cold water. The person that this remedy will suit will probably be irritable and have a thickly coated white tongue.

### *Antimonium tartaricum* (antimonium tartrate)

This remedy picture characteristically describes drowsiness, weakness and sweating, and these should be present when considering selecting this remedy. The skin picture of this remedy describes a pustular eruption, leaving a bluish-red mark.

### *Arsenicum album* (arsenic trioxide)

This remedy picture describes a blister-type eruption occurring in a person who is physically exhausted, very sensitive to the cold and very anxious.

### *Arum triphyllum* (Jack-in-the-pulpit)

This remedy picture has as its keynote acidity causing inflammation and destruction. It describes skin symptoms of pustular blister formation that is sensitive to the touch and may bleed. These symptoms are made worse in cold winds.

### *Mezereum* (spurge olive)

This remedy picture describes itchy, burning pimples in which pus can be found, and these are surrounded by fiery red haloes. These eruptions feel worse in the cold and when touched.

## Insect stings

For a simple *bee sting*, the first aid remedy is to rub on bicarbonate of soda. The homeopathic treatment is to give a single dose of the

30c potency of *Apis mellifica* (honey bee), the remedy picture of which describes localized swelling following a bite, giving a burning, stinging pain.

The picture also describes sudden swelling of the entire body. If a person has been stung by a bee before and it happens again, he or she can go into anaphylactic shock, a life-threatening condition in which the lips and throat swell, causing severe respiratory difficulties. This is an emergency and the conventional treatment is the administration of adrenaline and prednisolone (a steroid drug).

The first aid treatment for a *wasp sting* is to rub on vinegar. The homeopathic treatment is to give a single dose of the 30c potency of *Vespa crabro* (live wasp), the remedy picture of which describes intense itching and burning that is relieved by bathing in vinegar.

A general remedy that would be applicable to both bee and wasp stings is *Ledum* (marsh tea), the remedy picture of which describes any puncture wound that causes pain. Using the 6c potency, give one dose four times a day for the first day, reducing to one dose twice a day for five days.

# Nail problems

Looking at the nails can tell a lot about a person's health. Horizontal ridges indicate stresses that a person has been through – an illness, an accident or, in women, their monthly menstruation. Spoon-shaped nails indicate an iron deficiency anaemia. White flecks in the nails do not mean that the person is lacking in calcium but simply reflect injury to the nail bed.

### Ingrowing toe nails

These commonly occur on the big toe. To avoid ingrowing toe nails, it is important to wear well-fitting shoes. Toe nails should be cut carefully so that an edge of nail is left over the skin. Should the nail become ingrowing, a V-shaped wedge should be cut in the centre of the toe nail so that the nail is encouraged to grow away from the edge. Placing a cotton dressing underneath the toe nail that is ingrowing will also help the nail to grow upwards and not inwards.

The homeopathic treatment for a non-infected ingrowing toe nail involves the use of one of the following remedies. Using the 6c potency, give one dose twice a day for several weeks.

## *Magnetis polus australis* (south pole of magnet)

This remedy specifically helps ingrowing toe nails with sore pains on the inner aspect of the nail of the big toe, which are made worse by being touched and by walking.

## *Thuja occidentalis* (arbor vitae)

This remedy picture describes not only ingrowing toe nails but also nails that are ridged and brittle. Sufferers are aware that their joints "crack" whenever they stand up and that their feet have a tendency to sweat.

If an ingrowing toe nail – or, indeed, any nail – becomes infected, this condition is called *paronychia*, and if the nail bed is infected, it is called a *whitlow*. If an ingrowing toe nail becomes infected, the conventional treatment is to use antibiotic therapy combined with surgery to remove the toe nail as well as part of the nail bed. Known as Zadek's procedure, this will usually be carried out using a local anaesthetic rather than a general one.

Homeopathic remedies can also be used. Match the remedy picture to the physical symptoms. Using the 6c potency, give one dose four times a day until the condition improves.

## *Belladonna* (deadly nightshade)

This remedy picture describes a red, hot and tender nail and nail bed. It is useful in the early stages of an infection when the tip of the finger or toe begins to throb.

### *Hepar sulphuris* (Hahnemann's calcium sulphide)

This remedy picture describes an infection that is just beginning to form pus. The finger or toe is tender to touch, and squeezing its end releases pus.

### *Silicea* (pure flint)

This remedy picture describes an infection that is slow to heal up. This remedy will be used only if the other remedies have not resolved the infection. Using the 30c potency, give one dose twice a day for five days, reducing to one dose daily for five days.

#### *Fungal nail infections*

In these infections, whitish cheese-like material appears under the nail and the nail itself crumbles. The conventional treatment is to use antifungal drugs.

Homeopathic treatment is two-fold. First, the finger or toe is bathed in a *Calendula* (marigold) solution made by adding 10 drops of mother tincture to 1 litre of pure water. Then one of the following homeopathic remedies can be used. Select the remedy by matching the remedy picture with the physical symptoms. Using the 6c potency, give one dose four times a day for at least four weeks.

### *Antimonium crudum* (black sulphide of antimony)

This remedy picture describes brittle, deformed nails. Sufferers may also notice that their heels are painful, their feet feel very tender and the skin on them is thickened in many places.

### *Graphites* (black lead)

This remedy picture describes finger nails that are thick, black and rough, or toe nails that are brittle, crumbling, deformed and painful.

### *Silicea* (pure flint)

This remedy picture describes nails that are rough, brittle, deformed and may have white spots on them.

### *Thuja occidentalis* (arbor vitae)

This remedy picture describes brittle nails with surrounding skin that is red and tender to the touch.

### *Nail biting*

This condition occurs when a person bites his or her finger nails, occasionally down to the nail bed. This habit is usually the result of nervousness.

The conventional treatment is to offer reassurance and possibly psychotherapy and tranquillizers.

Homeopathic treatment is available. Select one of the following remedies and, using the 6c potency, give one dose twice a day.

### *Aconitum napellus* (monk's-hood)

This remedy picture describes people who are so anxious about life that they feel as if they want to die. They gnaw their fists and bite their finger nails.

### *Medorhinum* (gonorrhoea bacteria)

This remedy picture describes nervous individuals who not only bite their finger nails but also have a burning feeling in their hands and feet. Their legs feel heavy and ache all night, making them restless. They tend to get cramp in their legs.

### *Brittle nails*

This condition includes nails that crumble as well as being brittle.

The conventional treatment is to use moisturizing ointments.

The homeopathic treatment is to apply *Calendula* (marigold) ointment as frequently as necessary. The following homeopathic remedies can also be used at the same time. Using the 6c potency, give one dose twice a day.

### *Fluoricum acidum* (fluoric acid)

This remedy picture describes destruction in many tissues including the nails, which become distorted and crumble. It is an appropriate remedy for older people or those who have prematurely aged and look pale, miserable and broken down.

### *Graphites* (black lead)

This remedy picture describes individuals whose nails are thick, rough and crumbling and have a tendency to ingrow. The remedy suits those people who are overweight and who have a tendency to develop ECZEMA that exudes a honey-coloured fluid.

### *Senecio aureus* (golden ragwort)

This remedy picture describes brittle nails, and is particularly suited to women with menstrual difficulties associated with backache.

### *Silicea* (pure flint)

This remedy picture describes nails that are rough, yellow and brittle and are marked with white spots.

## Pityriasis rosea

This condition affects the skin mainly of young people. It is probably caused by a virus but is not an infectious illness. It starts with an oval patch on the skin, usually on the trunk, followed by a generalized rash on the rest of the body. It is usually non-itchy but is a cosmetic inconvenience. The illness is self-limiting, lasting for a few weeks only.

The conventional treatment is the prescribing of steroid creams or antihistamines to give relief from any itchiness.

For homeopathic treatment, select one of the following remedies by matching the remedy picture to the physical symptoms. Using the 6c potency, give one dose four times a day until the rash begins to fade. To soothe any itchiness, use *Urtica urens* (stinging nettle) ointment in conjunction with the homeopathic remedy.

### Arsenicum album (arsenic trioxide)

This remedy describes a red itchy rash, but the indications for prescribing it rely mainly on the general symptoms of the person. He or she is very anxious and very restless, feels the cold and wants repeated sips of cold water.

### Natrum muriaticum (sodium chloride)

This remedy picture describes red patches on a rough skin. Exercise and warmth make these patches itchy.

### Radium (radium bromide)

This remedy picture describes a red rash over the entire body, which is burning and very itchy and becomes moist if scratched.

## Prickly heat

This is an intensely itching skin condition particularly affecting fair skin. It occurs in tropical and subtropical climates where the skin sweats easily; when the sweat dries, it causes considerable itching that is relieved by scratching for a very few seconds only.

To prevent prickly heat from developing, it is important to wear loose-fitting cotton clothing, and to shower regularly to remove the dry sweat. There is anecdotal evidence that an effective preventative is an intramuscular injection of gamma globulin before travelling to an area where prickly heat is likely to be a problem.

The conventional treatment is to use steroid creams.

Suitable homeopathic remedies follow. As soon as the itching begins, use the 6c potency, giving one dose every three hours for a maximum of 12 doses. Then change to the 30c potency and give one dose twice a day for one week, reducing to one dose daily.

### Apis mellifica (honey bee)

This remedy picture describes itching of the skin associated with a burning feeling and possible swelling. The symptom is made worse from heat and from being scratched, and is made better from exposure to the open air, from being uncovered and from cold bathing.

### Cantharis (Spanish fly)

This remedy is characterized by intense irritation. The skin symptoms of burning and itching are made worse by exposure to the sun. An unusual symptom of this remedy is that sufferers may develop a burning sensation in their feet at night, and the symptoms are made worse when they urinate. The skin symptoms are improved by cold applications.

### Solidago virga (golden rod)

This remedy picture describes an itchy rash, mainly on the lower limbs, which may become swollen (oedema).

# Psoriasis

In this skin disease, which tends to run in families, the superficial layer of the skin (epidermis) is produced very quickly so that it piles up on itself, forming itchy lumps on different parts of the body. When these are scratched, the skin flakes off, revealing a raw surface underneath that may bleed. Nails can be affected as well, causing deformity, as can the joints, resulting in a form of arthritis.

Ultraviolet light therapy helps reduce the size and number of patches of psoriasis. This can be given artificially or the person can take part in controlled sun bathing. Diet is important. Excess alcohol and rich game meats should be avoided, and supplements of evening primrose oil should be taken, at least one gram each day.

Conventional treatment includes steroid therapy, coal tar skin creams and coal tar lotions to put in the bath to moisturize the skin.

To treat psoriasis homeopathically, select a remedy by matching one of the remedy pictures below to the physical symptoms. Using a 6c potency, give one dose three times a day as a long-term therapy.

### *Arsenicum album* (arsenic trioxide)

This remedy picture describes dry, rough, flaky skin that itches and burns. It is associated with restlessness, and the person feels icy cold and is very anxious.

### *Arsenicum iodatum* (arsenic iodide)

This remedy picture describes dry, scaly and itching skin. There is marked flaking that occurs in great quantity, revealing a raw, exuding surface underneath. The person may also suffer from night sweats which he or she finds exhausting.

### *Borax* (sodium borate)

This remedy picture describes an unhealthy-looking skin in which patches of psoriasis develop. Sufferers may also suffer from CHILBLAINS, which unusually are made better by exposure to the open air. They may also suffer from ERYSIPELAS. The unusual symptom of this remedy is fear of downward movement.

### *Kali arsenicum* (Fowler's solution)

This remedy picture describes psoriasis where there is intolerable itching made worse from warmth and when sufferers undress and walk about. They are restless and nervous and tend to be anaemic.

### *Kali bromatum* (potassium bromate)

This remedy picture describes psoriasis in a person who has generalized weakness, both physically and mentally.

### *Kali sulphuricum* (potassium sulphate)

This remedy picture describes psoriasis characterized by profuse flaking of the skin.

### *Mezereum* (spurge olive)

This remedy picture describes psoriasis in which thick, white crusts form on the skin. These are very itchy, a symptom that is made worse following a warm bath. The itchiness seems to change places when the person scratches a particular area. Following the scratching, the person generally feels cold.

### *Thyroidinum* (dried thyroid gland of sheep)

This remedy picture describes psoriasis associated with obesity. The person's hands and feet are generally cold.

## Shingles

This condition is caused by the same virus that causes CHICKEN POX (*herpes zoster*). This virus is thought to stay within the nerve, possibly from chicken pox infection years before, before revealing itself. Stress is thought to be a major cause of it reappearing. The symptoms start with pain in a strip of skin over the ribs, which radiates around one half of the body from the mid-line. This strip later develops a blistered rash that is both painful and itchy. If the affected strip of skin is on the face, the eye can become involved. The blister stage can last for two weeks.

The conventional treatment is to use anti-viral and pain-relieving drugs. Topical applications of calamine lotion help ease the irritation.

To treat shingles homeopathically, apply a lotion made from adding 10 drops of the mother tincture of both *Calendula* (marigold) and *Hypericum* (St John's wort) to 250 millilitres of pure water. Then use one of the following remedies, matching the remedy picture to the physical symptoms. Using the 6c potency, give one dose four times a day.

### *Arsenicum album* (arsenic trioxide)

This remedy picture describes shingles in which the burning pains are worse between midnight and 2.00 am. The rash is relieved by warm applications. The person is restless, anxious and inappropriately exhausted.

### *Lachesis* (bushmaster snake venom)

This remedy picture describes shingles affecting the left side of the body. The blisters have a bluish look to them, and the pain from them is relieved by cold applications.

### *Mezereum* (spurge olive)

This remedy picture describes shingles that are very sensitive to the slightest draught. The rash is intolerably itchy, which is made worse from a warm bath and by scratching. After the rash is scratched, the area feels cold. This remedy suits the older person.

### *Ranunculus bulbosus* (buttercup)

This remedy picture describes shingles giving intense burning and itching and particularly involves the palm of the hand. All the blistered areas are made worse from the slightest touch.

### Rhus toxicodendron (poison ivy)

This remedy picture describes shingles with a typical red, blistered appearance and which particularly affects the scalp. The symptoms are relieved when the person moves slowly about and from any warm applications.

Following an attack of shingles, a person can develop persistent nerve pain in the area of skin involved, medically called postherpetic pain. The conventional treatment is with an antidepressant. The homeopathic treatment is to give the nosode *Variolinum* (smallpox pustule): using the 30c potency, give one dose every 12 hours for a maximum of three doses. This nosode can also be given to people who have been in contact with a person who has shingles or chicken pox and wants to avoid catching these illnesses, particularly the older person or the person suffering from eczema.

# Urticaria

In urticaria – the medical name for nettle rash or hives – raised weals appear on the skin and itch intensely and swell. The cause of this condition is usually an allergy – to foods, notably shellfish, to certain drugs (e.g. aspirin) and to stress and to certain plants (e.g. nettles, poison ivy).

The conventional treatment for mild cases is antihistamine therapy and for the more serious cases, steroids. If the swelling occurs in the mouth and throat, this is called angioneurotic oedema, a potentially life-threatening condition that requires emergency medical attention. While awaiting medical help, *Apis mellifica* (honey bee) can be given every five minutes, using the 6c potency. Then an injection of adrenaline must be given by a medical practitioner.

For homeopathic treatment for milder cases of urticaria, take one of the following remedies, matching the remedy picture to the physical symptoms. Using the 30c potency, give one dose twice a day for five days, reducing to one dose daily for one week and finally to one dose twice a week until the symptoms subside. *Urtica urens* (stinging nettle) ointment can be applied as required in addition to the chosen homeopathic remedy.

### Apis mellifica (honey bee)

This remedy picture describes stinging, burning, itching skin eruptions, particularly on the lips and eyelids. These symptoms are made worse from warm applications.

### Antimonium crudum (black sulphide of antimony)

This remedy picture describes weals on the skin of a person who tends to have gastrointestinal upsets and has a thickly coated white tongue and is generally irritable with life.

### Calcarea carbonica (calcium carbonate)

This remedy picture describes urticaria that is improved in cold air. The person's skin visibly quivers from head to foot, which is followed by an attack of giddiness.

### Chloralum (chloral hydrate)

This describes urticaria that is worse at night and disappears during the day. It suddenly appears when the person becomes cold and is improved with warmth. Alcohol makes it much worse.

### Copaiva (balsam of copaiva)

This remedy picture describes hives associated with a fever and constipation. This remedy particularly suits children with long-standing urticaria.

### Dulcamara (bittersweet)

This remedy picture describes urticaria that comes on when the person is overheated in humid weather and when he or she has a stomach upset. The urticaria is improved in the cold.

### *Hepar sulphuris* (Hahnemann's calcium sulphide)

This remedy picture describes urticaria with weals on the skin and swelling of the eyelids and lips. The urticaria in this remedy picture has a tendency to recur. A peculiar symptom of this remedy is that the body gives out a strong odour.

### *Natrum muriaticum* (sodium chloride)

This remedy picture describes hives that may have a whitish appearance as well as the usual symptoms of itchiness and burning. The hives are made worse by exercise and by stress.

### *Polygonum punctatum* (smartweed)

This remedy picture describes urticaria that commonly causes small ulcers on the lower legs, particularly in women who are going through the menopause.

### *Rhus toxicodendron* (poison ivy)

This remedy picture describes urticaria particularly when the person gets wet. It is associated with rheumatism and with the person becoming chilled and subsequently developing a fever. The person is generally very restless.

### *Sepia* (inky juice of cuttlefish)

This remedy picture describes urticaria that is made worse in the open air and is improved in a warm room. Thick crusts sometimes form over sufferers' joints. The general symptoms of this remedy point to its use: sufferers' indifference to loved ones and their preference for their own space.

### *Urtica urens* (stinging nettle)

This remedy picture describes urticaria that gives rise to itchy red blotches that tend to appear in a seasonal manner (nettle rash). In addition, there are weals on the skin that are more elevated than the blotches, and these can occur with rheumatism, particularly after eating shellfish.

# Varicose ulcers

These ulcers form on the lower, inner aspect of the leg as a result of deficient circulation through the veins. They occur most frequently in women during pregnancy when the venous pressure in their lower legs increases and damages the valves in the deep-sited veins.

These ulcers take a long time to heal. The mainstay of treatment is suitable dressings to prevent infection, and pressure bandaging to help restore the venous circulation. This circulation is improved if the feet are raised high, ideally to the level of the heart, which is where the blood finally drains from the veins.

The ulcers should not have ointments applied to them; simple washing to keep them clean is sufficient, using a solution made of 10 drops of the mother tincture of *Hypericum* (St John's wort) in 1 litre of pure water. A daily supplement of at least 1 gram of vitamin C will help the healing process.

The following homeopathic remedies can also be used. Select the remedy by matching the remedy picture with the physical symptoms. Using the 6c potency, give one dose three times a day for as long as the ulcer continues.

### *Nitric acidum* (nitric acid)

This remedy picture describes a varicose ulcer that develops rapidly with severe splinter-like pains. The edges of the ulcer are not clean, and the base becomes easily infected.

### *Arnica* (leopard's bane)

This remedy picture describes an ulcer occurring over the site of a previous injury.

### Arsenicum album (arsenic trioxide)

This remedy picture describes an ulcer that develops a burning pain that is worse between midnight and 2.00 am. The discomfort is eased when anything warm is applied.

### Carbo vegetabilis (vegetable charcoal)

This remedy picture describes ulcers in an older person. They are commonly found to be infected, leaking a foul-smelling exudate that burns and possibly bleeds.

### Hamamelis virginica (witch hazel)

This remedy is a classical remedy for varicose veins. The remedy picture describes varicose ulcers that burn and have bloodstained bases.

### Kali bichromium (potassium bichromate)

This remedy picture describes ulcers that have clear-cut edges, as if a machine has punched them out. They do not usually become infected.

### Lachesis (bushmaster snake venom)

This remedy picture describes a leg with mottled marks into which ulcers eat. The ulcer edges are purple-blue in colour.

### Mercurius solubis (black oxide of mercury)

This remedy picture describes varicose ulcers that have irregular edges that spread out. They have shallow bases, tend to bleed and produce a cutting pain.

### Mezereum (spurge olive)

This remedy picture describes deep, painful varicose ulcers that feel worse when touched, at night, when exposed to warmth and in damp weather. Sometimes a thick scab forms over the ulcer under which pus forms.

### Phosphorus

This remedy picture describes varicose ulcers that bleed easily and profusely. This is particularly the case in women in the middle of their periods.

### Silicea (pure flint)

This remedy picture describes varicose ulcers that take longer than expected to heal, are painfully sensitive and commonly infected and have a spongy feel to them. There is a peculiar symptom: a sensation of coldness in the ulcer base.

# Warts and verrucas

These common benign growths on the skin are caused by viruses. *Verruca* is the Latin word for warts and is generally used to describe warts on the soles of the feet (properly called "plantar warts"). *Molluscum contagiosum* is a harmless viral infection characterized by shiny pearly small white lumps (papules) on the skin. All warts can spread within an individual and they can be passed on to others (particularly genital warts and verrucas) unless adequate precautions are taken. The wearing of a sock to cover verrucas when swimming is an easy example.

The conventional treatment is to use liquid nitrogen to burn the warts off the skin. This is simple and non-invasive but sometimes is unsuccessful.

The homeopathic treatment is to select one of the following remedies, matching the remedy picture with the physical symptoms. Using the 6c potency, give one dose four times a day until the wart disappears. In addition, bathe them with a solution of 10 drops of *Thuja occidentalis* (arbor vitae) mother tincture added to 1 litre of pure water, at least twice a day.

### *Nitric acidum* (nitric acid)

This remedy describes large, jagged warts that bleed easily when touched or from washing.

### *Antimonium crudum* (black sulphide of antimony)

This remedy picture describes horny-shaped warts on the hands and under the nails and verrucas on the feet.

### *Argentum nitricum* (silver nitrate)

This remedy picture describes warty granulations. The person as a whole is nervous, likes sugar and has a fear of heights.

### *Berberis vulgaris* (barberry)

This remedy picture describes flat warts that appear anywhere on the body. They are itchy and they burn and smart. They feel worse when scratched and better for cool applications.

### *Bovista* (puff ball)

This remedy picture describes warts that develop shooting pains.

### *Causticum* (Hahnemann's mixture of quicklime [calcium oxide] and potassium bisulphate)

This remedy picture describes warts that are large, bleed easily and can ulcerate. Typically they are found on the tips of the fingers, the end of the nose and on the eyelids and eyebrows.

### *Dulcamara* (bittersweet)

This remedy picture describes large, smooth warts on the face and on the palms of the hands. The palms are also prone to sweat easily.

### Kali carbonicum (potassium carbonate)

This remedy picture describes warts that itch.

### Magnesia sulphurica (Epsom salts)

This remedy picture describes large, soft warts which are usually solitary (symptom shared with *Dulcamara*).

### Mercurius iodatus flavum (proto iodide of mercury)

This remedy picture describes flat warts. The remedy will be chosen on the general characteristics of the person – those who develop recurrent sore throats, and whose tongues have a characteristic feature: it is thickly coated and yellow, but the edges and the tip are red. The tongue carries the imprint of the teeth.

### Natrum sulphuricum (sodium sulphate)

This remedy picture describes red, wart-like lumps on the body.

### Ruta graveolens (rue bitterwort)

This remedy picture describes flat, smooth warts on the palms. A peculiar symptom of this remedy is that these warts itch after the person eats meat.

### Silicea (pure flint)

This remedy picture describes warty growths on any part of the skin that never occur singly. The person as a whole prefers wet humid weather, and has sweaty feet.

### Staphysagria (stavesacre)

This remedy picture describes a large bulb-shaped wart with a short stalk – a "pedunculated wart", and a picture shared with *Thuja occidentalis*.

## *Thuja occidentalis* (arbor vitae)

This remedy picture describes warts attached to the body by short stalks (a symptom shared with *Staphysagria*). It also describes verrucas. The person may also suffer from INGROWING TOE NAILS and BRITTLE NAILS in general.

# Disorders of the Muscles and Skeleton

T his section covers problems of muscles, ligaments, bones and joints. It will include a review of conventional treatment as well as ways in which sufferers can help themselves, and it will reveal the way that homeopathy can offer another form of therapy.

## Ankle problems

*Sprained ankle*
The ankle joint is a hinge; it is unable to rotate. It is firmly held in position by ligaments that are so strong that, if the ankle is twisted, not only will the ligaments tear but the bones to which they are attached can be broken. Therefore, if the ankle is sprained, an accurate assessment, which may require an X-ray, must be made to exclude a fractured bone.

The ankle must be supported with suitable bandaging, and ice initially applied to the most tender area where the ligament has been torn (a bruise may be seen, a sign that blood has been lost from the torn ligament). The foot must also be elevated and the joint must not be allowed to bear weight.

Conventionally, pain-relieving tablets will also probably be given.

The homeopathic approach will include an accurate assessment (to exclude a fracture, which would mean placing the ankle in plaster of Paris). Assuming that there is no fracture, the management would be the same as for the conventional approach: bandaging, ice and elevation to avoid weight bearing as much as possible.

The following homeopathic remedies can be used as well:

### Arnica (leopard's bane)

This remedy is to be given immediately the ankle is injured. Using the 6c potency, give one dose every hour, for a maximum of ten doses.

### Bellis perennis (daisy)

This remedy picture describes muscular and joint soreness following a sprain, and can be used after *Ruta graveolens*. Using a 6c potency, give one dose twice a day.

### Natrum muriaticum (sodium chloride)

This remedy picture describes ankle joints that are weak with a tendency to turn inwards easily and therefore become sprained. Those whom this remedy will suit probably suffer from throbbing headaches, feel worse in hot weather and enjoy salty food. They also dislike any fuss being made of them, easily bear grudges and dislike extremes of temperature. This remedy can also be used to help prevent sprained ankles (in those who are likely to suffer from them). Using the 30c potency, give one dose once a week.

### Ruta graveolens (rue bitterwort)

This remedy picture particularly describes strained tendons, and should be used after *Arnica*. Using the 6c potency, give one dose twice a day for two weeks followed by *Bellis perennis* (see above).

### Fractured ankle
If the ankle is shown to be fractured on X-ray, give:

### Arnica (leopard's bane)

This remedy picture describes bruising from any cause. Using the 6c potency, give one dose every hour, for a maximum of six doses.

This is to be followed by:

### Symphytum (comfrey)

This remedy picture describes the healing of fractured bones. Using the 30c potency, give one dose daily for one week, reducing to one dose twice a week until the plaster of Paris is removed.

When the person has come out of plaster of Paris, the ankle will be stiff and will probably need physiotherapy in order to mobilize the joint. The following homeopathic remedy will help its recovery.

### Rhus toxicodendron (poison ivy)

This remedy picture describes a joint that has been previously damaged and has now developed a form of rheumatism. Sufferers find initial movement of the joint painful but subsequent movement makes the pain easier. They are therefore restless, knowing that gentle movement will help to alleviate the pain. These symptoms are made worse by the cold and improved by heat. Using the 6c potency, give one dose three times a day for five days, reducing to one dose a day for two weeks.

#### Other ankle problems

The following remedies apply to ankle problems that are not necessarily associated with any injury. Select the remedy by matching its picture with the physical symptoms.

### Apis mellifica (honey bee)

This remedy picture describes ankles that swell in the heat and probably ache with a stinging discomfort. Using the 30c potency, give one dose daily for three days, followed by a twice-daily dose of the 6c potency for ten days.

### Bryonia (wild hops)

This remedy picture describes a red, swollen and hot ankle giving a tearing and stitching sensation. The symptoms are worsened by the least movement. Using the 30c potency, give one dose daily for five days, then one dose on alternate days for two weeks.

## *Causticum* (Hahnemann's mixture of quicklime [calcium oxide] and potassium bisulphate)

This remedy picture describes pains in the ankle that are tearing and drawing, causing deformity. This results in a progressive loss of muscular strength. The symptoms are worse in dry, cold weather. Using the 6c potency, give one dose twice a day.

## *Hamamelis virginica* (witch hazel)

This remedy picture describes swollen ankles in association with VARICOSE VEINS. Using the 6c potency, give one dose twice a day.

## *Ledum* (marsh tea)

This remedy picture describes ankles that sprain easily. Sharp pains shoot through the foot and its joints. Sufferers' soles are so painful that they find it difficult to walk on them. The ankles are commonly swollen. These symptoms are worse in the heat and are better for anything cold (putting the feet in cold water is best of all). Using the 6c potency, give one dose twice a day for two weeks.

## *Staphysagria* (stavesacre)

This remedy picture describes stiff joints (including the ankle), and the ankle feels beaten and painful. These symptoms come on following an episode of indignation or grief. Using the 6c potency, give one dose twice a day for two weeks.

## *Viscum album* (mistletoe)

This remedy picture describes shooting, tearing pains in the ankle and knee that alternate with similar pains in the elbow and shoulder. Sufferers also feel a glow rising from the feet to the head so that they feel as if they are on fire. Using the 6c potency, give one dose twice a day.

## Ankylosing spondylitis

This disease is caused by autoimmunity (where sufferers' immune systems attack their own bodies), resulting in inflammation and stiffness of the small joints of the spine. Eventually these joints become fused together so that the spine becomes rigid. This disease usually starts at the junction of the spine with the pelvis (specifically the sacroiliac joints).

This is a disease that must be managed by conventional therapy. This will include physiotherapy and probably steroid therapy as well as nonsteroidal anti-inflammatory drugs.

General advice is to keep the spine as supple as possible with appropriate exercises including physiotherapy and yoga. By lying on the abdomen rather than the back, the spine assumes its correct posture.

Homeopathy uses physiotherapy and constitutional remedy therapy (from a specialist homeopath who will match sufferers' symptoms with their general features). If this is not possible, the following remedy may be taken. Using the 30c potency, give one dose daily for one week and thereafter one dose twice a week.

### Aesculus hippocastanum (horse chestnut)

This remedy picture describes backache affecting the pelvis and hips, which is made worse by walking or by bending over. When walking, the feet have a tendency to turn inwards, the soles of the feet feel sore and tired and the feet swell.

## Arthritis

This term describes a disease of any joint. See GOUT, INFECTIVE ARTHRITIS, OSTEOARTHRITIS, PSORIATIC ARTHRITIS, RHEUMATOID ARTHRITIS, TUBERCULAR ARTHRITIS.

# Backache

This section includes prolapsed intervertebral discs, in which the pads between the vertebra of the spine are pushed out and trap a nerve. If this occurs in the lower lumbar spine, it gives symptoms of *sciatica*, pain shooting down the back of the leg to the sole of the foot; if in the cervical spine in the neck, it gives symptoms of pain radiating down one or both arms. A sprained ligament in the vertebral column can lead to a stiff back that may make it impossible for the person to move: this is commonly known as *lumbago*. Backache may also be caused by arthritis of the joints in between each vertebral body, and it can (rarely) arise from a secondary (metastatic) deposit from a primary cancer.

Because of all these possible causes, it is important to obtain advice from a medical practitioner before treating backache. Tests will be done following a physical examination. These may include X-rays and blood tests.

### Arthritis of the spine

This condition is treated conventionally with nonsteroidal anti-inflammatory drugs. In both conventional and homeopathic methods of therapy, it is important to maintain the suppleness of the back with appropriate exercises from a physiotherapist, osteopath or chiropractor; yoga is also very helpful. Homeopathic remedies that can be used can be found in the section on osteoarthritis (*below*).

### Lumbago

This condition gives symptoms of backache that occasionally cause the person to "lock up", unable to move. It is important to check that there is no underlying bony abnormality by careful physical examination, which may include an X-ray. This condition is treated conventionally with pain-relieving drugs and nonsteroidal anti-inflammatory drugs, together with physiotherapy, osteopathy or chiropractic. The aim of these treatments is to give pain-free back movement.

Attention must also be paid to the general condition of sufferers and, in particular, their weight, as obesity can aggravate back problems.

The following homeopathic remedies can be used as a complementary form of therapy or on their own to alleviate the problem. It is important to follow the initial diagnostic approach mentioned above for conventional treatment, as well as paying attention to body weight. Select the homeopathic remedy by matching its picture with the physical symptoms. Using the 6c potency, give one dose three times a day for five days, or less if the condition improves.

### *Aesculus hippocastanum* (horse chestnut)

This remedy picture describes a continual dull pain in the lumbar region of the back. Occasionally sufferers feel as if their backs will give out and break and have to make repeated efforts to rise up from the sitting position. This pain is made worse from walking or from stooping and is referred downwards into the hips and pelvis.

### *Antimonium tartaricum* (antimonium tartrate)

This remedy picture describes such severe pains in the lumbar region that the slightest effort causes retching and sufferers come out in a cold sweat. Generally they feel as if a weight is attached to the end of their spine (coccyx), which is dragging them downwards. They also feel as if the vertebrae in their spines are rubbing against each another.

### *Graphites* (black lead)

This remedy picture describes lumbago giving a crawling sensation over sufferers' buttocks. They feel as if their lumbar vertebrae are broken.

### *Nux vomica* (poison-nut)

This remedy describes acute lumbago. Sufferers have a generalized ache in the lumbar region with a feeling that the lumbar spine will break. They also have an urge to sit up in bed in order to turn over, as well as a crawling sensation running up their spine. This remedy is particularly useful for women who suffer from lumbar backache following labour.

### Rhus toxicodendron (poison ivy)

This remedy describes lumbago that is relieved by hard pressure, by resting on a hard surface, by walking about slowly and by bending over backwards.

### Sepia (inky juice of cuttlefish)

This remedy describes a "weak" back, with sufferers liable to get a sudden pain in their backs as if struck by a hammer. This pain is made worse and even brought on by stooping or by kneeling. The pains in the back are improved by pressing against something hard and from passing wind.

### Prolapsed intervertebral discs

The conventional treatment for a diagnosis of prolapsed intervertebral disc in the lumbar region is pain relief, and it may also include emergency surgery to remove the intervertebral disc that is pressing on the sciatic nerve (causing sciatica). Back-strengthening exercises are also encouraged (this may also include yoga).

If the prolapsed disc is in the cervical region of the neck, the treatment will include the wearing of a cervical neck collar to straighten the cervical vertebrae and so lift the intervertebral disc that is protruding and pressing on the brachial nerve. Pain-relieving drugs may also be prescribed.

Homeopathy can be used as a truly complementary form of therapy working alongside the conventional treatment, but never exclusively. Select the remedy by matching its picture with the physical symptoms. Using the 6c potency, give one dose four times a day.

FOR THE TREATMENT OF SCIATICA

### *Arsenicum album* (arsenic trioxide)

This remedy picture describes sciatica that is improved by gentle walking and from warm applications. It also describes a drawing pain from the armpit to the elbow, associated with tingling of the fingers.

### *Bryonia* (wild hops)

This remedy picture describes sciatica with a sensation of pins and needles in the sole of the foot. These symptoms are made worse from the least movement and from any weather change.

### *Kali bichromium* (potassium bichromate)

This remedy picture describes sciatica where the pain is made worse when the person urinates. The pains also radiate through the coccyx, making walking difficult.

### *Tellurium*

This remedy describes sciatica that is worse on the right side and is made worse by coughing, laughing and straining to defecate.

FOR THE TREATMENT OF PROLAPSED CERVICAL DISC

### *Belladonna* (deadly nightshade)

This remedy picture describes a stiff neck with stiff shoulders, particularly the right one. There is often a swollen gland in the back of the neck.

### *Berberis vulgaris* (barberry)

This remedy picture describes stitching pains in the neck that are made worse from breathing. There is a sore spot underneath the shoulder blade, usually on the right side.

### *Bryonia* (wild hops)

This remedy picture describes a stiff neck and numbness and pain between the two shoulder blades radiating down to the stomach area and from the left shoulder blade towards the heart.

### *Causticum* (Hahnemann's mixture of quicklime [calcium oxide] with potassium bisulphate)

This remedy picture describes such stiffness in the neck that any neck movement becomes almost impossible. This pain is made worse when the person swallows.

### *Graphites* (black lead)

This remedy picture describes neck pains that are worse when the person looks up and down.

### *Kali bichromium* (potassium bisulphate)

This remedy picture describes neck stiffness made worse by movement of the head backwards and forwards. Cutting pains radiate downwards to the kidneys, making it impossible for the person to walk.

### *Nux vomica* (poison-nut)

This remedy picture describes a dull, gnawing pain, starting from a stiff neck and radiating down the arms (mainly on the right side). These pains are made worse by being touched, and the stiff neck is made worse from anything cold and from nervous shocks.

### *Tellurium*

This remedy describes numb and painful sensations from the last cervical vertebra down to the fifth thoracic vertebra. These sensations also extend upwards to the back of the head (occiput).

# Bone pain

This rare symptom needs careful assessment. It can be associated with influenza, with primary and secondary cancer of the bone, with infection of the bone (osteomyelitis) and with hairline fractures of the bone. The conventional therapy is pain relief and the appropriate treatment of the underlying condition.

The following homeopathic remedies can be used to give relief, but bear in mind the importance of obtaining a precise diagnosis. Select the remedy by matching its picture with the physical symptoms. Using the 6c potency, give one dose three times a day for ten days.

### *Asafoetida* (gum of the stinkasand)

This remedy picture describes bone pain mainly in the lower leg and particularly in the main bone of the lower leg, the tibia.

### *Eupatorium perfoliatum* (thoroughwort)

This remedy is commonly known as "bone set" because of its promptness in helping to alleviate the violent aching bone pains that accompany certain illnesses with fevers, notably influenza and malaria.

# Cervical spondylitis

In this condition, a vertebra presses on nerves leaving the spine. The resulting symptoms – stiffness, pain or pins and needles – are referred to the back of the head, down each arm (one or the other or both) and down the spine and lower limbs.

The conventional treatment is the use of nonsteroidal anti-inflammatory drugs, with physiotherapy and possibly a cervical collar.

The homeopathic treatment is to consider physiotherapy and a cervical collar, together with remedies applicable to osteoarthritis (*see* p. 321) and prolapsed intervertebral cervical disc problems (*see above*).

# Cramps

These are painful muscular spasms that come on from vigorous exercise (which probably causes dehydration and salt loss), and are also common in older people where the peripheral arterial circulation has become blocked by ATHEROSCLEROSIS.

The immediate treatment is to massage the muscle involved and to stretch it. Where salt loss is a probable precipitating factor in people who sweat easily and profusely, daily salt supplements are necessary.

The conventional treatment is to give quinine sulphate, baclofen or diazepam on a daily basis for those people who suffer from recurrent cramps.

The following homeopathic remedies can be used on a daily basis to prevent cramps. Using the 6c potency, give one dose twice a day. For an acute attack of cramp, these remedies can be given, using the 6c potency, every ten minutes for a maximum of six doses.

### *Agaricus muscarius* (toadstool)

This remedy picture describes cramps in the soles of sufferers' feet. These individuals will probably feel stiff all over and have painful contractions in their calves. This remedy also describes trembling and shaking, and sufferers may well walk unsteadily, and when they hold objects in their hands, their fingers may shake. Their toes and feet may have an itchy feeling, as if frozen.

### *Arnica* (leopard's bane)

This remedy picture describes cramp in muscles that have been overexerted. The muscles in this state are very sensitive to the touch and to anything wet and cold.

### *Calcarea carbonica* (calcium carbonate)

This remedy picture describes cramps of the calf muscles when sufferers stretch out their legs, particularly at night. They may also feel that their lower legs are damp and cold, as if they are wearing damp stockings.

### *Causticum* (Hahnemann's mixture of quicklime [calcium oxide] and potassium bisulphate)

This remedy picture describes cramps in the calf muscles, feet and toes. Sufferers may also note tearing rheumatic pains in their limbs, which are improved by bed warmth.

### *Chamomilla* (camomile)

This remedy describes cramps that occur in the calf muscles at night, which are so severe that the person leaps out of bed to walk around.

### *Colocynthis* (bitter cucumber)

This remedy picture describes cramps in muscles during sexual intercourse. It also describes cramps around the hip area and in the right shoulder.

### *Cuprum metallicum* (copper)

This remedy picture describes cramps in the palms of the hand, calf muscles and soles of the feet. Sufferers may also have a tendency to grip their thumbs in the palms of their hands.

### *Dioscorea villosa* (wild yam)

This remedy picture describes cramps in the flexor muscles (those that bring the joints closer to the body) of the fingers and toes. The person may also complain of a weak back, sciatica (*see* p. 302) and BRITTLE NAILS.

### *Graphites* (black lead)

This remedy picture describes cramps that can occur in any muscle group of the body. The person that this remedy will suit tends to be overweight, has offensive-smelling feet and has ECZE-MA that has a tendency to weep a honey-coloured exudate.

### *Hyoscyamus* (henbane)

This remedy picture describes cramps in the toes and calf muscles that occur when the person is walking upstairs.

### *Ignatia* (St Ignatius' bean)

This remedy picture describes cramps in the calf muscles, and is particularly suited to the person who is undergoing a grief reaction.

### *Lachesis* (bushmaster snake venom)

This remedy picture describes cramps in the calf muscles whenever the person becomes fearful.

### *Lycopodium* (club moss)

This remedy picture describes cramps in the calf muscles that occur when the person is walking about at night, and in their toes at night.

### *Magnesia muriatica* (muriate of magnesium)

This remedy picture describes cramps in the thigh muscles that are worse when sufferers are sitting down. They may also find that their arms commonly "go to sleep".

### *Natrum muriaticum* (sodium chloride)

This remedy picture describes cramps of the hamstring muscles (on the underside of the thigh), which feel as if they are too short. It is common for sufferers to have numbness and a sensation of tingling in their fingers and lower extremities. Their joints have a tendency to crack on motion.

### Nux vomica (poison-nut)

This remedy picture describes cramps in the feet and calf muscles that make sufferers stand up to stretch their muscles. This cramp can also come on while they are walking, in which case they are forced to stand still. Their arms commonly "go to sleep".

### Platina (platinum)

This remedy picture describes cramps of the calf muscles associated with a sensation of tightness around the thighs as if they are wrapped too tightly by a bandage.

### Secale cornutum (ergot)

This remedy picture describes violent cramps in the hands, legs and feet. All the limbs are icy cold. Sufferers walk unsteadily, their feet appearing to be dragged along. The person in this remedy picture has a ravenous hunger.

### Stannum (tin)

This remedy picture describes cramps in the hands so that the person is unable to let go of a broom handle.

### Sulphur

This remedy picture describes cramp mainly in the left calf muscle. The person that this remedy will suit enjoys beer and fatty foods, is sociable and enjoys a joke and has a definite point of view about all matters.

### *Veratrum album* (white hellebore)

This remedy picture describes cramps in the calf muscles whenever the person defecates.

### *Viburnum opulus* (high cranberry)

This remedy picture describes cramps in the calf muscles that occur in women at the time of menstruation.

# Writer's cramp

In this condition, cramp occurs in the finger muscles whenever a writing implement is held by the fingers and writing continues for a long time. It can also occur when using typewriters or word processors or carrying out any other repetitive task involving the fingers.

Conventional treatment involves the use of drugs such as diazepam, which affect generalized cramps.

Homeopathic treatment involves the use of one of the following remedies. Select the remedy by matching its picture with the physical symptoms. Using the 6c potency, give one dose immediately before carrying out the task that is known to cause cramp; this should prevent the cramp from occurring. However, if the cramp does occur, give one dose of 6c potency every 30 minutes, for a maximum of five doses.

### *Anacardium* (marking nut)

This remedy picture not only describes writer's cramp but also cramps from the toes to the instep of the foot and from the heel to the calf muscle. The person may also have warts on the palms of their hands.

### *Argentum metallicum* (silver)

This remedy describes writer's cramp and upper arm weakness.

The legs also feel weak and tremble, particularly when going downstairs.

### *Arnica* (leopard's bane)

This remedy picture describes pain in muscles from over-exertion and particularly cramp in the finger muscles. Sufferers have pain in their arms that is improved when the arms are allowed to hang down.

### *Causticum* (Hahnemann's mixture of quicklime [calcium oxide] with potassium bisulphate)

This remedy picture describes a paralysis of the right hand and of the tongue. The person suffers from writer's cramp as well as cramps in the calf muscles, feet and toes. Warts on the fingertips are a common occurrence.

### *Cyclamen* (sow bread)

This remedy picture describes cramp-like contractions between the right thumb and the right index finger – the only way to separate them is by using force. The person suffers from writer's cramp.

### *Magnesium phosphoricum* (magnesium phosphate)

This remedy picture describes trembling hands with cramps in the fingers caused by exertion and prolonged use of any tools. These people suffer from writer's cramp.

### *Picric acidum* (picric acid)

This remedy has a profound effect on the nervous system, causing an inability to think clearly as well as muscular weakness, which leads on to writer's cramp.

### *Stannum* (tin)

This remedy picture describes a paralytic weakness of the person's hands so that they have a tendency to drop things. The fingers jerk when holding a writing implement, and then the fingers and thumbs go into contractions, leading to writer's cramp.

### *Sulphuricum acidum* (sulphuric acid)

This remedy picture describes fingers that jerk whenever the person falls asleep or begins to write. In this state, he or she develops writer's cramp.

# Dupuytren's contracture

This condition is a thickening of the fibrous layer under the skin of the palm of the hand, which causes the little finger and the one immediately next to it to curl inwards. It occurs most commonly in middle-aged men. It is associated with alcoholism but can be an inherited problem.

The conventional treatment is surgical correction, which is the best option.

Physiotherapy and homeopathy can be used in the early stages to help prevent the condition from worsening. Select the homeopathic remedy by matching its picture with the physical symptoms.

### *Calcarea fluorica* (calcium fluoride)

This remedy picture describes an ability to dissolve hard, thickened tissues. It can be used in either the 6c potency – in which case give one dose four times a day for two weeks – or more preferably in the 30c potency, when one daily dose should be given for two weeks, reducing to one dose twice a week.

*Causticum* (Hahnemann's mixture of quicklime [calcium oxide] with potassium bisulphate)

This remedy picture describes painful contractions of muscular tendons. Use the same dosage schedule as for the previous remedy.

*Veratrum album* (white hellebore)

This remedy picture describes a thickening of the skin of the palm of the hand. The person feels sleepy and is liable to faint. Using the 6c potency, give one dose a day.

# Elbow disorders

This joint is both a hinge and a ball-and-socket joint so that it can rotate and move up and down. It is prone to GOUT, RHEUMATOID ARTHRITIS and OSTEOARTHRITIS.

# Fibrositis

This condition is caused by individual muscle fibres sticking together and causing stiffness and a dull, nagging, painful discomfort.

Conventionally the treatment is to relieve the symptoms with muscle relaxants (diazepam) and with massage.

Massage is also used homeopathically, together with one of the following remedies. Select one by matching the remedy picture with the physical symptoms. Using the 6c potency, give one dose three times a day.

*Aconitum napellus* (monk's-hood)

This remedy picture describes fibrositis that comes on suddenly and usually in dry, cold weather. The person is very anxious and restless.

### Arnica (leopard's bane)

This remedy picture describes pains in the muscles as if they have been beaten and bruised. The muscles are worse when touched and from any movement. The pains improve when the person lies down.

### Bryonia (wild hops)

This remedy picture describes pain in any muscle group that is made worse by the slightest movement and by dry cold wind. The pains are eased by firm pressure.

### Ledum (marsh tea)

This remedy picture describes muscular stiffness, beginning in the lower limbs and ascending to other muscle groups higher in the body. The symptoms are eased by cold applications.

### Rhus toxicodendron (poison ivy)

This remedy picture describes stiffness and pain that is worse on initial movement and is eased by subsequent movement. For this reason, the person is continually restless, as gentle movement eases his or her discomfort. Warmth also helps with the stiffness and pain.

## Fractures

When these occur, they must be treated conventionally. However, the following homeopathic remedies can be used in a complementary way.

### Aconitum napellus (monk's-hood)

This remedy can be given immediately as a single 30c potency dose while awaiting medical attention. It will help alleviate anxiety.

Following the conventional treatment, the following homeo-pathic remedies can be given to help the fractured bone to re-cover.

### Eupatorium perfoliatum (thoroughwort)

This remedy is known as "bone set" and is useful for helping to alleviate the pains in bones that have been fractured. Using the 6c potency, give one dose three times a day for two weeks.

### Symphytum (comfrey)

This remedy is particularly useful for helping fractured bones to heal. Using the 6c potency, give one dose daily for one month. This remedy can be used together with Eupatorium perfoliatum.

## Ganglion

This is a cystic swelling of a tendon sheath or joint lining, filled with a jelly-like substance. It is usually pain free but can be tender when pressed.

The conventional treatment is to remove the ganglion surgi-cally or to apply extreme pressure to burst it.

There are several homeopathic remedies that can be used to help disperse a ganglion. Select a remedy by matching its picture with the physical symptoms. Using the 6c potency, give one dose twice a day for as long as necessary.

### Ammonium carbonicum (carbonate of ammonium)

This remedy picture describes obese persons who feel weak and who generally have heart problems. Ganglions are a common feature in this type of person.

### Benzoicum acidum (benzoic acid)

This remedy picture describes the formation of a ganglion in the wrist area. The person that this remedy suits will also probably suffer from GOUT and have strong-smelling urine.

### *Ruta graveolens* (rue bitterwort)

This remedy acts on the flexor tendons (i.e. the tendons attached to the muscles that bring the open palm towards the body), particularly of the wrist where ganglions are commonly found. The wrist and fingers are usually stiff.

### *Silicea* (pure flint)

This remedy picture describes ganglion formation, particularly around the knee cap.

### *Sticta* (lungwort)

This remedy picture describes rheumatic complaints, catarrhal conditions and influenza. The person with this cocktail of symptoms commonly develops ganglions around the knees.

### *Sulphur*

This remedy picture includes ganglion formation in a person who has a strong desire for sweets, is a strong character with a definite point of view, enjoys humour and is emotionally demonstrative.

# Gout

This disease is due to the accumulation in the blood of excess uric acid, the breakdown product of protein metabolism, which is usually excreted from the body via the kidneys. This metabolic pathway can be disrupted by an inherited predisposition, because of certain drugs (notably the diuretic drugs that encourage the kidneys to excrete more water), by impaired kidney function and by certain illnesses (PSORIASIS and leukaemia). Uric acid crystals are then deposited within one or more joints, to cause a form of arthritis. The joints involved are usually the big toe, the knuckles, the knees and the elbows. Usually the first attack of gout affects one joint only, causing severe pain that is made worse from the slightest touch; it may also cause a fever.

The conventional treatment is divided into the treatment of the acute attack and the treatment of long-term gout. The acute attack is managed by keeping the very tender joint away from anything that could touch it and therefore increase the pain. Pain-relieving drugs are given, mainly the nonsteroidal anti-inflammatory drugs.

The conventional long-term treatment is to reduce the uric acid level in the blood, using the drug allopurinol, and to continue to reduce pain by using nonsteroidal anti-inflammatory drugs.

Dietary advice is important both from a conventional and a homeopathic point of view. As uric acid is the breakdown product of protein metabolism, it is advisable not to eat protein-rich red meat but to confine the diet to white meat. Alcohol consumption should be restricted to white wine and preferably to only one glass a day. Red wine and spirits should be avoided. Cheese consumption should be reduced to mild cheeses only and preferably goat's cheese.

The homeopathic management of the acute attack is to protect the joint from any physical contact and to use one of the following remedies. Select one by matching the physical symptoms to a remedy picture. Using the 6c potency, give one dose every 15 minutes, for a maximum of 12 doses, reducing to one dose an hour for six doses, and finally one dose four times a day for two days.

### Colchicum (meadow saffron)

This remedy picture describes a red, hot, swollen joint that produces tearing, throbbing pains that are worse in the evening and at night. Touch causes excruciating pain. The person feels very ill and will probably have a fever. An unusual symptom is that the person commonly dreams of mice.

317

## *Sabina* (savine)

This remedy picture describes arthritic pains associated with red, shining swellings that are worse when exposed to heat. Sufferers want their windows wide open to obtain cool fresh air. They are aware of violent pulsations in their bodies.

## *Urtica urens* (stinging nettle)

This remedy picture describes acute gout with stinging pains that are associated with itching.

The following homeopathic remedies are particularly useful for helping arthritis caused by long-term gout. Using the 6c potency, give one dose twice a day.

## *Benzoicum acidum* (benzoic acid)

This remedy picture describes tender nodules from uric acid deposits, and joints that have become tender and stiff due to gout.

## *Guaiacum* (resin of lignum vitae)

This remedy picture describes tearing pains particularly in the ankles, where the pains extend upwards to the knees. The symptoms also include stiffness, redness and swelling. The joints that are affected are intolerant of pressure and heat.

## *Lycopodium* (club moss)

This remedy picture describes sufferers with recurrent attacks of gout and who also develop arthritis in their joints, particularly the shoulder and elbow joints. It is common for them to develop cramps in their calves and toes in bed at night.

## *Rhododendron* (snow rose)

This remedy picture describes tearing pains in all limbs, but especially those on the right side. The big toe is frequently inflamed from gout. All symptoms are made worse at the onset of stormy weather.

## Hip disorders

This joint is of the ball-and-socket variety. It is prone to develop OSTEOARTHRITIS, for which, conventionally, nonsteroidal anti-inflammatory drugs are commonly prescribed and ultimately a replacement of the hip joint is surgically performed.

Instead of nonsteroidal anti-inflammatory drugs, homeopathic remedies can be selected. See the remedies described for ANKLE PROBLEMS.

## Infective arthritis

This is a very serious condition for which medical advice is essential. It is caused by the invasion of bacteria into a joint from a nearby infected wound or from an injection in the blood-stream.

Conventional treatment with antibiotics is the main choice of therapy, which may have to be given intravenously.

Homeopathic treatment can be used but only as a form of complementary therapy. The following homeopathic remedies can be given using the 6c potency.

### Aconitum napellus (monk's-hood)

This remedy should be given in the first place. The picture describes suddenness of symptoms, a hot and swollen joint and a fever. The person is apprehensive and fearful of dying. The remedy should be given hourly, for a maximum of 12 doses. Following this remedy, another from the list below can be used.

### Belladonna (deadly nightshade)

This remedy picture describes a joint that is hot, red and tender to the touch. Any jarring movement causes a lot of pain. The fever is so high that the person may become delirious. The face is red and the eyes are widely dilated and staring. Give one dose four times a day.

### Bryonia (wild hops)

The characteristic feature of this remedy is pain in the joint from the slightest movement, which is relieved by rest. The joint is red and swollen. Give one dose four times a day.

### Hepar sulphuris (Hahnemann's calcium sulphide)

This remedy picture describes an infection that is beginning to form pus. Give one dose four times a day.

## Knee problems

This joint can develop arthritis, mainly of the OSTEOARTHRITIS variety. The conventional treatment is weight reduction if necessary, nonsteroidal anti-inflammatory drugs and ultimately replacement of the knee joint. A new complementary treatment involves taping the knee joint in such a way that the acupressure points are pressed therapeutically.

### Housemaid's knee

The swelling, pain and stiffness of the knee joint was given the name "housemaid's knee" because women used to get on their knees to scrub floors. It represents an underlying OSTEOARTHRITIS. Weight reduction is important if the person is overweight, and thigh-strengthening exercises will help.

The conventional treatment is with nonsteroidal anti-inflammatory drugs. If the fluid in the knee joint is excessive, this can be aspirated (sucked out through a syringe).

There are several homeopathic remedies that are useful in treating this condition. Select the remedy picture that matches the physical situation, and give one dose of the 6c potency twice a day.

### Kali iodatum (potassium iodide)

This remedy picture describes swollen, painful knee joints. The symptoms are worse at night and in damp weather.

### Rhus toxicodendron (poison ivy)

This remedy picture describes tender knee joints. The lower limbs feel stiff, and cold fresh air is not tolerated as it makes the skin painful. Overwork makes the pains worse, but heat and gentle movement improve the pain.

### Sticta (lungwort)

This remedy picture describes swelling, tenderness and heat over the knee joints, which are painful. These pains come in spasms.

# Osteoarthritis

This joint condition is one of wear and tear. The joint surfaces become roughened and develop spikes of bone that cause pain on movement. This is usually a problem of ageing, but it can also occur following a previous fracture through a joint surface, and in menopausal women who are losing the lubricating function of oestrogen and find that their joints begin to ache.

The conventional treatment is to reduce body weight if necessary, which will help take the pressure off the weight-bearing joint surfaces. The mainstay of conventional treatment is the use of nonsteroidal anti-inflammatory drugs. Surgical joint replacement is common for hips, knees and possibly shoulders. In menopausal women, hormone replacement therapy may help reduce joint problems, including OSTEOPOROSIS.

The homeopathic approach similarly recommends weight reduction, but extra dietary advice is given. Caffeine, red meat and red wine are omitted from the diet. Alcohol consumption is reduced to one unit (one glass of wine, half a pint of lager or beer, one pub measure of spirits or sherry) a day.

The following homeopathic remedies can be used in either a complementary way with conventional therapy or on their own. Select the remedy that matches the physical symptoms. Except where otherwise directed, give one dose of the 6c potency three times a day.

### *Arnica* (leopard's bane)

This remedy can be used when there is a history of traumatic damage to a joint. Using the 30c potency, give one dose every 12 hours for three doses once a month. This remedy can be given simultaneously with another remedy if the latter's remedy picture fits the overall physical situation. Use the 6c potency and give one dose three times a day.

### *Bryonia* (wild hops)

This remedy picture describes joint pains that are made worse from the slightest movement. The pains are made better from rest and from cold applications.

### *Calcarea phosphorica* (calcium phosphate)

This remedy picture describes weakness and pain in the hips, particularly when climbing stairs. The small joints of the hand are sore, with pain along the edges of the finger nails. The fingertips feel sore as if splinters are under the nails. All these symptoms are worse in damp, cold weather, particularly in melting snow, and are improved in the dry, warm weather of summer.

### *Ledum* (marsh tea)

This remedy picture describes osteoarthritis that starts in the lower limbs and ascends to the joints of the upper body. All joints are heard to crack on movement. The pains are relieved by cold applications.

### Pulsatilla (wind flower)

This remedy picture describes joint pains that rapidly shift about. The arms feel broken and dislocated, the elbows feel numb and other joints are red and swollen. The person's legs feel heavy, and there are sticking pains in the lower leg (tibia) that are worse when the person lies down and from heat. These symptoms are improved on exposure to cool, fresh air.

### Rhododendron (snow rose)

This remedy picture describes pains and stiffness in joints that are made worse before a storm. These symptoms improve after the storm has broken, from warmth and when the person has something to eat.

### Rhus toxicodendron (poison ivy)

This remedy picture describes acute pain on any initial movement but which is improved by subsequent movement until sufferers become tired and the pain returns. They are restless because their pain is relieved by subsequent movement. The symptoms are improved by warmth.

## Poliomyelitis

This is a viral condition that attacks the motor nerves, leading to headache, a fever, muscular weakness and eventual long-term paralysis. The illness is spread by personal contact and through the mouth–faecal route, but it is slowly being eradicated thanks to worldwide immunization funded by Rotary International. However, there are still some pockets of active poliomyelitis left in the developing world.

Babies are routinely immunised against this disease with an oral vaccine. The conventional treatment is for the person who is suspected of having poliomyelitis to rest in a darkened, quiet room.

Initially, the homeopathic treatment involves giving:

### *Aconitum napellus* (monk's-hood)

This remedy describes an illness of sudden onset associated with a fever, much anxiety and a fear of dying. Using the 6c potency, give one dose every 15 minutes, for a maximum of ten doses.

When it is apparent that poliomyelitis is the diagnosis, switch the homeopathic remedy to one of the following, matching the physical symptoms with the remedy picture. Using the 6c potency, give one dose every four hours for two days, reducing to one dose twice a day for two weeks.

### *Kali phosphoricum* (potassium phosphate)

This remedy picture describes paralysis of the extremities that is made worse from exercise. The person's limbs become painful and he or she starts to feel exhausted.

### *Lathyrus* (chickpea)

This remedy picture describes paralysis of the lower limbs. The limbs are very stiff (spastic) and they feel very heavy. There is a peculiar symptom: the tip of the person's tongue feels as if it has been scalded.

The following remedy picture is so close to poliomyelitis that it can be used not only to treat the disease but also as a preventative. It is important to state, however, that the conventional oral (Sabin) polio immunization is the preferred way of preventing poliomyelitis.

*Bungarus krait* (unspecified snake venom)

This remedy picture describes poliomyelitis exactly. Using the 30c potency, give one dose every 12 hours, for a maximum of three doses (as a means of prevention as well as for therapy).

## Polymyalgia rheumatica

This autoimmune illness causes stiffness, particularly of the shoulder and neck muscles. It is most common in women over the age of 50. It may be associated with a mild fever, weight loss and anaemia. It is diagnosed by the person's medical history and a blood test.

The conventional treatment with steroid therapy is the best choice.

The homeopathic approach is to discover the particular constitutional remedy for the individual, which will mean a consultation with a specialist homeopath. Dietary supplements of the anti-oxidant type (*see* p. 25) will be helpful.

## Psoriatic arthritis

The skin condition PSORIASIS can also be associated with a form of arthritis. The symptoms are similar to those of OSTEOARTHRITIS and the homeopathic remedies are the same.

## Reiter's syndrome

This syndrome comprises a combination of arthritis, URETHRITIS and CONJUNCTIVITIS. It usually develops after sufferers contract NON-SPECIFIC URETHRITIS, but it can occur after an attack of bacillary dysentery. However, it normally only develops in people with a genetic predisposition, and these are usually men. In fact, Reiter's syndrome is the most common cause of arthritis in young men. It usually starts with a urethral discharge, followed by conjunctivitis and then arthritis, which commonly only affects one or two joints.

The conventional treatment involves antibiotic drops for the conjunctivitis, nonsteroidal anti-inflammatory drugs for the arthritis and antibiotics for the urethritis.

The ideal homeopathic treatment is a constitutional remedy that will embrace the characteristics of the sufferer as well as his (or, more rarely, her) specific symptoms. This constitutional remedy can only be obtained after a consultation with a specialist homeopath. If this is not possible, select the appropriate remedy from the remedy pictures for CONJUNCTIVITIS (see p. 86), for OSTEOARTHRITIS (see p. 321) and for URETHRITIS (see p. 213).

# Repetitive strain injury (RSI)

This condition gives pain in various joints as a result of continually performing the same repetitive movements. It is particularly well known in people who use computers and word processors, but it can also strike those engaged in other occupations, such as chicken pluckers.

The conventional treatment is to exclude any physical injury by X-ray assessment and then treat the person with nonsteroidal anti-inflammatory drugs as well as advising him or her to stop doing the work that has caused the problem or at least to investigate more ergonomic ways of doing it.

The homeopathic approach is to make an accurate diagnosis with X-ray and to give the following homeopathic remedies:

### *Staphysagria* (stavesacre)

This remedy picture describes indignation and is therefore useful to give as those suffering from this problem are clearly irritated. Using the 30c potency, give one dose a day for three days.

Following this remedy, the following may be considered. Select one by matching the remedy picture with the physical symptoms. Using the 6c potency, give one dose three times a day for two weeks.

### *Bryonia* (wild hops)

This remedy picture describes pains that are made worse by any movement and eased by rest.

### *Causticum* (Hahnemann's mixture of quicklime [calcium oxide] with potassium bisulphate)

This remedy picture describes tearing, drawing pains in the muscles and joints, particularly of the arms. These symptoms are made worse in dry, cold winds and are improved in warmth and, paradoxically, in damp, wet weather.

### *Rhus toxicodendron* (poison ivy)

This remedy picture describes pains that are worse on initial movement but improve on subsequent movement, only to become painful again as the muscle begins to tire.

## Restless limbs

Restlessness of the arms, hands, legs and/or feet can have several important diagnoses for which a medical consultation is important. The movements could represent medically serious conditions such as chorea, clonus, Parkinson's disease or a neurotic tendency. If none of these causes fits the diagnosis, the cause remains unknown.

The conventional treatment is to use the appropriate treatment for the medical condition if one is found or, if no diagnosis is established, a muscle relaxant such as diazepam.

General relaxation exercises are helpful and are used both conventionally and homeopathically.

The following homeopathic remedies can be used to alleviate

the restlessness. Using the 6c potency, give one dose twice a day, reducing to one dose daily as the restlessness improves.

## Upper arms

### Aconitum napellus (monk's-hood)

This remedy picture describes trembling of the upper arms brought on by fear or from a previous situation that causes the person to remain fearful.

### Agaricus muscarius (toadstool)

This remedy picture describes twitching and trembling which is worse in hurried movements and is better for slow movement.

### Causticum (Hahnemann's mixture of quicklime [calcium oxide] with potassium bisulphate)

This remedy picture describes restlessness of the upper limbs, which is worse at night. It is usually associated with joint pains.

## Hands

### Kali bromatum (potassium bromide)

This remedy picture describes fidgety hands with sufferers busy twitching their fingers. There is generalized twitching and jerking movements of the hands, which are better when sufferers are occupied mentally or physically.

### Tarentula cubensis (Cuban spider)

This remedy picture describes hands that tremble and are associated with fidgety feet. These symptoms are worse at night and are improved whenever the person smokes a cigarette.

### *Tarentula hispania* (Spanish spider)

This remedy picture describes restless hands that the person always keeps busy, and the fingers are sucked and bitten. The symptoms are made worse with motion and noise and are improved in the open air and with music.

*Lower limbs*

### *Arsenicum album* (arsenic trioxide)

This remedy picture describes trembling, twitching movements that become particularly violent during sleep at night. The person is very anxious and drinks little but often.

### *Causticum* (Hahnemann's mixture of quicklime [calcium oxide] and potassium bisulphate)

This remedy picture describes restlessness of the lower limbs that is worse in bed in the morning and at night.

### *Kali carbonicum* (potassium carbonate)

This remedy picture describes tearing pains in the thigh with possible sciatica but definitely with jerking movements of the leg. The person feels the cold a great deal and is better in warm conditions. The symptoms tend to be at their worse at about 3.00 am, and begin to come on as soon as the person begins to fall asleep.

### *Lachesis* (bushmaster snake venom)

This remedy picture describes restlessness of the lower limbs, which is caused by the warmth of the bed.

### *Medorhinum* (gonorrhoea bacteria)

This remedy picture describes a person who cannot keep their legs still. Their legs feel heavy and ache all night. They may develop cramps in them, which are improved by stretching the leg.

### Rhus toxicodendron (poison ivy)

This remedy picture describes restlessness of the legs that comes on while the person is sitting. They are improved by gentle movement and by warm conditions.

### Tarentula hispania (Spanish spider)

This remedy picture describes restless legs where sufferers have an impulse to walk, although they can run better than walk. They find kneeling difficult.

### Zincum metallicum (zinc)

This remedy picture describes sufferers who cannot keep their legs and feet still. They develop cramps in their leg muscles when they get cold.

*Feet*

### Medorhinum (gonorrhoea bacteria)

This remedy picture describes sufferers who cannot keep their feet still nor their legs. The person as a whole has an anticipatory anxiety and feels better by the sea.

### Sulphur

This remedy picture describes restless feet after the person has drunk beer, while lying down in bed and particularly from the warmth of the bed.

### Zincum metallicum (zinc)

This remedy picture describes sufferers who cannot keep either their feet or their legs still. The symptoms of restlessness occur while they are sitting and particularly when they are in bed.

# Rheumatoid arthritis

This condition causes pain and stiffness of any joint, but particularly those of the fingers leading to deformity. It is a disease that usually occurs in midlife but can occur much earlier in children and adolescents (when it is called Still's disease).

It is an autoimmune disease that requires detailed investigation from which a treatment plan can be worked out. The disease runs a course of progressive deterioration, although occasionally it disappears for a while (a remission) or burns itself out. The aim of therapy, both conventional and homeopathic, is to induce a remission as well as to minimize the symptoms.

The conventional treatment may include steroid therapy and nonsteroidal anti-inflammatory drugs as the first-line drug therapy, as well as physiotherapy (including gentle exercises and wax baths for the hands). If these drugs do not improve the disease, second-line drugs will be used, including sulphasalazine, gold, penicillinamine and methotrexate, taken in sequence. If these do not help, a third line of drug therapy is introduced: azathioprine and cyclophosphamide.

Homeopathic treatment includes physiotherapy, dietary supplements of evening primrose oil (at least 1,500 milligrams per day) and a diet low in red meat and alcohol (one unit of white wine a day only) and high in vegetables. Autoimmune diseases involve the formation of free radicals ($O^3$ molecules instead of $O^2$ molecules). These rogue molecules upset the normal metabolic pathways, making the illness worse. The body has naturally occurring enzymes that can deactivate free radicals, and to stimulate these enzymes, the following food supplements are indicated: probiotic therapy (see p. 27), vitamin E with selenium, vitamin C (at least 1 gram each day), magnesium and zinc, as well as raw organic carrots: these are known collectively as the anti-oxidant therapy, and are to be used in all autoimmune illnesses, including MULTIPLE SCLEROSIS, MYALGIC ENCEPHALOMYELITIS, CROHN'S DISEASE, ULCERATIVE COLITIS, NEPHRITIS and acute illnesses like influenza and PYELONEPHRITIS.

The principal homeopathic treatment is a constitutional remedy (which will include miasm assessment, see p. 95) for which the advice of a specialist homeopath is needed. If this is not possible, the following homeopathic remedies can be used to help alleviate symptoms of rheumatoid arthritis. Select the remedy by matching its picture with the physical symptoms.

### Apis mellifica (honey bee)

This remedy picture describes painful, hot, swollen and stiff joints, particularly of the fingers and ankles. These symptoms are made worse by exposure to heat. Using the 6c potency, give one dose four times a day.

### Bryonia (wild hops)

This remedy picture describes joints that are red, swollen and hot, with stitching and tearing pains that are made worse from the slightest movement and/or pressure and from heat. Using the 6c potency, give one dose three times a day.

### Causticum (Hahnemann's mixture of quicklime [calcium oxide] with potassium bisulphate)

This remedy picture describes severe pains in the joints, particularly of the hands and feet. Sufferers are unable to walk or to use their hands without considerable pain. The symptoms are worse in the cold and are improved by warmth, particularly by the heat of the bed. Humid weather is ideal for improving the symptoms. Using the 6c potency, give one dose four times a day.

*Rhus toxicodendron* (poison ivy)

This remedy picture describes swollen stiff joints that are painful on initial movement and eased by subsequent movement. Sufferers tend to be restless as they know that repeated movement eases the pain. The symptoms are also improved by heat. Using the 6c potency, give one dose four times a day.

# Shoulder joint

This joint is of the ball-and-socket variety, and is held in position by the strength of the attached ligaments and muscles. It can become dislocated fairly easily, and when this happens, emergency treatment is required. Repeated dislocations will need surgery to tighten up the ligaments. It can also develop OSTEOAR-THRITIS and RHEUMATOID ARTHRITIS. Conventionally it is now possible to replace the shoulder joint surgically.

The following homeopathic remedies are also suitable for problems of the shoulder joint. Using the 6c potency, give one dose twice a day.

*Chelidonium majus* (celandine)

This remedy picture describes a fixed pain under the lower angle of the right shoulder blade (scapula). This pain may extend into the chest and stomach, causing nausea or vomiting.

*Ferrum metallicum* (iron)

This remedy picture describes pain in the shoulder that is improved when the person walks around slowly and is worse when sitting, from exposure to the cold and from getting too hot. The symptoms become much worse towards midnight.

*Ferrum phosphoricum* (iron phosphate)

This remedy picture describes pains in the shoulder that extend

333

into the wrist and chest. The symptoms are worse for being touched or jarred and are relieved by cold applications. The symptoms are at their very worst at night and between 4.00 and 6.00 am.

### *Rhus toxicodendron* (poison ivy)

This remedy picture describes pains in the shoulder that are made worse on the initial movement but are improved by subsequent movements. Heat also helps alleviate the pain, and the person tends to be restless in order to create the gentle movement that is known to alleviate the pain.

### *Sanguinaria* (blood root)

This remedy picture describes pain in the right shoulder that is made worse when in bed at night.

### *Sulphur*

This remedy picture describes heaviness of sufferers' shoulders, with pains particularly in the left shoulder. They tend to walk with stooped shoulders, finding it difficult to walk erect.

## Frozen shoulder

This condition occurs during middle age in women more often than in men. It causes a limitation of movement of the arm, particularly raising it and attempting to put the hand behind the back.

The conventional treatment is physiotherapy with or without nonsteroidal anti-inflammatory drugs.

The homeopathic approach includes physiotherapy with one of the following remedies. Select the remedy according to its picture, matching this with the physical symptoms. Using the 6c potency, give one dose four times a day for one week, reducing to one dose twice a day.

### *Chelidonium majus* (celandine)

This remedy picture describes pain in the arms and shoulders so that sufferers find it difficult to twist their arm behind them. This remedy is the classical liver remedy.

### *Ferrum metallicum* (iron)

This remedy picture describes sufferers who have an irresistible desire to bend their elbows, an action that causes considerable pain.

### *Ferrum phosphoricum* (iron phosphate)

This remedy picture describes pain in the shoulders that extends into the chest and wrists. The slightest movement makes the pain worse, particularly when sufferers attempt to put their hands behind them.

### *Ledum* (marsh tea)

This remedy picture describes pressure in the right shoulder particularly, which is also throbbing. Any movement makes this discomfort worse. Heat makes these symptoms worse, and they are marginally improved from cold applications.

### *Phytolacca* (poke root)

This remedy picture describes shooting pains in the right shoulder, with stiffness and an inability to raise the arm. The pains are like electric shocks and can fly into other joints.

### *Rhus toxicodendron* (poison ivy)

This remedy picture describes joint symptoms and specifically pain on moving the hands behind the body. Sufferers are generally restless as they find it is the initial movement that is painful and that repeated movements become less painful. Heat also improves the symptoms.

### *Rumex crispus* (yellow dock)

This remedy picture is characterized by pain in the left shoulder on coughing and whenever the hands are raised. The hands are cold whenever sufferers cough. They may also get spasmodic cramps in their ankles and feet.

### *Sanguinaria* (blood root)

This remedy picture describes pain in the shoulders, worse on the right side, which is made worse whenever sufferers try to raise their arms or to put them behind their backs. This remedy in particular would suit a woman of menopausal age.

### *Sanicula (aqua)* (water of Sanicula Springs, Ottawa)

This remedy picture describes emaciated children who are unable to put their hands on their heads. In people of all ages, there is stiffness that is made worse when the arms are raised and are put behind the back. The back, too, is so stiff that sufferers must turn the whole body around in order to look behind them. They sit with their heads forwards to alleviate the pain and stiffness.

## Tenosynovitis

This condition is an irritative "inflammation" of the tendon sheath, which causes pain on movement. When gentle pressure is put on the affected tendon sheath, it is possible to feel a grating sensation.

The primary treatment, both conventional and homeopathic, is to rest the muscle and its tendon. Conventionally, pain-relieving drugs are given, usually the nonsteroidal anti-inflammatory variety.

The following homeopathic remedies can also be used. Select the remedy picture that matches the physical situation, and using the 6c potency, give one dose three times a day for seven to ten days.

### Apis mellifica (honey bee)

This remedy picture describes a pain that is stinging and burning and is made worse from any hot application.

### Belladonna (deadly nightshade)

This remedy describes a burning hot tendon sheath that throbs with pain. This pain is made much worse by the slightest jarring movement.

### Bryonia (wild hops)

This remedy picture describes pain that is made immediately much worse from the slightest movement and is improved when the muscle and tendon are not moved at all. Heat also makes the condition worse.

### Kali iodatum (potassium iodide)

This remedy picture describes pains in the tendons that occur long after an injury and which are worse at night.

### Pulsatilla (wind flower)

This remedy picture describes a tightness and a dragging sensation over the muscle and its tendon. This is made worse when the affected limb hangs down. Heat makes the condition worse, and the person cries easily and often.

### Rhus toxicodendron (poison ivy)

This remedy picture describes a tearing pain that is made worse from the initial movement and eased by subsequent movement until the muscle becomes fatigued. The tendon is stiff and swollen and is made worse from cold, damp weather and improved by heat.

### *Ruta graveolens* (rue bitterwort)

This remedy picture describes tendons that feel sore. Sufferers totter about and stumble easily and often. Their thighs feel broken, a symptom that is made worse whenever they stretch their legs.

### *Sticta* (lungwort)

This remedy picture describes shooting pains in the tendons.

## Tubercular arthritis

This condition must be treated using conventional medicine. When the tubercular disease has been eradicated and symptoms of arthritis persist, use the remedies described for OSTEOARTHRITIS.

# Problems of the Nervous System

## Physical problems

This section will cover the physical illnesses due to problems in the nervous system.

## Bell's palsy

This is a paralysis of one side of the face due to damage to or inflammation of the seventh cranial nerve. This may affect the eyelid, preventing it from closing properly and possibly leading to CONJUNCTIVITIS. The cause is unknown, although a virus is suspected: as it goes from the brain to the face, the nerve passes through the middle ear and an earache is a common feature of this illness.

Conventional treatment is with steroid drugs and antibiotic eyedrops for any conjunctivitis that may develop in the eye where the eyelid doesn't work properly. This eye should have an eye patch put over it.

Homeopathic treatment is with the following remedies. Select one by matching its picture with the physical symptoms. If conjunctivitis develops, *see* p. 86 for homeopathic remedies applicable for this condition.

### *Aconitum napellus* (monk's-hood)

This remedy picture describes sudden onset of a problem, especially if brought on by a cold wind. Using the 6c potency, give one dose four times a day for two days.

Then follow with:

### *Causticum* (Hahnemann's mixture of quicklime [calcium oxide] with potassium bisulphate)

This remedy picture describes sufferers with paralysis on one side of their faces and difficulty in opening their mouths. Using the 6c potency, give one dose twice a day.

## Chorea (including Huntington's chorea)

This condition consists of violent, unpredictable movements of all limbs, which are not painful. Huntington's chorea is an inherited terminal illness that causes these movements and progressive dementia. There is no known cure for Huntington's chorea, and the movements of chorea are treated conventionally with muscle relaxants such as diazepam.

The homeopathic treatment is best supervised by a specialist homeopath. The following remedies may be used if this consultation is not possible. Select the remedy by matching its picture with the physical symptoms. Using the 6c potency, give one dose four times each day.

### *Agaricus muscarius* (toadstool)

This remedy picture describes limb movements that are so unpredictable that sufferers don't feel as if their limbs belong to them. The symptoms are worse in the cold and before a thunderstorm. They are better for slow movement.

### *Causticum* (Hahnemann's mixture of quicklime [calcium oxide] with potassium bisulphate)

This remedy picture describes sufferers who have twisting and jerking movements of their body, and they notice that their joints crack. These symptoms are better in the warmth, particularly from the heat of their beds. The symptoms are worse in dry, cold winds.

### *Cuprum metallicum* (copper)

This remedy picture describes spontaneous jerking movements mainly in the person's hands and feet.

### *Lachesis* (bushmaster snake venom)

This remedy picture describes jerking movements of sufferers' limbs, and these movements are worse on their left sides. The symptoms are always worse after sleeping.

### *Stramonium* (thorn apple)

This remedy picture describes violent movements of all the sufferers' limbs, giving them a staggering walk. The symptoms are much worse in the dark.

### *Tarentula hispania* (Spanish spider)

This remedy picture describes nervous people who just cannot keep still. Their limbs keep jerking in an unpredictable way. They are very sensitive to the needs of others.

# Epilepsy

This condition is caused by an abnormal electrical brain discharge resulting in convulsive movements of the limbs that makes sufferers become unconscious. (The febrile convulsions that occur in children when they have a fever are discussed on p. 412.) While having a fit, sufferers may bite their tongues and be incontinent of urine.

If you encounter a person having a fit, check that his or her airway is clear and move any furniture out of the way so that the person with the fit won't be physically injured. Following a first attack, the person needs a full medical work-up (brain scan, electroencephalogram [EEG]) to check that there is no predisposing cause.

The immediate conventional treatment for a person who is having a fit is to give rectal diazepam, which will stop the fit. The long-term management is with anti-convulsant medication.

The homeopathic treatment for the immediate attack is:

### Aconitum napellus (monk's-hood)

This remedy picture describes sudden onset of any illness. Using 6c potency in liquid form, give two drops every ten minutes.

The conventional detailed investigation is recommended by the homeopath. Ideally the person should consult a specialist homeopath for an all-embracing remedy that will include the rest of their constitution as well as their epilepsy. If this is not possible, the following remedies can be used. Select one by matching its picture with the physical symptoms. (The person's fits usually follow the same pattern so it is possible to make an accurate assessment in selecting a remedy.) Using the 6c potency, give one dose daily.

### Aethusa cynapium (fool's parsley)

This remedy picture describes an epileptic fit where sufferers clench their thumbs and have red faces. Their teeth are tightly clenched and their pupils are dilated, staring and slow to react. The sequence of events is usually drowsiness after vomiting or defecation, followed by the fit.

### Argentum nitricum (silver nitrate)

This remedy picture describes sufferers whose pupils are permanently dilated several days before a fit, which is also preceded by much restlessness. The fits usually occur at night. The remedy picture also describes people who dislike heat, fear heights and crave salt and sweets.

### Bufo (poison of the toad)

This remedy picture describes sufferers whose pupils are widely dilated and unresponsive to light before a fit (a symptom shared with *Argentum nitricum*). Just before an attack, their eyeballs roll upwards and to the left, their heads are drawn to one side and then back, and they make licking movements with their tongue, feel their faces and rub their noses. The fit starts with twitching of the face and then extends to the rest of the body. During the attack, the face is bathed in sweat.

## *Causticum* (Hahnemann's mixture of quicklime [calcium oxide] with potassium bisulphate)

This remedy picture describes epileptic fits occurring at the time of puberty. They happen as a result of a fright and when the person has become chilled. They occur at night, leaving the body icy cold, and tend to occur mainly on the right side. Urine flows profusely during a fit.

## *Cicuta virosa* (water hemlock)

This remedy picture describes excessively violent fits during which sufferers are thrown into odd positions. The most consistent position is for the head, neck and spine to be bent backwards (the medical term for this is the "opishotonos position"). The fits are brought on by touch and by draughts. During a fit, the head is hot while the extremities are cold. In between attacks, the person is mild, gentle, placid and yielding (the opposite of *Cuprum* and *Nux vomica* where the person is irritable, spiteful and violent).

## *Cuprum metallicum* (copper)

This remedy picture describes a fit that starts when sufferers begin to draw in their fingers, clenching their thumbs, or when their muscles begin to twitch gently. As the fit starts in earnest, they fall to the ground with a shriek and are incontinent of urine and faeces. During the fit, their thumbs are drawn into their palms and their fingers are closed over them with great violence, and there is such rigidity of the jaw muscles that it is impossible to give any medicines. The face and lips turn blue, and the eyes jerk and roll. Between attacks, sufferers are spiteful, violent and weepy and cry out with a shriek (the opposite of *Cicuta virosa*).

### *Glonoine* (nitroglycerine)

This remedy picture describes a fit during which sufferers' fingers and toes spread apart (the opposite of *Cuprum metallicum*) and there is a glowing redness of the face. The head develops a congested headache just before a fit, and the heart starts to beat violently and irregularly as well. The fit is set off following exposure to the sun. After a fit, the pupils are contracted (a symptom shared with *Ignatia* and *Opium*).

### *Ignatia* (St Ignatius' bean)

This remedy picture describes a fit brought on by fear or grief. A characteristic feature of this remedy picture is that, following a fit, the face is deathly pale and the pupils are contracted (a symptom shared with *Glonoine* and *Opium*). The convulsions coincide with the eruption of teeth.

### *Ipecacuanha* (ipecac root)

This remedy picture describes a person who suffers from nausea and possible vomiting before and during a fit. The fit characteristically affects the left side.

### *Lyssin* (saliva of rabid dog)

This remedy picture describes a fit that is preceded by an increased sense of smell, taste and touch. The convulsion is always associated with throat symptoms and starts as a result of a reflex (an attempt to swallow or to speak, a draught of air, the sight and sound of running water, bright light, a loud noise or strong odours).

### *Nux vomica* (poison-nut)

This remedy picture describes a fit that occurs in sufferers who become very angry. They are nervous, oversensitive and irritable. The fit is made worse from the slightest touch, noise and draught (a symptom shared with *Cicuta virosa*).

### *Opium* (dried latex of poppy)

This remedy picture describes sufferers who have a fit if the room is too hot. They kick off their bed clothes, and their skin is red and mottled, particularly on their faces. The fit starts with facial twitching (like *Ignatia* except that the face is red) and proceeds to a convulsion when the body goes into a spasm such that the head bends backwards towards the heels (opishotonos), a symptom shared with *Glonoine* and *Platinum*. The pupils are constricted following a fit.

### *Platina* (platinum)

This remedy picture describes those who have fits but don't lose consciousness (a symptom shared with *Nux vomica*). During the fit, they lie on their backs with their heads extending backwards to their heels (like *Glonoine* and *Opium* except that, in this remedy picture, the knees are widely separated).

### *Plumbum metallicum* (lead)

This remedy picture describes sufferers whose legs feel heavy and go numb and whose tongues become swollen just before an attack. They also have a marked sensitivity to touch, associated with a loss of muscular power. When the fit does occur, it takes a long time for them to regain consciousness, and even when consciousness returns, the limbs affected by the fit remain paralysed for quite a time.

### *Pulsatilla* (wind flower)

This remedy picture describes a person whose fit is followed by relaxation and a tendency to vomit (a symptom shared with *Ipecacuanha*). The distinguishing feature of this remedy is that the person as a whole is mild but changeable, and can become irritable with easy weeping.

### *Silicea* (pure flint)

This remedy picture describes people who have fits at night at about the time of the new moon. Before the fit, they are aware of a cold sensation on their left side and a twisting of their left arms.

### *Stramonium* (thorn apple)

This remedy picture describes a person whose fits are triggered by bright lights or dazzling objects (a symptom shared with *Lyssin*). If liquid touches the sufferers' lips, the convulsions start again. Paradoxically, although very aware of their sensitivity to lights, these people fear the dark. When the fit is taking place, one side of the body is paralysed while the other is convulsing.

### *Tarentula hispania* (Spanish spider)

This remedy picture describes sufferers who, when they have fits, fall to the ground unconscious without warning. Their eyes remain open and seem to be squinting. They are generally overactive and find music soothing.

### *Zincum metallicum* (zinc)

This remedy picture describes a person who has a fit during a current illness (a symptom shared with *Cuprum metallicum*). Sufferers become unusually cross before a fit, and are generally restless, especially their feet. Their whole body is seen to jerk during sleep (this is not a fit).

# Migraine

It is important to have a correct diagnosis for this, to rule out any underlying physical cause. This is done by consultation with a medical practitioner who may order a CT brain scan, a blood test to exclude temporal arteritis (inflammation of the lining of the arteries in the scalp over the temples) and a plain X-ray of the cervical spine to exclude arthritis.

If all these tests are normal, migraine can be diagnosed. The symptoms are: a preceding aura ("warning" sensation such as a feeling of elation, thirst, a craving for sweet foods, distinctive flashing lights), followed by a headache of varying quality and severity, which may be associated with nausea and vomiting as well as temporary paralysis of a limb. The person usually feels exhausted after the attack, which can last for up to 24 hours.

Cluster headaches are recurrent localized headaches, usually occurring behind one eye and primarily in men. These attacks don't last for very long but can recur several times a day. The same detailed investigation as described for migraine is necessary, and they are also treated in the same way.

The conventional treatment is with painkilling drugs. The simple drugs are paracetamol, aspirin and codeine. If these are not successful, stronger nonsteroidal anti-inflammatory drugs are used. A new line of conventional drug therapy has emerged with the selective 5-HT agonists, which have been successful in treating migraine. The conventional treatment for managing recurrent attacks is with a daily dose of a beta-blocker (propranolol) and pizotifen (Sanomigran). Methysergide is the oldest drug available for preventing recurrent attacks of migraine.

Certain foods can be important triggering factors for both migraines and cluster headaches. Cheese, chocolate, citrus fruits and red wine should be excluded from the person's diet. Emotional factors also have to be considered.

Homeopathic treatment involves the same detailed investigations as described for the conventional approach. Both migraine and cluster headaches are treated by constitutional therapy, prescribing an all-embracing remedy. This is best obtained by consultation with a specialist homeopath, who will also assess dietary and emotional factors.

If this is not possible, the following specific remedies are applicable for treating an acute migraine or cluster headache. Select the remedy by matching its picture with the physical symptoms. Using the 30c potency, give one dose every hour for a maximum of three doses. If there is no improvement, switch to the 6c potency and give one dose every hour until the headache subsides.

### *Argentum nitricum* (silver nitrate)

This remedy picture describes a headache that makes the head feel as if it is in a clamp. It is associated with temporary blindness and a crawling sensation over the scalp. Sufferers feel as if the bones of their skull are separating, and the headache always ends with them vomiting. It can start from an emotional disturbance, is made worse from warmth and is made better from cold applications and from firm pressure.

### *Belladonna* (deadly nightshade)

This remedy picture describes a throbbing, hammering headache that is worse on the sides of the head (temples) and is made worse from movement. Sufferers have a feeling in their brain like water – the symptoms come and go in waves. They also have a cold sensation in the middle of their foreheads.

### *Bryonia* (wild hops)

This remedy feature describes a splitting headache that makes sufferers feel as though they have been hit on the head with a hammer. The headache is mainly sited in the back of the head (occiput). There is also a sensation that the brain is being squeezed out. Any movement, even the movement of the eyeballs, makes the headache worse.

### *Ferrum metallicum* (iron)

This remedy picture describes a throbbing, hammering headache that starts in the sides of the head (temples) and then extends to the back of the head (occiput). It is made worse when sufferers cough, stoop or descend stairs, and it is improved when they let their hair down. They are liable to get a sudden pain in the left eye, and their heads feel hot while their feet feel cold. While they have the headache, they suffer from giddiness (vertigo). When the headache has gone, any writing will cause it to return.

### Glonoine (nitroglycerine)

This remedy picture describes a headache that comes in waves of terrible pounding and bursting pains, as though sufferers were standing on their heads. The symptoms are brought on by exposure to the sun, and are improved by sufferers holding their heads tightly – they feel as if their brains are too small for their skulls, which will explode. The headache is also improved when they lie down to go to sleep.

### Iris versicolor (blue flag)

This remedy picture describes a sick headache associated with nausea and blurred vision. The headache is sited in the sides of the head (temples) and is usually worse on the right side. The scalp feels constricted. These symptoms occur following relaxation after a period of hard mental work.

### Lycopodium (club moss)

This remedy picture describes a headache at the sides of the head (temples) as if they are being screwed together, or a pressing headache on the top of the head (vertex), or a headache in the back of the head (occiput). All of these headaches are worse between 4.00 and 8.00 pm and when sufferers stoop, cough and are hungry. They have frown lines on their foreheads. The headaches improve in the fresh air and from regular warm foods and drinks, particularly if they are sweet.

### Mercurius corrosivus (corrosive sublimate of mercury)

This remedy picture describes a congestive headache with a burning sensation in the cheeks. Sufferers feel a drawing pain in the bones of the skull, and they have an offensive-smelling sweat.

### Natrum muriaticum (sodium chloride)

This remedy picture describes a throbbing headache, as if someone is hammering inside the person's skull trying to get out. This headache is worse premenstrually, and causes nausea and vomiting. Before the headache begins, the person may notice tingling in the lips or in the limbs causing possible temporary paralysis. The symptoms are helped by sleep.

### Nux vomica (poison-nut)

This remedy picture describes a headache that feels as if a nail is being driven through the person's head. It is brought on by over-indulgence in alcohol and tobacco, and is associated with giddiness as though the person is about to lose consciousness. This remedy is the classic one for a "hung-over" feeling.

### Petroleum (crude rock oil)

This remedy picture describes a severe headache that is relieved by the person pressing on the side of the head (temple). It is started by the person shaking while coughing. The head feels numb, as if made of wood, and also feels sensitive as if a cold breeze is blowing on it.

### Pulsatilla (wind flower)

This remedy picture describes a headache brought on by over-work and after sufferers have eaten a fatty meal. The pains start on the right side of the face (the right temple) and cause painful tear production on the same side. The pains may extend into the teeth. Sufferers feel better from being in the fresh air and out of a warm environment.

### *Sanguinaria* (blood root)

This remedy picture describes a headache that starts in the back of the head (occiput) quite suddenly like a "flash of lightning" and spreads over the scalp to settle over one of the eyes (usually the right). These headaches can be triggered by exposure to the sun and are common in women at the start of the menopause. The veins on the temples are usually dilated. The person feels better after lying down and having a sleep.

### *Silicea* (pure flint)

This remedy picture describes a throbbing headache that starts in the back of the head (occiput) and spreads over the scalp, settling over the eyes. Sufferers have temporary blindness, and they urinate profusely, a symptom that improves when the headache starts. The headache is made worse by physical exertion, studying, noise and cold air, and it is improved by the person wrapping up the head warmly and by applying pressure on the head. The person's head and neck sweat profusely and offensively.

### *Spigelia* (pinkroot)

This remedy picture describes a headache that feels like a tight band around the head, which usually settles in the left eye. The quality of the headache is described as throbbing and violent. The sense of hearing is heightened. The headache is made worse from movement, touch and from noise, and is improved when the person lies on the right side and with the head held high.

### *Stramonium* (thorn apple)

This remedy picture describes a headache that causes the person to speak incoherently. It starts early in the morning, improving towards the middle of the day. The pain is sited in the forehead, particularly over the eyebrows. The pain is described as a boring pain, and it is preceded by blurred vision. The headache makes the person stagger, with a tendency to fall forward and to the left.

### Sulphur

This remedy picture describes a throbbing headache that is improved when the person lies on the right side and applies pressure to the head. It is worsened and may be brought on whenever the person washes his or her hair.

### Veratrum album (white hellebore)

This remedy picture describes a headache with nausea, vomiting and diarrhoea. Sufferers have a cold sweat on their foreheads and their faces are pale. They find that their necks are too weak to hold up their heads. They have a sensation as though there is a lump of ice on the top of their head.

### Veratrum viride (white American hellebore)

This remedy picture describes a congested headache of such intensity that it almost makes sufferers unconscious. The head feels hot and bloated as though full of throbbing arteries, and the eyes are bloodshot. The pupils are dilated, and sufferers have double vision. They find it difficult to hold their heads up, and they also feel dizzy and nauseous.

# Motor neurone disease

This terminal disease causes a degeneration of the nerves within the central nervous system that control the muscles; there is no known cause. The limbs are floppy and the muscles show spontaneous twitches and slowly loose their bulk (atrophy). The disease gradually spreads upwards from the feet (making walking awkward) and finally causes sufferers to have difficulty in swallowing and to develop chest infections, from which they usually die.

There is no conventional curative therapy. Treatment is entirely supportive.

Homeopathic treatment is also not curative but it can be helpful in a general way. Consultation with a specialist homeopath is necessary to give an overview of the person and the illness. However, if this is not possible, the following homeopathic remedy can be given:

### *Conium* (poison hemlock)

This remedy picture describes heavy, weary limbs, especially the legs. This weakness begins in the lower limbs and spreads upwards. Using the 6c potency, give one dose three times a day. When the person finds it difficult to move the tongue, the remedy should be given in liquid form (one dose equals two drops).

## Multiple sclerosis

This is a condition in which the myelin sheath that surrounds nerve fibres is eaten away. This causes short circuiting within the nervous system so that it doesn't function properly. Typical early symptoms are pins and needles in the limbs, urgency and frequency of urination, one hand that doesn't function properly (a "useless hand") and a painful eye (retrobulbar neuritis). These early symptoms disappear after a short period, and often the diagnosis is not made because of this. Multiple sclerosis is notorious for its relapse–remission pattern.

The cause of multiple sclerosis is still a mystery. The immune system is inevitably involved, for the T-cell lymphocytes have been shown to attack the myelin around the nerve fibres. The trigger for this attack appears to have a genetic basis, and this predisposition may itself be triggered by a long-term viral illness.

The diagnosis is established by specialized magnetic resonant X-rays, which show the areas of demyelination within the nervous system. Examination of the cerebrospinal fluid (by a lumbar puncture) also reveals significant changes in multiple sclerosis.

When people are confronted with this diagnosis, their energies are directed into attempting to maintain their health for as long as possible as the disease progresses to chronic progressive multiple sclerosis. In this final stage, sufferers will need wheelchairs (as they will be unable to walk), urine incontinence aids and, finally, nursing care. However, not everyone with multiple sclerosis progresses to this. Some remain apparently completely healthy and active with no disability.

When the diagnosis is made, sufferers show obvious anxiety, asking, "What is going to happen to me?" During this time of uncertainty, they may search for the ultimate cure.

Hyperbaric oxygen therapy became fashionable a while ago, and there is some evidence that urine symptoms are improved with hyperbaric oxygen. Applied kinesiology has been used to work out the "allergies" that sufferers may have – such as allergies to the mercury in their teeth fillings and in their wrist watches and wheat, cow dairy products and yeasts in their diet. Correction of these "allergies" has not been proven to be significant, although there are anecdotal stories of success, particularly with gluten-free and macrobiotic diets. Reflexology, massage and acupuncture have been claimed to be helpful but not curative.

Conventional treatment to help control muscle spasms is with diazepam and baclofen. Urine infections are common as sufferers are unable to empty their bladders properly, and these are treated with antibiotics. Any infection affects the tone of the muscles, increasing the person's disability. A relatively new drug called beta interferon has just been licensed. It is given by injection to people in the relapse–remission phase. Trials have shown a 30–40 per cent reduction in the number of relapses. Some people using this therapy have noted a side-effect of flu-like symptoms.

Active physiotherapy has a proven beneficial effect on muscle function. This form of physiotherapy encourages muscle groups that are not affected by demyelination to work at their best and discourages muscle groups that have been overactive (the extensor group), which reduces spasms of these muscles. Stretching exercises help reduce muscle spasm, particularly of the lower limbs.

This helps physical transfer movements. Cannabis has been shown anecdotally to reduce muscle spasms, but as it is an illegal substance, no medical trials can be conducted to test its efficacy.

Diet has been shown to reduce the number of relapses significantly. Sufferers should avoid eating a diet with saturated fats (found in butter, animal fats and dairy products) and should eat one rich in unsaturated and polyunsaturated fats (found in seeds, fish oils, green leafy vegetables, liver, kidneys, heart, brain, sweetbreads, lean meat, shellfish, mackerel and other oily fish). A diet low in refined sugar is also important as is a diet without caffeine or nicotine, both of which cause an increase in muscular sensitivity.

Supplements of gamma linoleic acid are essential. Found in evening primrose oil, at least 2 grams should be consumed each day.

Other ways of boosting the immune system are with probiotic therapy (*see* p. 27) and antioxidant therapy (*see* p. 25). To the vitamins in the antioxidant therapy regime, add magnesium, zinc and manganese. These can be found in multi-mineral tablet form.

Heat and tiredness make the condition worse, and therefore sufferers should take adequate rest and avoid heat (by air conditioning). They should also be encouraged to lead a stress-free life but to keep their brains as active as possible and to maintain a social life.

Homeopathy can add to overall well-being. A specialist homeopath, who will be able to treat the person constitutionally, should be consulted. If this is not possible, the following homeopathic remedies may be used. Select the remedy by matching its picture with the physical symptoms. Using the 6c potency, give one dose twice a day.


### *Aurum muriaticum* (sodium chloroaurate)

This remedy picture describes people who walk uncertainly, needing a walking aid or to hang on to pieces of furniture. They are worse when climbing stairs and better from cold washing and cold weather.

### *Lathyrus* (chick pea)

This remedy picture describes extreme stiffness of the legs; sufferers cannot bend or cross their legs when sitting. If they are able to stand up straight, their heels do not touch the floor. If they sit or bend forward, they have difficulty in straightening up. The picture also describes an increased bladder irritability so that sufferers have to urinate more frequently and urgently to avoid incontinence. A peculiar symptom of this remedy picture is soreness on the tip of the tongue.

### *Tarentula hispania* (Spanish spider)

This remedy picture describes people who have jerking movements of their lower limbs, associated with muscular weakness. They have sudden mood swings and must always be busy. They are very sensitive and are made worse by seeing other people in trouble. They feel better after a massage, when outside and from exposure to bright colours and music. To avoid a urinary infection, they should be encouraged to drink cranberry juice (at least 1 litre per day) and to attend to personal hygiene (this has been discussed under CYSTITIS, pp. 222–3). If a urinary infection does occur, the conventional treatment is antibiotic therapy. The homeopathic approach is to encourage the person to drink as much barley water as possible (at least 1 litre per day), together with the homeopathic remedies on pp. 217–22.

## Parkinson's disease

This condition is a chronic, progressive degeneration of the central nervous system, characterized by slowness, poor movement, muscular rigidity and a muscular tremor. Sufferers have a characteristically blank expression, a shuffling walk and a characteristic tremor of the hands called "pill-rolling". The disease usually occurs in the middle-aged and the elderly, and is due to the degeneration of a specific part of the brain (the *substantia nigra*) and a decrease in a chemical transmitter called dopamine.

The cause for this degeneration is unknown, although certain drugs (notably the major tranquillizers) can cause similar symptoms as a side-effect. The illness progresses slowly without necessarily hastening death. Some people with this disease develop dementia and others become depressed.

The conventional treatment is with anticholinergic drugs.

Treatment of depression with homeopathic remedies is discussed on p. 369, and the homeopathic treatment of dementia is dealt with on p. 541. Homeopathic treatment of the Parkinson's disease itself involves consultation with a specialist homeopath who will be able to give an overall assessment of the person. If this is not possible, the following remedies may be given to help control the symptoms. Match the remedy picture with the physical symptoms. Using the 6c potency, give one dose twice a day.

### *Agaricus muscarius* (toadstool)

This remedy picture describes jerking, twitching and trembling movements and generalized weakness. Mentally there is a slow progression from increased cheerfulness to a final stage of depression. The picture also describes facial muscles that feel stiff. In addition, the extremities feel stiff all over, with trembling causing an unsteady walk.

### *Gelsemium* (yellow jasmine)

This remedy picture describes sufferers who can become nervous when asked to do a new task. Their limbs slowly lose muscular power and become obviously weak and there is much trembling. Sufferers become tired with the slightest effort. Their facial muscles become contracted, especially around their mouths, their chins quiver and finally their lower jaws droop. Their tongues tremble and become coated.

### *Hyoscyamus* (henbane)

This remedy picture describes sufferers who mentally are very suspicious. They speak obscenities and have a tendency to laugh at everything. Their tongues are dry, red, cracked and immovable. Their lower jaw drops. Their pupils are dilated and sparkling even though they are downcast and don't pay attention to anyone. Their hands are always moving, picking at objects. Their muscles are generally very twitchy.

### Mercurius solubis (black oxide of mercury)

This remedy picture describes weakness and trembling of all limbs but especially the hands. The fingers feel numb and the feet sweat in bed in the morning. Sufferers have a metallic taste in their mouths, which produces a lot of saliva. They stammer, and have violent thoughts with an uncontrollable desire to run away.

### Rhus toxicodendron (poison ivy)

This remedy picture describes people who are restless and cannot rest in any position. Their muscles twitch and tremble. They have muscular stiffness and suffer from CRAMPS. These symptoms are worse in the damp but are improved in the warmth and when sufferers move around. This is the reason for the restlessness seen in this picture.

# Trigeminal neuralgia

In this condition, there is a nagging pain on one side of the face (along the line of the fifth cranial nerve). The cause is unknown; the recovery is gradual and spontaneous. The person is left with a minimal weakness in the affected muscles.

The conventional treatment is with painkilling drugs.

There are several homeopathic remedies that may be used. Select one by matching its picture with the physical symptoms. Using the 6c potency, give one dose three times a day.

### *Aconitum napellus* (monk's-hood)

This remedy picture describes neuralgic pain in the cheeks mainly on the left, associated with pain in the jaws and with tingling and numbness. Affected individuals are very anxious and restless, and commonly fear death.

### *Spigelia* (pinkroot)

This remedy picture describes neuralgic pain in the cheek, extending into the teeth. It is made worse when sufferers stoop and when they touch their faces.

### *Verbascum* (mullein)

This remedy has a pronounced action on the fifth cranial nerve. The picture describes neuralgic pains affecting the cheeks, particularly the left one, with tear formation and a sensation as if the parts are being crushed by a pair of pliers. The symptoms are made worse whenever sufferers talk, sneeze or move into a room with a different temperature. The pains come in flashes, being particularly precipitated by the least movement, including when sufferers clench their teeth.

# *Mental problems*

## Alcoholism

When a person becomes addicted to alcohol, this creates problems not only for the alcoholic (cirrhosis of the liver) but also for those close to him or her (social and financial loss). The immediate help needed by alcoholics is to join a self-help group; this, combined with psychotherapy, will help them avoid alcohol. There are also self-help groups for families and others close to alcoholics.

As sufferers stop drinking, their diet needs careful attention because the balance between the intake of carbohydrates and protein must be re-established. They will also probably be deficient in minerals and vitamins, and so they should have supplements of both.

When very heavy drinkers stop drinking alcohol, they can develop delirium tremens ("the DTs"). In this frightening condition, affected individuals develop visual hallucinations of grotesque proportions, and they sweat and walk in an irregular fashion.

The conventional treatment is usually carried out within a specialized unit that will support alcoholics while they "dry out". They may need sedation during this period. In order to stay off alcohol, some alcoholics need to take a drug that will cause them to vomit violently if they ever drink alcohol.

Homeopathic treatment is ideally obtained from a specialist homeopath, who will give the person the appropriate constitutional remedy as well as focusing on specific local symptoms as they emerge during detoxification. However, if this is not possible, there are certain homeopathic remedies that are specifically helpful for people addicted to alcohol; these can also be used with the constitutional remedy. Select the remedy by matching its picture with the physical symptoms. Using the 6c potency, give one dose twice a day.

### *Avena sativa* (common oat)

This remedy picture describes people who find it difficult to keep their minds focused on any subject, and sometimes feel at the end of their tether. They are known to be alcoholics.

### *Capsicum annuum* (cayenne pepper)

This remedy picture describes people who crave an alcoholic stimulant. This, however, causes an upset stomach. They have a peculiar symptom of a burning sensation on the tips of their tongues.

### *Cimicifuga racemosa* (black snake root)

This remedy picture describes people who have early morning

nausea from drinking too much alcohol. Their tongues are pointed and tremble.

### Hyoscyamus (henbane)

This remedy picture describes suspicious, talkative people who are inclined to laugh at everything. Alcohol upsets their stomach, causing hiccups (which leave a bitter taste in their mouths) and occasionally vomiting, which may contain blood (haematemesis).

### Lachesis (bushmaster snake venom)

This remedy picture describes very chatty people who crave alcohol (and oysters). They develop a gnawing pain in their stomachs unless they have something to eat. They don't like tight clothing around their neck or their stomachs.

### Nux vomica (poison-nut)

This remedy picture describes people who are irritable, ambitious and fault-finding. They drink alcohol to excess and smoke too much. They suffer from giddiness with lapses of unconsciousness, and from headaches that start in the back of their heads and spread over their scalps and into their eyes. All of these symptoms are worse in the morning.

### Opium (dried latex of poppy)

This remedy picture describes people who suffer from delirium tremens associated with terribly frightening visions. Following alcoholic binges, they have periods of unconsciousness.

### Ranunculus bulbosus (buttercup)

This remedy picture describes people suffering from the ill-effects of alcohol. Their hands shake uncontrollably (a symptom of delirium tremens). They are irritable, with a creeping sensation on their scalp, and they suffer from pressing headaches as though something is about to burst through their foreheads and eyes.

### *Stramonium* (thorn apple)

This remedy picture describes people with delirium tremens whose general behaviour is extraordinarily loud. They speak, laugh, sing and dance and behave and speak inappropriately.

# Anger

This emotion expresses negative feelings that can boil over into a loss of temper. This can be verbal or physical.

Both the conventional and the homeopathic approach is to understand the reason for the anger and to redirect this negative energy into a more positive direction. This will include psychotherapy and, possibly, psychoanalytic therapy.

The best homeopathic treatment is through consultation with a specialist homeopath who will prescribe the person's constitutional remedy. If this is not possible, the following remedies may be used following an outburst of anger. Using the 30c potency, give one dose as required.

### *Aconitum napellus* (monk's-hood)

This remedy picture describes a sudden outburst of emotion for no obvious reason. The person is usually very nervous and has a fear of dying.

### *Anacardium* (marking nut)

This remedy picture describes people who easily lose their tempers and seem bent on acts of wickedness, lacking all moral restraint.

### *Arsenicum album* (arsenic trioxide)

This remedy picture describes people who are restless and anxious and easily become exhausted. They like order so, whenever there is confusion, they become angry.

### *Aurum metallicum* (gold)

This remedy picture describes people who feel utterly worthless and become angry at the slightest contradiction. They are constantly and rapidly questioning without waiting for a reply. They cannot do things fast enough and become oversensitive to noise, excitement and confusion.

### *Bryonia* (wild hops)

This remedy picture describes people who are exceedingly irritable so that the slightest thing can make them angry. They are very determined, wanting objects that, when offered, are immediately rejected. They are always talking about business.

### *Hepar sulphuris* (calcium sulphide)

This remedy picture describes people who can become violently angry at the slightest cause if it irritates them. They feel terrible in the evening, when they even contemplate suicide.

### *Kali carbonicum* (potassium carbonate)

This remedy picture describes people who are generally miserable, yet can become very irritable and angry. They are full of fear, don't want to be left on their own, are never quiet or contented and are obstinate, with a hypersensitive reaction to pain, noise and touch.

### *Nitric acidum* (nitric acid)

This remedy picture describes irritable, hateful, vindictive and headstrong people who easily become angry. They can get themselves into a state of despair when they fear death. They feel worse in the evening and better when being driven about.

### Nux vomica (poison-nut)

This remedy picture describes people who are like bulls: they charge in without thinking, full of their own ambitions. They indulge to excess in alcohol, caffeine and nicotine, and easily become angry when things don't go their way.

### Sepia (inky juice from cuttlefish)

This remedy describes people who can become very angry when criticized. They become sad and withdraw into themselves, away from their loved ones and their occupation.

### Sulphur

This remedy picture describes people who can suddenly explode with anger, which can equally quickly subside and they forget everything about it. They are sociable, enjoying company, alcohol and a joke. They have a definite point of view, which is strongly held, and can become angry with anyone who disagrees with them.

### Tarentula hispania (Spanish spider)

This remedy picture describes people whose mood can suddenly change from happiness to anger. Their angry mood is physically destructive, making them violent and rude. Paradoxically they want to be on their own and yet want someone to be around. They are ungrateful and discontented. Their life is directed by whims, and they must constantly be on the move. They are sensitive to music.

## Anxiety and phobias

Anxiety becomes a problem if it continues for a long period of time. It is like taking an examination every day of your life. The heart and breathing rates are raised, even though sufferers are unaware of this. They are unable to function properly and feel stressed out. Sometimes something in particular provokes the anxiety, and this is known as a *phobia*.

The conventional treatment is with tranquillizers and, possibly, psychotherapy.

The homeopathic approach is, first, to adjust sufferers' diet so that caffeine (found in coffee, chocolate and cola drinks) is absolutely avoided. Aromatherapy, massage, reflexology and meditation can usefully be used in conjunction with homeopathy. Consultation with a specialist homeopath is recommended as he or she will be able to recommend a constitutional remedy for the particular person. If this is not possible, the following remedies may be used.

For a phobia that has been clearly identified, start the homeopathic treatment with:

## Syphilinum (syphilis spirochete)

The remedy picture includes a phobic tendency. This remedy is a nosode (a remedy made from diseased tissue) as well as a basic miasmic remedy (*see* p. 95). Using the 30c potency, give one dose every 12 hours, for a maximum of three doses. Then do nothing for three weeks and then proceed with the remedy for the particular phobia, as set out below.

For generalized anxiety as well as a particular phobia, select one of the following remedies by matching its picture with the physical symptoms. For anxiety, use the 6c potency and give one dose twice a day. For a phobia, use the 6c potency and give one dose immediately when an attack occurs, repeating this every ten minutes for a maximum of ten doses, then reducing to one dose twice a day.

## Aconitum napellus (monk's-hood)

This remedy picture describes a situation in which the person suddenly becomes very frightened, anxious and fearful of dying.

### *Argentum nitricum* (silver nitrate)

This remedy picture describes anxious people who feel worse in crowds (*claustrophobia*) and in high places. They have an impulse to jump out of windows. They also have a peculiar symptom of feeling fearful just as they are entering a church or going to the opera.

### *Arnica* (leopard's bane)

This remedy picture describes people who have a phobia of being touched or being approached by anyone. They also have a fear of open spaces (*agoraphobia*).

### *Arsenicum album* (arsenic trioxide)

This describes anxious people who feel much worse towards the late evening (typically at midnight) and when they are left on their own. They are very restless, excessively neat and tidy and, whenever ill, feel and act much worse than expected. They also feel the cold.

### *Belladonna* (deadly nightshade)

This remedy picture describes a person who has a particular phobia of dogs (a symptom shared with *Tuberculinum*). The person that this remedy will suit is hyperactive, has a vivid imagination and easily becomes flushed in the face, with widely dilated pupils and a fast heart rate.

### *Calcarea carbonica* (calcium carbonate)

This remedy picture describes people who become increasingly anxious towards the early evening. They feel that they are losing their minds, that some misfortune will happen to them, or that they may catch some infectious disease. This anxiety increases their heart rate. The heads of these people sweat easily, and these individuals are obstinate, with a tendency to become constipated.

### *Carbo animalis* (animal charcoal)

This remedy picture describes people who are made anxious by the dark, a symptom that is made worse when they shut their eyes. They can easily become homesick.

### *Carbo vegetabilis* (vegetable charcoal)

This remedy picture describes a person who is particularly anxious about the appearance of ghosts.

### *Gelsemium* (yellow jasmine)

This remedy picture describes people who suffer from stage fright and examination nerves. They prefer to be left on their own and are fearful in open spaces (*agoraphobia*) (a symptom shared with *Arnica*).

### *Ignatia* (St Ignatius' bean)

This remedy picture describes people who develop extreme nervousness following a shock, grief or a disappointment.

### *Iodum* (iodine)

This remedy picture describes people who are anxious about themselves in the present situation but not for future events. They become cross and are restless. They occasionally get the urge to run and also to do something violent. They complain that they feel exhausted and yet feel better by being busy. They have a tendency to weep and to feel sorry for themselves. They dislike meeting people, especially medical practitioners.

### *Kali arsenicum* (Fowler's solution)

This remedy picture describes people who are so jumpy and anxious that they are easily startled by the slightest noise and/or touch.

### Kali carbonicum (potassium carbonate)

This remedy picture describes people who become anxious and fearful whenever left on their own. They weep easily, are never sure how to express themselves, and become irritable and quarrelsome with everything and everyone. They worry about their own condition, which they realize is not normal.

### Lac caninum (dog's milk)

This remedy picture describes people who are anxious that they are going to faint.

### Lycopodium (club moss)

This remedy picture describes people who are anxious about attempting anything new for fear of failure, yet when they finally tackle the problem, they are successful. They are fearful of being on their own in their own homes. They feel at their worst between 4.00 and 8.00 pm.

### Lyssin (saliva from a rabid dog)

This remedy picture describes people who have a considerable fear of water (*hydrophobia*). They also have a fear that they are going mad. They speak rapidly, are impatient and have a violent temper that impels them to do reckless things.

### Medorhinum (gonorrhoea bacteria)

This remedy picture describes people who feel uncomfortable in crowded places (*claustrophobia*), only feeling better by the seaside. They also have an underlying feeling of anxiety.

### Natrum muriaticum (sodium chloride)

This remedy picture describes people who have lost self-confidence, becoming nervous, anxious and worried. This follows the break-up of a close physical relationship.

### Phosphorus

This remedy picture describes people who become very anxious before and during thunderstorms.

### Pulsatilla (wind flower)

This remedy picture describes people who dislike crowded places (*claustrophobia*), which make them anxious, and prefer the fresh air outside.

### Silicea (pure flint)

This remedy picture describes people who have a phobia of pointed objects (and particularly dislike injections) and are pre-occupied with pins and needles.

### Stramonium (thorn apple)

This remedy picture describes people who go into a violent spasm whenever water is seen (*hydrophobia*). They generally behave crazily.

### Tuberculinum (nucleo-protein from tubercular abscess)

This remedy picture describes people who have a phobia of animals and of dogs in particular. They vacillate between happiness and sadness at quick intervals. They can behave well one moment and then suddenly change and behave badly.

## Depression

This is broadly classified into *reactive depression* (where there is a specific cause for the person to be depressed) and *endogenous depression* (where there is no specific cause). In both cases, people become sluggish mentally and physically. They lose the will to do anything, and some will choose suicide as an option.

The conventional treatment for endogenous depression is with antidepressant medication and, possibly, psychiatric assessment that may lead to hospital admission to protect such individuals from harming themselves.

Homeopathy must be a second choice of therapy. It can, however, be used in a complementary way with antidepressants; the effect will be additive. It is best to consult a specialist homeopath to help this serious condition. If this is not possible, the following remedies may be used. Select the appropriate one by matching its picture with the physical symptoms. Give one dose of the 30c potency daily for five days, then the 6c potency at one dose twice a day until the person begins to improve.

### Aconitum napellus (monk's-hood)

This remedy picture describes people who suddenly become sad and anxious. Music in particular makes them feel sad. They are also full of fears, particularly about their own mortality, and of being in a crowd and crossing the street. They are restless and keep tossing about.

### Agaricus muscarius (toadstool)

This remedy picture describes sad individuals who also are stubborn, yet have moments of extraordinary extrovert behaviour when they embrace strangers and kiss their hands.

### Agnus castus (chaste tree)

This remedy picture describes people who have a nervous depression accompanied with mental forebodings, particularly of their speedy death. They also have a peculiar symptom of apparently always smelling herrings.

### Ambra grisea (amber, a morbid secretion of the whale)

This remedy picture describes people who are full of despair and have lost their love of life. They dread meeting people, and want to be left alone. Being intensely shy, they can't do anything in the presence of other people. They blush easily.

### Arsenicum album (arsenic trioxide)

This remedy picture describes people who despair of their life, feeling that they are going to die, so they refuse to take treatment. They are usually very neat and tidy and restless. Their despair makes them move from place to place without being able to settle.

### Aurum metallicum (gold)

This remedy picture describes people who feel worthless, can do nothing right and feel suicidal, yet paradoxically fear death. Their symptoms are made worse in cold weather and when they have a cold.

### Calcarea arsenica (calcium arsenate)

This remedy picture describes a fat woman around the time of her menopause. She is depressed and anxious, and desires the company of other people.

### Calcarea carbonica (calcium carbonate)

This remedy picture describes obese, sad people who just sit thinking about nothing and aimlessly break matchsticks. They have a tendency towards constipation and towards sweating, particularly on their heads.

### Carbo animalis (animal charcoal)

This remedy picture describes sad, reflective people who wish to be left on their own. They avoid all conversation, are easily frightened, have a fear of the dark (a symptom that is made worse when they close their eyes) and can easily become homesick. They tend to weep whenever they eat a meal.

### *Carbo vegetabilis* (vegetable charcoal)

This remedy picture describes unhappy people who are also anxious and irritable. They have a specific fear of ghosts and therefore dislike darkness.

### *Causticum* (Hahnemann's mixture of quicklime [calcium oxide] with potassium bisulphate)

This remedy picture describes people who feel sad and cry easily. They are intensely sensitive about the sufferings of fellow human beings and of animals.

### *Cimicifuga racemosa* (black snake root)

This remedy picture describes depressed people who have a feeling of some impending evil event. They feel as though there is a cloud surrounding them. They have a particular fear of riding in a car and feeling obliged to jump out. They also have a recurrent vision of rats and mice.

### *Cinchona officinalis (China)* (Peruvian bark)

This remedy picture describes sad people whose worries crowd into their minds, preventing sleep. They suddenly cry out, throwing themselves about. They have a specific desire to hurt other people's feelings.

### *Coffea cruda* (unroasted coffee)

This remedy picture describes people who are overactive. They can be joyous one moment and immensely sad the next. When sad, they can be driven to utter despair.

### *Crotalus horridus* (rattlesnake)

This remedy picture describes sad people who are also very chatty and yet have a desire to escape from their lives and from the people around them. They are impatient and tend to weep. They imagine that their brains are beginning to fail them.

### *Ferrum metallicum* (iron)

This remedy picture describes a woman who becomes particularly sad following her menstrual period. She feels that she is always in the right, is sensitive and excitable (more so whenever she is contradicted) and weeps and laughs to excess. She finds the slightest noise intolerable.

### *Gelsemium* (yellow jasmine)

This remedy picture describes people who cannot cry even though grief-stricken, and consequently brood and become sad.

### *Graphites* (black lead)

This remedy picture describes sad people who weep without cause and find that music can make them weep particularly easily. While sitting at work, they are fidgety, feeling miserable and unhappy. They become forgetful, making mistakes when speaking and writing.

### *Hellebore* (Christmas rose)

This remedy picture describes people who have black moods that are worse between 4.00 and 8.00 pm. They are slow in answering questions, stare blankly into the distance and sigh involuntarily. They pick at their lips and clothes, and feel better when wrapped up warmly.

### *Heloderma* (gila monster)

This remedy picture describes people who are severely depressed and have a sensation of falling over on to their right side. They have a feeling of a cold band around their head, a pain that starts in their right ear and extends around the back of their head and into their left ear.

### *Helonias* (unicorn root)

This remedy picture describes people who are profoundly depressed. They feel better when kept busy so that their minds are kept off their depression. They are irritable and cannot tolerate any contradiction.

### *Ignatia* (St Ignatius' bean)

This remedy picture describes people whose moods are changeable, yet they are generally introspective, tearful and non-communicative and privately brood, feeling full of despair.

### *Iodum* (iodine)

This remedy picture describes sad people who have sudden impulses to run and do something violent. They tend to do strange things without any cause. They may kill someone or themselves. They have the feeling that all is well and yet fear meeting people, particularly medical practitioners.

### *Kali bromatum* (potassium bromate)

This remedy picture describes sad people who feel that they are being followed or that they may be poisoned. They therefore fear people, yet cannot remain on their own.

### *Kali phosphoricum* (potassium phosphate)

This remedy picture describes people who become sad over business and religious matters.

### *Lac caninum* (dog's milk)

This remedy picture describes despondent individuals who are cross and irritable and scream all the time and more so at night. They are full of fears, of falling downstairs and of disease. They have a vivid imagination, seeing snakes and vermin.

### *Lachesis* (bushmaster snake venom)

This remedy picture describes people who are normally very chatty but become obsessed with religious matters, which fill their minds with despair. They think that others are planning their funerals.

### *Lilium tigrinum* (tiger lily)

This remedy picture describes people who feel that a terrible illness is about to come into their bodies and despair for their own religious salvation.

### *Lycopodium* (club moss)

This remedy picture describes people who easily become sad when left on their own. They easily lose self-confidence and are therefore not at all keen to undertake new tasks. They become confused over words that have just been written, and even find difficulty in reading what they have just written.

### *Mercurius solubis* (black oxide of mercury)

This remedy picture describes sad people who are so apathetic that eating becomes an irrelevance. They sweat easily with a smelly odour. They do everything in a hurry, and have an uncontrollable desire to travel far away. Such women have suicidal thoughts during their periods, which diminish whenever they cry.

### *Murex* (purple fish)

This remedy is particularly applicable to women. If they find themselves in a very despondent state, this symptom is improved when there is an increase in their vaginal discharge. In this state, women become anxious about their health in general and find that their memory plays tricks on them so that they find it difficult to find the correct word.

### *Natrum carbonicum* (sodium carbonate)

This remedy picture describes depressed people who find comprehension difficult and therefore frustrating. They are very sensitive to noise, cold, music and changes in the weather (particularly thunder).

### *Natrum muriaticum* (sodium chloride)

This remedy picture describes sad, depressed people following a grief reaction, particularly the break-up of a close relationship. They want to cry on their own, finding emotional and physical support difficult to handle.

### *Natrum phosphoricum* (sodium phosphate)

This remedy picture describes despondent individuals who develop frightening fears. At night, they imagine that pieces of furniture are people and "hear" footsteps in the next room.

### *Nitric acidum* (nitric acid)

This remedy picture describes irritable, hateful, vindictive people who can get into such a rage that they tremble. Following these outbursts, they feel very sad but refuse consolation from those that have been abused.

### *Psorinum* (scabies vesicle)

This remedy picture describes people who are full of despair and feel that nothing is going to go right and that they are never going to improve. They feel emotionally and physically very cold.

### *Rhus toxicodendron* (poison ivy)

This remedy picture describes people who feel anxious, sad and helpless with a profound sense of despondency. These symptoms are all worse in the evening. They fear being poisoned and have thoughts of suicide by drowning.

### Sepia (inky juice from cuttlefish)

This remedy picture describes sad people who want to retreat into their own space, getting away from the people around them. In this mood, they don't want to be touched.

### Stramonium (thorn apple)

This remedy picture describes people whose have mood swings between extreme sadness and extreme excitement.

### Sulphur

This remedy picture describes people who cry for no reason. This is made worse by any form of consolation. They have fixed ideas on philosophy, politics and religious matters.

### Veratrum album (white hellebore)

This remedy picture describes people who despair because of some impending misfortune from which there will be no salvation. They sit in a stupor, noticing nothing, then suddenly have an urge to cut and tear things.

### Zincum metallicum (zinc)

This remedy picture describes people who cry when angry. They repeat all questions before answering them. They also fear that they are going to be arrested for a supposed crime, which makes them depressed. They start on waking up, as if frightened, and roll their heads from side to side. They are sensitive to noise and particularly to people talking.

# Grief

This emotion, which can cause depression (*see above*), can be due to the death of a loved one (a person or a pet) or from the break-up of a close emotional relationship.

The conventional treatment is with tranquillizers and, possibly, psychotherapy.

The homeopathic approach is with a constitutional remedy prescribed by a specialist homeopath. If this is not possible, the following remedies can be given. Select one by matching the remedy picture with the physical symptoms. Using the 30c potency, give one dose daily for one week, then change to the 6c potency and give one dose twice a day until the person begins to improve.

### *Aurum metallicum* (gold)

This remedy picture describes people who become very depressed following a grief reaction when someone close to them has died. They become very sensitive to noise and hide their grief by making themselves very busy.

### *Ignatia* (St Ignatius' bean)

This remedy picture describes people who are profoundly disturbed through personal grief. They weep openly and frequently.

### *Natrum muriaticum* (sodium chloride)

This remedy picture describes a grief reaction following the break-up of a close personal relationship. This person dislikes extremes of temperature (both hot and cold), likes salty foods and is able to bear a grudge.

### *Phosphoricum acidum* (phosphoric acid)

This remedy picture describes people who become profoundly

depressed following grief, the depression causing them to be physically unwell. The depression is so severe that suicide is considered an option. They feel better by keeping warm and are made worse from physical exertion.

### Pulsatilla (wind flower)

This remedy picture describes people who react badly to emotions of grief. They cry easily and often need a lot of emotional and physical support. They feel better outside in the fresh air, and positively dislike fatty foods.

### Staphysagria (stavesacre)

This remedy picture describes people who suffer a grief reaction and develop an indignant attitude towards everyone around them: "Why did this happen to me?" They feel slightly better from warmth, after breakfast and from rest in bed at night.

## Homesickness

This condition can occur in people of all ages. The old saying "Home is where the heart is" is a truism. The following homeopathic remedies can help alleviate some (if not all) of the symptoms. Select the remedy by matching its picture with the physical symptoms. Using the 30c potency, give one dose as required.

### Capsicum annuum (cayenne pepper)

This remedy picture describes people whose homesickness is associated with sleeplessness and a tendency to feel like committing suicide. They feel better while eating and from warmth. They usually have red cheeks.

### Carbo animalis (animal charcoal)

This remedy picture describes people who, as well as feeling homesick, fear the dark (a symptom that is made worse when they close their eyes) and are easily frightened. They want to be left on their own, feeling sad and reflective. They avoid conversation, and have a tendency to weep during a meal. They feel worse in the morning.

### *Phosphoricum acidum* (phosphoric acid)

This remedy picture describes people who feel homesick, have a tendency to weep and dread the future. They sit quietly on their own, brooding over their situation.

## Jealousy and envy

This powerful emotion, which can lead to violence, is usually caused by a broken love partnership, when one partner finds a new love, or is suspected of doing so. On a lesser scale, a person can feel envy about another's material possessions.

Occasionally tranquillizers or antidepressant medication are indicated. Psychotherapy may be recommended.

The homeopathic approach is to prescribe the person's constitutional remedy which is obtained by consulting a specialist homeopath. If this is not possible, one of the following remedies may be given. Select it by matching its picture with the physical symptoms. Using the 30c potency, give one dose daily for one week, then reduce the potency to 6c and give one dose twice a day.

### *Apis mellifica* (honey bee)

This remedy picture describes jealous people who are fidgety and hard to please. They are apathetic, finding it difficult to contemplate anything, but then suddenly cry out with apparent stinging pains.

### Hyoscyamus (henbane)

This remedy picture describes jealous people who are also very suspicious. Their mood varies between hilarity, when they laugh at everything, to despair, when they want to run away.

### Lachesis (bushmaster snake venom)

This remedy picture describes jealous people who feel foolish at having this emotion. They are always talking and prefer clothing that does not fit tightly around the neck or abdomen. The symptoms are always worse in the early morning.

### Nux vomica (poison-nut)

This ambitious person is liable to become very jealous of anyone when things don't go the way he or she would like.

### Pulsatilla (wind flower)

This remedy picture describes people who are very emotional anyway. They cry easily and often, and when a relationship ends, they become jealous and crave fuss and caresses even more.

# Mania

In this condition, people become so overactive that they need no sleep, they forget to eat and, unless untreated, they become seriously physically ill.

The conventional treatment is the correct choice, involving psychiatric help and possibly hospital admission. The therapy given is a combination of major tranquillizers and lithium carbonate.

Homeopathic treatment should only be used in a complementary way with the conventional therapy. Consultation with a specialist homeopath is ideal, in order to work out the constitutional profile of the person. The following remedies can be considered if this consultation is impossible. Select one by matching its picture with the physical symptoms. Using the 30c potency, give one dose once a week, reducing to one dose a month as the person begins to improve.

### *Arsenicum album* (arsenic trioxide)

This remedy picture describes people who feel driven to move from place to place in a fruitless attempt to find peace. They are very anxious, feeling worse in the cold and towards the middle of the night.

### *Belladonna* (deadly nightshade)

This remedy picture describes people who live in a world of their own, totally unaware of the reality of life around them. They have auditory and visual hallucinations, that tell them what to do. The person that this remedy suits typically has a red face and widely dilated pupils.

### *Hyoscyamus* (henbane)

This remedy picture describes people who are very suspicious of others, prefer to undress in inappropriate circumstances and always laugh. They talk very rapidly and their speech is crude.

### *Kali bromatum* (potassium bromide)

This remedy picture describes people who feel that they have been singled out as an object of divine wrath. They feel that they must do something and so continually move about. They suffer from night terrors.

### *Mercurius solubis* (black oxide of mercury)

This remedy picture describes people who have hurried speech that makes them stammer, and they are restless and sweaty. They have an uncontrollable urge to travel far away. They also have violent impulses for homicide (they want to punch strangers on the nose) and suicide. This creates fear in them so that escape is the only possibility. They become so indifferent to everything that food is considered an irrelevance.

### *Nux vomica* (poison-nut)

This remedy picture describes people who are workaholics. They are perfectionists who attempt to get everything right. They stay up all night, drinking caffeine and alcohol and probably smoking cigarettes as well.

### *Stramonium* (thorn apple)

This remedy picture describes people who talk continuously about religious matters. They are earnest and beseeching in their speech, and nothing will stop them from talking. They have delusions about their identity, feeling that they are someone else. Physical as well as verbal activity is continual.

### *Veratrum album* (white hellebore)

This remedy picture describes people who have an uncontrollable urge to cut things up. They have a frenzied way of expressing themselves, and it is not uncommon for them to shriek and curse. They finally become sad, sitting in a stupor, noticing nothing.

## Manic depression

This condition is a combination of mania and depression. The person usually begins with a manic phase, which is treated conventionally as stated in the section on mania, and this is followed by a prolonged depression (*see above*).

In the manic phase, these individuals feel that nothing is wrong with them – they feel so good and manage everything so well. In fact, they need to be protected from themselves with treatment. Similarly, in the depressed phase, they are so low that they need treatment in order to protect themselves. In both of these situations, the conventional treatment is essential as enforced admission to a psychiatric hospital may be required.

Homeopathic treatment is very much the second choice, but can be used in a complementary way with the conventional treatment. Select the appropriate remedies in the sections on DESPAIR and MANIA, depending on the condition of the person, and follow the dosage schedules described for each remedy.

# Mischievous behaviour

This emotion occurs when a person plays deliberate tricks on another. This can sometimes lead the mischievous person to get into trouble.

Ideally, homeopathic treatment should involve consultation with a specialist homeopath who will assess the person constitutionally. If this is not possible, the following remedies may be considered. Match the remedy picture with the physical symptoms. Using the 6c potency, give one dose three times a day for two weeks.

### *Anacardium* (marking nut)

This remedy picture describes people who have fixed ideas and believe that they are two people and have two minds. They suffer from impaired memory, giving the impression of being absentminded. They are very easily offended and, on occasion, have bursts of mischievousness.

### *Lac caninum* (dog's milk)

This remedy picture describes people who have a poor opinion of themselves, have visions of snakes and have become absentminded. They think that they have someone else's nose and that everything that another says is a lie. In this mood, they become mischievous.

### Nux vomica (poison-nut)

This remedy picture describes ambitious people who can be devious in their business dealings, which they say is just themselves being mischievous.

## Quarrelsome behaviour

This emotion describes individuals who pick arguments with anyone about anything. It makes them feel unhappy, and certainly makes those around them unhappy.

Homeopathic treatment involves checking that the diet is not influencing their behaviour and also the prescribing of their constitutional remedy by a specialist homeopath. If this is not possible, the following remedies can be used. Select one by matching its picture with the physical symptoms. Using the 30c potency, give one dose daily for one week, reducing to the 6c potency and giving one dose twice a day.

### Aurum metallicum (gold)

This remedy picture describes people who feel hateful and are quarrelsome. Basically they are seriously depressed, thinking that they have done something wrong. They are very sensitive to the least contradiction.

### Ignatia (St Ignatius' bean)

This remedy picture describes people whose emotional behaviour is seriously disturbed from a recent grief. Their behaviour becomes unpredictable, making them alternately quarrelsome and sympathetic.

### Nux vomica (poison-nut)

This remedy picture describes ambitious people who are workaholics and perfectionists. They strive for success and, in this mode, become quarrelsome with anyone who stands in their way.

### Petroleum (crude rock oil)

This remedy picture describes people who are irritable and easily offended and worry about everything. They feel that their death is near and that they must settle their affairs as quickly as possible. They become disturbed from any extra mental pressure, and this makes them quarrelsome.

### Sulphur

This remedy picture describes people who enjoy an argument, which is interpreted as them being quarrelsome. They are not neat and tidy, and enjoy alcohol and fatty food.

### Tarentula hispania (Spanish spider)

This remedy picture describes disgruntled, ungrateful people who are guided by the whim of the moment. They have sudden changes in mood and, in their destructive phase, become quarrelsome. They are sensitive to music, and paradoxically, although adverse to company, they want someone to be with them. They must be constantly busy.

### Tuberculinum (nucleo-protein from tubercular abscess)

This remedy picture describes people who are irritable and contradictory, especially when they first wake up. Their mood varies between overactivity and despair. They frequently use foul language, cursing and swearing when irritated.

## Schizophrenia

This is a serious mental condition in which the person may be at risk to themselves and to others. For this reason, psychiatric assessment is urgent as affected individuals may need to be admitted to hospital compulsorily. This is not only for the person's benefit but also for those people around him or her.

The conventional treatment is with major tranquillizers.

Homeopathic treatment, which is very much a second choice, should be supervised by a specialist homeopath. If this is not possible, the following remedies can be used in a complementary way with conventional drugs. Select one matching the picture with the physical symptoms. Using the 30c potency, give one dose twice a week (but not on consecutive days).

### *Belladonna* (deadly nightshade)

This remedy picture describes people who live in a world of their own. They have visions and are oblivious of the reality around them. These visions are of terrifying monsters which the affected individuals will not believe are not real.

### *Hyoscyamus* (henbane)

This remedy picture describes very talkative people who are also very suspicious and jealous of other people. They behave obscenely in speech and by undressing in inappropriate circumstances. They laugh at everything and at inappropriate times. They attempt to run away.

### *Stramonium* (thorn apple)

This remedy picture describes people who are violent verbally and physically. Their minds make them think that what they are doing is what they have been told to do. They speak earnestly and ceaselessly.

# PART II

# *Problems of Newborn Babies, Infants, Children and Adolescents*

This section shows how homeopathy can be used in a totally safe way to help treat certain illnesses. It is important to remember that a correct diagnosis must be established as conventional medical therapy may be the optimum way to treat the condition. However, homeopathy can work alongside conventional treatments, giving a boost to the therapeutic options, and in certain circumstances, homeopathic remedies can be used on their own.

# Newborn Babies

This section deals with problems in the immediate period following delivery up until the first few weeks of life. Remedies can be given either in the granular form or as a liquid. Approximately 10 granules equals one dose of the granular form. One drop is equal to one dose of the liquid form. Both of these preparations can be given while a baby is asleep, by applying the medication to their lips or on to their exposed tongue.

## Birthmarks

These marks – medically called *naevus* (singular) and *naevi* (plural) – cause considerable parental anxiety. There are two types. *Café au lait* spots are caused by localized pigmentation of the skin and are permanent marks on the skin. They are like moles, only larger, and eventually will have hairs growing out from them.

The other type of birthmark is caused by an accumulation of tiny blood vessels. *Capillary naevi* are flat and pink, usually fade within 18 months and need no treatment. *Strawberry naevi* are red, raised from the skin surface and about 2.5 cm (1 in) in diameter. They grow in size with the child and begin to fade at about the age of three. Occasionally this type of naevus can bleed. The first aid measure is to press firmly on it and to give one dose of **Phosphorus** 6c potency every five minutes until the bleeding stops, then give one dose of 30c potency every 12 hours, for a maximum of three doses. For a *strawberry naevus* that doesn't bleed, a monthly dose of **Thuja occidentalis** using the 30c potency is helpful.

*Port wine stains* are a deeper shade of pink than capillary naevi, are slightly raised above the skin surface, are quite large and generally persist well into adult life. They are found on the face and limbs. The modern conventional treatment is with laser therapy, which slowly obliterates the capillaries that cause this naevus.

There is no homeopathic treatment other than constitutional therapy to support the person as a whole. This can be obtained from a specialist homeopath.

# Circumcision

This surgical procedure is carried out very early in a male baby's life, usually for religious reasons, but in countries such as the United States, it is done for (spurious) hygiene reasons. The procedure involves cutting off the foreskin from the tip of the penis (the glans penis), after which a paraffin gauze dressing is applied to the penis.

The homeopathic treatment involves applying a *Calendula* (marigold) and *Hypericum* (St John's wort) lotion. This is made by adding ten drops of the mother tincture of each remedy to 250 millilitres of pure water, putting some on to clean lint and applying this to the glans penis at least twice a day. This will help heal the skin and alleviate the discomfort.

# Colic

The diagnosis is important as the symptoms of spasmodic abdominal pain can mask serious surgical emergencies. Having established that this is not the case (and many babies suffer from innocent infantile colic), the following homeopathic remedies are helpful. Select one by matching the remedy picture as closely as possible with the physical symptoms.

### *Bryonia* (wild hops)

This remedy picture describes pain in the abdomen that is made worse from any pressure but is eased by the baby lying absolutely still. Using the 6c potency, give one dose as required.

### *Carbo vegetabilis* (vegetable charcoal)

This remedy picture describes infantile colic that may have been brought on by a car journey. The baby is excessively windy from both upward wind (flatulence) and downward wind (flatus). Using the 6c potency, give one dose as required.

### *Chamomilla* (camomile)

This remedy picture describes infantile colic causing restlessness and irritability that can only be settled by carrying the babies around and even pushing them around in their buggies or driving them around in cars. Their abdomens are bloated and very windy. Characteristically one cheek is red while the other is pale. Using the 6c potency, give one dose as required.

### *Colocynthis* (bitter cucumber)

This remedy picture describes colicky pains in the abdomen, and this remedy is the most widely used one for infantile colic where babies draw up their legs in response to the spasmodic pain. The pain is relieved by firm pressure (which occurs naturally when babies draw up their legs). Using the 6c potency, give one dose as required.

### *Ignatia* (St Ignatius' bean)

This remedy picture describes colicky pains in babies whose mothers are undergoing a grief reaction. This is particularly applicable to breastfed babies. Using the 6c potency, give one dose twice a day.

### *Magnesia phosphoricum* (magnesium phosphate)

This remedy picture describes infantile colic similar to that seen in *Colocynthis* but the pain is relieved more by heat than by pressure. Using the 6c potency, give one dose as required.

### *Nux vomica* (poison-nut)

This remedy picture describes babies who develop infantile colic particularly when they are overtired. They also show difficulty in defecation, but the colic is improved when they manage to pass a stool. It is a common feature of this remedy that the babies have an umbilical hernia. Using the 6c potency, give one dose four times a day for as long as required.

# Difficult delivery

The following remedies can be given to a newborn baby following a difficult delivery.

### *Arnica* (leopard's bane)

This remedy should be considered in all cases of prolonged labour where there has been excessive moulding of the head. Using the 6c potency, give one dose four times a day, for a maximum of ten doses.

### *Natrum sulphuricum* (sodium sulphate)

This remedy should be considered whenever a baby has been delivered by forceps, ventouse extraction or Caesarean section, when the head has been subjected to a traumatic event. Using the 30c potency, give one dose only.

# Feeding difficulties

This condition is medically important because, if babies' food intake is not sufficient, they will fail to thrive. If they suffer from projectile vomiting, pyloric stenosis (when the outlet from the stomach to the small intestines is blocked in some way) is a possible diagnosis and must be excluded by a medical consultation.

If the baby is being breastfed, the following homeopathic remedies can be used. Select one from the remedy picture that most closely matches the physical situation. For bottle-fed babies, consider switching to a different formula feed.

### *Aethusa cynapium* (fool's parsley)

This remedy describes babies who regurgitate their feed as soon as it has been swallowed. As a result, they remain hungry and become distressed. Using the 6c potency, give one dose four times a day until the baby shows signs of improvement, when the dosage can be gradually reduced.

### *Calcarea carbonica* (calcium carbonate)

This remedy picture describes larger-sized babies who have large heads. They sweat easily, particularly over their scalp. They are greedy for their food but tend to vomit after a feed. Using the 30c potency, give one dose daily for one week.

### *Natrum carbonicum* (sodium carbonate)

This remedy picture describes babies who find that any form of milk disagrees with them, causing much regurgitation and diarrhoea. Their abdomens become bloated, leading to a lot of wind, both up (flatulence) and down (flatus). Using the 30c potency, give one dose daily for one week.

### *Phosphoricum acidum* (phosphoric acid)

This describes babies who are slow feeders and fail to thrive. Their skin is pale and waxy so that the overall appearance is unhealthy. They tend to lie awake with their eyes open but not crying. Using the 6c potency, give one dose four times a day, slowly reducing the frequency once they begin to improve.

### *Silicea* (pure flint)

This remedy picture describes smaller babies with fine hair. Their feet in particular have a tendency to sweat easily. Paradoxically, they refuse to suckle the breast and yet want to suckle. They appear to be thirsty and readily accept a bottle but disappointingly vomit as soon as they have drunk from it. Using the 30c potency, give one dose daily for one week.

# Fever

This symptom is very distressing to parents: What does it mean? Should I call the doctor? Will my baby be harmed?

The vast majority of babies with fevers have no serious medical condition. It has recently been shown that a fever stimulates the immune system, which means that the fever is the natural way that the body defends itself.

The immediate conventional advice is to give babies some liquid paracetamol, encourage the intake of fluid and sponge them down with tepid water. Should the fever continue for more than 24 hours, seek medical help.

The immediate homeopathic treatment is to give *Aconitum napellus* (monk's-hood). Using the 6c potency, give one dose every 15 minutes, for a maximum of ten doses. If the baby's temperature does not go down, give *Belladonna* (deadly nightshade). Using the 6c potency, give one dose every 15 minutes, for a maximum of ten doses. If the baby still has a fever after this, seek medical help.

# Gastroenteritis

This condition is very serious in babies as dehydration can occur very quickly. The symptoms are profuse diarrhoea and vomiting. Dehydration produces floppy skin and a sunken fontanelle (the "soft spot" on the top of the head) and sunken eyes. The cause of this illness is bacterial infection and is uncommon in breastfed babies: the bacteria get into the feeding utensils of the bottle-fed baby.

Conventional treatment is to admit affected babies to hospital in order to rehydrate them by intravenous fluid therapy.

At the beginning of this illness, the following homeopathic remedies can be used to help the baby recover before becoming dehydrated. Using the 6c potency, give one dose every ten minutes for a maximum of one hour. Then, if there is no improvement, seek medical advice.

*Aethusa cynapium* (fool's parsley)

This remedy picture describes gastroenteritis in bottle-fed babies who vomit up the milk as soon as it is swallowed. They are hungry again as soon as vomiting has occurred. They also vomit up white frothy matter, and they sweat.

*Colocynthis* (bitter cucumber)

This remedy picture describes babies who have a spasmodic pain in their abdomens, which makes them draw up their legs. This successfully reduces the pain, as does localized firm pressure. The babies vomit while the pain occurs.

*Phosphorus*

This remedy picture describes vomiting in babies after drinking cool liquid, as soon as it has warmed up in the stomach. (This applies to bottle-fed babies only, where the feed hasn't been warmed up sufficiently.)


# Nappy rash

This condition is a reaction of babies' skin to their urine and faeces. It causes redness, bleeding, itchiness and blister formation, and occurs on the buttocks, genital area and inner thighs. There may be an added yeast infection of *Candida albicans,* particularly if the babies have had antibiotic therapy or, if they are being breastfed, their mothers have received antibiotics.

The best treatment for this condition is to expose the affected skin to the air, without any nappy. The babies should be washed with water only (no soap), and if their nappies are not disposable, consideration should be made to using disposable nappies. Cloth nappies should certainly be washed thoroughly and rinsed completely in order to remove any soap.

The conventional treatment is to use creams on the buttock area that will act as a barrier or to use antibiotic or anti-*Candida* creams with or without a steroid component.

The homeopathic treatment is to encourage parents to allow their babies to lie exposed to the open air as much as possible and to consider one of the following remedies, matching the remedy picture with the physical symptoms. Using the 6c potency, give one dose four times a day, for a maximum of 12 doses.

### Calcarea carbonica (calcium carbonate)

This remedy picture describes nappy rash in fat babies who tend to sweat a lot on their scalps, particularly at night.

### Mercurius solubis (black oxide of mercury)

This remedy picture describes a moist, raw nappy rash in a baby who produces more saliva than expected.

### Medorhinum (gonorrhoea bacteria)

This remedy picture describes a sore, red and itchy buttock area that bleeds easily.

### Rhus toxicodendron (poison ivy)

This remedy picture describes a nappy rash that is not only red and raw but also has many small blisters on the skin.

### Sulphur

This remedy picture describes a nappy rash that is red, itchy but dry and the skin is scaly.

## Jaundice

This condition is common in babies, particularly if they are premature. The skin becomes yellowish as do the whites of the eyes. This is due to the immaturity of the liver, which is unable to cope with the natural breakdown products in the blood.

The conventional treatment is to expose these babies to ultra-violet light, which breaks down the products causing the jaundice. They are encouraged to drink as much water as possible. Should the amount of bilirubin (which causes the jaundice) in the blood rise too high, there is a risk of brain damage, and to avoid this, an exchange blood transfusion is given.

The homeopathic approach is the same as the conventional approach except that the following remedies can be given.

### Chamomilla (camomile)

This remedy should be given in the first instance. Using the 6c potency, give one dose every hour, for a maximum of six doses.

### Mercurius solubis (black oxide of mercury)

This is useful for detoxifying the blood of bilirubin. Use it after *Chamomilla* if the jaundice is not fading. Using the 6c potency, give one dose every hour, for a maximum of six doses.

## Night crying

This is a situation where babies are unable to settle down to sleep. Having excluded pain as a cause, and indeed boredom, the following homeopathic remedies can be used. Select one by matching its picture with the physical symptoms.

### Chamomilla (camomile)

This remedy picture describes babies who can only be settled by being carried around, pushed around in their buggies or even taken out for a car ride. Using the 6c potency, give one dose as required but with a maximum of two doses each night.

### Ignatia (St Ignatius' bean)

This remedy picture describes crying babies, especially when their mothers are going through a grief reaction. This is especially true in breastfed babies. Using the 6c potency, give one dose twice a day.

### Nux vomica (poison-nut)

This remedy picture describes babies who wake up, crying and apparently hungry, in the early hours of the night and yet are not pacified by being fed. Their crying usually diminishes by the passage of wind (flatus) or by a bowel action. Using the 30c potency, give one dose daily for a maximum of ten doses.

### Phosphorus

This remedy picture describes babies who take short naps during the day and night but are unable to settle for a longer sleep. This results in them having prolonged periods of night crying without being in pain or being hungry. Using the 30c potency, give one dose once a day, for a maximum of ten doses.

## Seborrhoeic eczema

This form of eczema is common in the first few months of life and appears on the face, trunk, limbs and scalp. It comprises red blotches with dry flaky skin, which can become yellow crusts that ooze yellow liquid. When on the scalp, it is known as "cradle cap".

The conventional treatment for this condition is aqueous creams with or without steroid creams.

The homeopathic approach is to bathe babies in water without using any soap. The following homeopathic remedies can also be used. Using the 6c potency, give one dose four times a day.

### Calendula ointment (marigold)

This ointment can be applied to any dry skin area.

### *Vinca minor* (lesser periwinkle)

This remedy picture describes spots on the scalp that ooze a liquid that causes the hair to mat together. The skin in general is red in patches and is made worse from the slightest rubbing.

### *Viola tricolor* (pansy)

This remedy picture describes "cradle cap": crusts on the face and scalp that can ooze yellow fluid.

Seborrhoeic eczema can lead on to eczema, for which treatments, both conventional and homeopathic, can be found on p. 267.

# Septic spots

These are quite common in newborn babies. They arise as crops of pustular spots with red margins.

The conventional treatment is to use an antibiotic. The following homeopathic remedies can be used instead with therapeutic success. They should be taken in the following sequence:

1. *Belladonna* (deadly nightshade): This remedy picture describes the skin of a baby with red papules but without any pus, representing the onset of septic spots. Using the 30c potency, give one dose.
2. *Hepar sulphuris* (calcium sulphide): This remedy picture describes a later stage in the formation of septic spots and follows on from *Belladonna* when the papules have developed pus within them. Using the 30c potency, give one dose twice a day, for a maximum of two days.
3. *Silicea* (pure flint): This remedy follows on from *Belladonna* and *Hepar sulphuris* in resolving the septic spots should the healing progress become static. Using the 30c potency, give one dose twice a day, for a maximum of five days.

## Sticky eyes

This is an infection of the conjunctiva of the eyes in which the eyelids become stuck together with dried pus.

The conventional treatment is to use antibiotic eye drops. The homeopathic treatment involves the use of the following remedies.

### *Apis mellifica* (honey bee)

This remedy picture describes eyelids that have become swollen, a condition called *blepharitis*. Using the 30c potency, give one dose at night, for a maximum of five nights.

### *Argentum nitricum* (silver nitrate)

This remedy picture describes pus being discharged from the conjunctiva. The conjunctiva also becomes swollen. Using the 30c potency, give one dose daily, for a maximum of five doses.

## Umbilical hernia

This hernia is a protrusion from the tummy button that can reach at least 2.5 cm (1 in) in length. There is no risk that it will burst, and commonly these hernias resolve naturally.

The conventional treatment is surgery when the child is about four or five years old.

While awaiting surgery, the following homeopathic remedies can be used. Using the 6c potency, give one dose twice a day.

### *Calcarea carbonica* (calcium carbonate)

This remedy picture describes babies with large heads that sweat easily. They find defecation difficult, and whenever they strain, an umbilical hernia appears.

### *Lachesis* (bushmaster snake venom)

This remedy picture describes babies whose abdomens swell with wind, are sensitive to the touch and develop umbilical hernias.

### Nux moschata (nutmeg)

This remedy describes babies whose tummy buttons are sore, possibly infected, and from which umbilical hernias develop.

### Nux vomica (poison-nut)

This remedy picture describes babies who find sleep difficult, particularly at night. Those whom this remedy will suit tend to develop colic when they are uncovered. Umbilical hernias occur in this type of baby.

### Opium (dried latex of poppy)

This remedy picture describes drowsy babies with hard, bloated abdomens, who find defecation almost impossible. Their faeces are rock hard. With this picture, an umbilical hernia is common.

### Plumbum metallicum (lead)

This remedy picture describes babies who have excessive bouts of colic, giving pain that they try to scratch away. They appear to have a lot of wind in their abdomens, but they are unable to pass any of it. With this picture, umbilical hernias are a common feature.

# Urinary tract infections

These infections cause babies to develop a fever but no particular cause for this is ever found. It is important to fully investigate such babies, particularly boys, as the infection may be due to an abnormality of the urinary tract. Depending on the precise diagnosis, the treatment is determined accordingly. Generally a high fluid intake is indicated in order to prevent recurrent urinary infections. Cranberry juice acts as an antiseptic drink.

# *Infants*

This section covers children between the ages of six weeks and five years. Many of the problems of infants at least up to the age of one year will be the same as for babies (*see above*) and the same remedies will apply.

## Balanitis

This is an infection of the glans penis that results in a pustular discharge from the foreskin.

The conventional treatment is to use antibiotics.

The homeopathic treatment is to use one of the following remedies. Select the one whose picture matches the physical symptoms; this may be difficult as the presence of pus will mask any early signs. Using the 6c potency, give one dose four times a day, for a maximum of ten doses.

### *Causticum* (Hahnemann's mixture of quicklime [calcium oxide] and potassium bisulphate)

This remedy picture describes red spots on the glans penis with a discharge from this area.

### *Rhus toxicodendron* (poison ivy)

This remedy picture describes a swollen foreskin with pus coming out from the glans penis. The body of the penis may also be swollen. Using the 6c potency, give one dose four times a day, for a maximum of ten doses.

If these infections become recurrent, a surgical procedure – CIRCUMCISION – is indicated, for which post-operative homeopathic treatment is available.

# Bedwetting

Most infants should have bladder control by the age of 18 months, although about 10 per cent of five-year-olds still wet their beds. The homeopathic treatment available for this condition is discussed in the section on ENURESIS on p. 226.

# Bronchiolitis

This is a viral infection that causes infants to wheeze, and often occurs after they have caught a COLD. It is uncommon after the age of 18 months. It is potentially dangerous in infants under the age of six months when it can cause HEART FAILURE and PNEUMONIA.

The conventional treatment is to put the infant into a warm, steamy environment.

The homeopathic treatment is to deal with the symptoms of the primary cold (see p. 9), particularly the A, B, C treatment: using the 6c potency, give one dose of each remedy in rotation every ten minutes.

If the infant is not responding and is becoming even more distressed, summon medical help. In the meantime, give one of the following remedies by matching the pictures with the physical symptoms.

### *Antimonium tartaricum* (antimonium tartrate)

This remedy picture describes exhausted infants who have difficulty breathing because they feel too weak. They suck in their nostrils with the effort of breathing, and they are too weak to cough up any phlegm. They may also vomit. Using the 6c potency, give one dose every five minutes.

### *Carbo vegetabilis* (vegetable charcoal)

This remedy picture describes infants who look ill and have cold sweat on their bodies. Their lips may be blue and their breathing wheezy. Using the 6c potency, give one dose every five minutes.

# Constipation

The definition of constipation is not the absence of a daily bowel movement but the difficult passage of a hard, small stool. The treatment (conventional and homeopathic) has been discussed in the section on constipation on p. 000. When using the homeopathic remedies outlined there, the broad guidelines about diet and probiotic therapy still apply. The recommended dosage is to use the 6c potency and give one dose twice a day for as long as necessary. Give this in liquid form: one dose is two drops (for babies over 5.4kg (12 lb) in weight).

Breastfed babies are never constipated unless there is a medical problem, primarily Hirschsprung's disease where the nerve supply to the lowest section of the bowel is absent. The conventional treatment for this condition is surgery. However, bottle-fed babies can become constipated. It is important to exclude any pathological reason for constipation in babies.

If babies become constipated and there is no disease or other condition, give them as much water-based liquid as possible. The natural laxatives can also be considered but great care must be taken not to overdose them.

The only homeopathic remedy that can be used is **Senna** (cassia acutifolia), which has a remedy picture that describes a constipated baby who suffers from a lot of wind colic and flatulence.Using the 6c potency, give one drop three times a day until the constipation begins to resolve, at which stage the frequency of doses can be reduced.

# Coughs

This distressing symptom is one of the commonest in infants seen by general practitioners. It may represent an upper respiratory tract illness that produces catarrh, which infants attempt to keep off their lungs by coughing. More seriously, however, it may represent a lower respiratory tract infection and the infants attempt to cough up infected mucus from their lungs. Or it may just be that a person within the home is smoking cigarettes. In any event, a precise diagnosis must be established before embarking on any treatment.

Homeopathic treatments for COUGHS are discussed on p. 11. Other remedies can be found for LARYNGITIS (p. 111), BRONCHITIS (p. 109) and ASTHMA (p. 94).

# Croup

This distressing illness affects babies and young children, and is usually caused by a virus, and can follow a COLD. A spasm of the vocal cords makes inhaling difficult, causing a feeling of suffocation and an abnormal breathing noise called "stridor", which causes anxiety not only in the child but also in the parents. **This illness must be taken seriously. If the lips of the child with croup begin to go blue, it is vital to summon immediate medical help.**

The air that affected children breathe must be made as humid as possible, by creating a lot of steam in the room. This can be done by boiling a kettle or saucepan full of water. Alternatively, placing the child in a bathroom with the hot water running in the tub or shower will be beneficial.

The following remedies are useful to help alleviate the croup. These can given as either a powder or liquid and placed on the lips or exposed tongue of the affected child. Tablets can be crushed to reduce them to a powder. Use these remedies only if the child's lips remain pink; if they begin to go blue (indicating that there is insufficient oxygen in the bloodstream), it is imperative that immediate medical attention is sought.

### *Aconitum napellus* (monk's-hood)

This is the remedy of first choice, to be used as soon as the croup starts. Using the 30c potency, give one dose, then repeat in 15 minutes. (Parents can also take this remedy to alleviate their entirely suitable anxiety.)

If there is no improvement in the child, go on to:

## *Hepar sulphuris* (Hahnemann's calcium sulphide)

This follows *Aconitum napellus*. It describes symptoms that are made worse in a cold environment and where there are cold draughts, reinforcing the importance of keeping the child in a warm, humid environment. Using the 30c potency, give one dose and repeat in one hour's time if there is no improvement and providing that the child's lips are still pink.

If there is still no improvement in the croup and the child's lips are pink, go on to:

## *Spongia tosta* (roasted sponge)

This remedy picture describes affected children who wake up with the croupy cough, which is worse when their heads are low and when they try to talk. Using the 30c potency, give one dose and then repeat after one hour.

Following this, if there is no improvement and the lips are still pink, give two more doses of *Hepar sulphuris*, rotating with *Spongia tosta* for two doses and so on.

# Dental problems

These problems (including fear of going to the dentist) are discussed on p. 60. The following remedies are indicated for children. Using the 30c potency, give one dose daily.

## *Cina* (worm seed)

This remedy picture describes whining children who are spiteful, cross, oversensitive to pain and uncooperative, and do not want to be touched, carried around the room or even looked at. The children that this remedy suits may have suffered from THREAD-WORMS in the past.

### *Chamomilla* (camomile)

This remedy picture describes children who whine and are cross and oversensitive to pain but can be quietened by being carried around or cuddled. The characteristic feature of this remedy picture is that the child has one red cheek while the other is normal in colour.

It is recommended that *Arnica* (leopard's bane) is given after any dental procedure: using the 30c potency, give one dose every three hours, for a maximum of ten doses. However, if an injection is to be given, *Arnica* should not be given beforehand, as this will make the pain of the dental procedure worse.

# Dyslexia

This difficulty in coping with written symbols, both letters and numbers, often leads to affected children being inappropriately labelled under-achievers. They find both reading and writing difficult and, as a result, lose confidence.

Once a correct diagnosis/assessment of dyslexia has been made, the conventional approach is special education.

Children with this difficulty will benefit from consulting a specialist homeopath who will be able to offer them a comprehensive homeopathic workup. If this is not possible, there is one homeopathic remedy that can also help. Using the 6c potency, give one dose daily.

### *Lycopodium* (club moss)

This remedy picture describes children who become confused over simple daily affairs and are fearful of starting new ventures. They have lost self-confidence and are in constant fear of breaking down under stress. They spell or write the wrong words or syllables, and are unable to read what they have just written. They commonly feel sad on waking up in the morning, and are afraid to be left alone. Using the 6c potency, give one dose twice a day for three weeks, stop the remedy for one week, and then repeat.

# Ear infections

These are common in children, giving symptoms of crying, fever and pain in the ear. Sometimes the infection causes the eardrum to burst as the build-up of pressure from the pus becomes greater than the strength of the eardrum membrane.

For the treatment of acute ear infections (*otitis media*), both conventional and homeopathic, *see* p. 39.

Some children develop recurring ear infections, in which case they should be taken to see a homeopathic specialist who will give advice about diet and prescribe constitutional homeopathic remedies. The conventional treatment for recurring ear infections is long-term antibiotic therapy. Recently, however, it has been shown that this therapy may be a factor in causing glue ear (*serous otitis media*). *See* p. 44 for remedies for treating this condition.

# Encopresis

This term describes the soiling of underwear with faeces by children who have been toilet trained. The usual cause is CON-STIPATION (*see* p. 406). It may also result from emotional difficulties, which will need psychological support. In this situation, the advice from a specialist homeopath, who will look at all the issues involved, can be invaluable.

# Feeding difficulties

Feeding difficulties can be a problem up to the age of one, and it is important to establish a correct diagnosis as these infants come into the category of "failure to thrive". For breastfed infants who are having some difficulty in retaining their feed, and provided that they are gaining weight satisfactorily, the homeopathic remedies discussed under "Feeding difficulties" in the "New-born babies" section (*see above*) will also apply to infants. The homeopathic remedies can also be used for bottle-fed infants, provided that weight gain is satisfactory; then a switch to a different preparation is indicated. (It was usual to switch to a soya milk substitute, but this practice has now been called into question because of soya milk's oestrogen content. Therefore soya milk should only be used under medical guidance.)

As children grow up, other factors that may cause feeding difficulties become important: food fads and food allergies, as well as medical conditions such as *pyloric stenosis* (a condition that begins with projectile vomiting caused by an obstruction of the outlet from the stomach) and, rarely, CROHN'S DISEASE. Food allergies can be diagnosed from an accurate medical history and from muscle testing (applied kinesiology). For bottle-fed infants, it is not uncommon to discover an allergy to cow's dairy products – milk, cheese and yoghurt. For them, a switch to goat's dairy products is indicated.

To treat feeding difficulties in general, the following remedies may help. Choose one by matching the remedy picture to the child's physical symptoms. Using the 6c potency, give one dose four times a day for one week, reducing to one dose twice a day until the child begins to feed properly.

### *Anacardium* (marking nut)

This remedy picture describes an infant whose appetite varies between no appetite and ravenous hunger.

### *Hellebore* (Christmas rose)

This remedy picture describes loss of appetite particularly for vegetables and meat. This remedy is associated with brain damage.

### *Hyoscyamus* (henbane)

This remedy picture describes children who dislike drinking water. They are also prone to attacks of hiccups.

### *Phosphoricum acidum* (phosphoric acid)

This remedy picture describes loss of appetite in children who crave juicy fluids and cold milk. They feel as if there is a weight in their stomachs.

### *Zincum chromatum* (zinc chromate)

This remedy picture describes conflict in that the children crave something but do not know what and, at the same time, have an aversion to even thinking about food.

# Febrile convulsions

This condition is *not* EPILEPSY, but a physical condition that causes similar symptoms to those of epilepsy but are brought on by a rapid rise in body temperature. It is not the height of the temperature that gives febrile convulsions (fits) but the rapidity with which the temperature rises. The first time this happens understandably causes much parental concern and anxiety. However, children who have febrile convulsions are no more likely to develop epilepsy than children who have no previous history of febrile convulsions.

The immediate first aid measure to take is to make sure that the airways of the children are clear so that they are able to breathe in an unobstructed way. They should also be sponged down with tepid water to bring their temperature down. Putting them near a fan will help as well.

The immediate conventional medical therapy is to give rectal diazepam when the fits last for more than a few minutes.

When an infant has been assessed as having a tendency to suffer from febrile convulsions, it is possible to use homeopathic remedies after following the aforementioned first aid advice. Select the remedy by matching its picture to the physical symptoms (a child who suffers from febrile convulsions tends to have the same type of fit on each occasion).

### *Aconitum napellus* (monk's-hood)

This is the remedy of first choice and is used in all cases at the first sign of any fever. It is then followed by the selective and more specific remedy. Give one dose of the 30c potency.

Having given this remedy, one of the following can be given five minutes later. Using the 30c potency, give one dose.

### *Aethusa cynapium* (fool's parsley)

This remedy picture describes electrical disturbances in the brain and nervous system associated with gastrointestinal disturbances. During the convulsions children's thumbs are clenched, their faces become red, their eyes turn downwards, their pupils dilate and become staring, and their mouths begin to foam.

### *Belladonna* (deadly nightshade)

This remedy picture describes febrile convulsions that are followed by a prolonged period of unconsciousness, which is then followed by nausea and vomiting.

### *Cina* (worm seed)

This remedy picture describes febrile convulsions in children who are fat, hungry and cross. Teeth grinding is a common feature. Before the convulsions occur, the children scream out. When they do occur, there are violent movements of arms and legs.

### *Hyoscyamus* (henbane)

This describes children who act in an unseemly way by frequently undressing themselves and exposing their genitals. They have difficulty in coordinating their arm movements.

### Nux vomica (poison-nut)

This remedy picture describes thin, overactive, nervous and irritable children who may have a liking for cola drinks (which contain caffeine).

### Opium (dried latex of poppy)

This remedy picture describes children whose febrile convulsions occur only at night. As well as the rapidly rising temperature, glaring lights, nightmares and being frightened by the sudden appearance of somebody in their bedrooms can all be precipitating causes.

## Gastroenteritis

**This is a serious condition because of the possibility of the infant becoming dehydrated, which will require hospitalization and intravenous rehydration.**

This condition has already been discussed in the section on newborn babies (see p. 396), and the homeopathic remedies discussed there will also apply to infants. In addition, because infants are beginning to eat solid food, the following remedies can also be used. Select one by matching its picture to the physical symptoms. Using the 6c potency, give one dose every 15 minutes, for a maximum of eight doses. If there is no improvement, call for medical help.

### Arsenicum album (arsenic trioxide)

This remedy picture describes children who vomit and have diarrhoea at the same time. They are cold and physically distressed.

### Cinchona officinalis (China) (Peruvian bark)

This remedy picture describes children with gastroenteritis who are very sensitive to the slightest touch. They are cold and vomit undigested food. Their faeces contain undigested food and are yellow and frothy. There is a lot of wind (flatus).

### *Dulcamara* (bittersweet)

This remedy picture describes gastroenteritis occurring in damp wet weather or if the children become chilled. The faeces are green-yellow, and blood or slime is present.

### *Phosphoricum acidum* (phosphoric acid)

This remedy picture describes gastroenteritis in an already weak infant. The diarrhoea is painless, profuse, yellow and contains undigested food particles.

### *Podophyllum* (may apple)

This remedy picture describes profuse, offensive stools that seem to drain affected children dry. This remedy particularly suits young children when their stool output appears greater than their food input, as the remedy picture describes children who have a desire for a lot of water but none for food. There is marked gurgling in the abdomen. The diarrhoea is worse in the morning. The children's heads sweat easily during sleep.

## Head banging

This condition, in which children bang their heads against a wall or against the side of their cots, is an expression of anger, possibly against their parents who may not be showing them affection.

The first thing to do is to show undiluted affection to these children.

The conventional treatment is to see a child psychiatrist.

The homeopathic approach is to see a specialist homeopath. If this is not possible, the following homeopathic remedies may help. Select one by matching its picture to the physical symptoms. Using the 6c potency, give one dose twice a day.

### *Chamomilla* (camomile)

This remedy picture describes angry infants who indulge in head banging. The only way to settle them is by carrying them around. A common feature of this remedy is for one cheek of the infant to be red while the other is pale.

### *Millefolium* (yarrow)

This is the remedy of first choice as its picture describes head banging against a wall.

### *Silicea* (pure flint)

This remedy picture describes withdrawn infants who bang their heads against anything in order to attract attention.

# Infectious diseases

This section includes the common infectious illnesses that infants typically suffer.

---

## Immunization

In the Western world, there is a routine schedule of immunization against the following diseases:

- DIPHTHERIA, pertussis (WHOOPING COUGH) and TETANUS – the DPT vaccine
- HAEMOPHILUS INFLUENZA b (Hib) – against one form of bacterial MENINGITIS
- MEASLES, MUMPS and RUBELLA (German measles) – the MMR vaccine
- POLIOMYELITIS

Recently there have been discussions about including the vaccine against HEPATITIS B. The incidence of this serious form of hepatitis is increasing at an alarming

---

rate worldwide. The vaccine is already included in the cocktail of immunizations in continental Europe but not in the United Kingdom, where it is only offered routinely to those babies considered at risk – i.e. those born to mothers who already have hepatitis B.

While there are homeopathic nosode preparations available for these illnesses, which some people may prefer (to avoid possible side-effects of the immunization and to strengthen babies' immune systems naturally), it is the author's opinion that these should not be used and that the conventional immunization schedule should be followed. For those who disagree with this, the alternative homeopathic nosode treatment will be mentioned after each infectious disease in the text.

Following these immunizations, infants may develop a fever. This is managed conventionally by giving liquid paracetamol. The homeopathic approach has already been discussed under "Fever" in the section on newborn babies (see above). If a fever develops, give a single dose of **Thuja occidentalis (arbor vitae)**, using the 30c potency.

### Chicken pox

This infectious illness is caused by the *herpes zoster* virus and is spread – via droplets from the mouth – quickly among groups of children. The incubation period is between 13 and 17 days, and the illness lasts about 10 days. It starts with the child feeling unwell with a possible mild fever. The following day, a blister-type, intensely itchy rash appears all over the body. Should an individual spot be scratched off, a permanent scar will remain. The child remains infectious while the blisters are present and is not infectious when they have formed scabs.

The *herpes zoster* virus that causes chicken pox also causes SHINGLES. The crossover of these two illnesses is uncertain, and it is not possible to say that an adult can catch shingles from being in contact with an infant who has chicken pox or vice versa.

The conventional treatment for chicken pox is to cool the skin down as much as possible to stop the itchiness. This is done by using calamine lotion.

The following homeopathic remedies can be used instead. Using the 6c potency, give one dose every hour as necessary, reducing to one dose every four hours as soon as possible.

### *Antimonium tartaricum* (antimonium tartrate)

This remedy picture describes a blister-type rash in children who whine every time they are touched. They may feel as if there is a band around their forehead.

### *Pulsatilla* (wind flower)

This remedy picture describes a blister-type rash in children who are exceptionally clingy and not very thirsty. They feel noticeably better in a cooler environment.

### *Rhus toxicodendron* (poison ivy)

This remedy picture describes a blister-type rash in children who are particularly restless. This remedy is probably the first choice in treating chicken pox.

### *Diphtheria*

This highly infectious condition is caused by the diphtheria bacillus. It is very rare nowadays because of the successful immunization programme. The incubation period is two to six days. The initial symptoms are a fever, sore throat and swollen glands in the neck. Slowly a membrane spreads over the tonsils and palate and possibly down to the larynx (voicebox), so that breathing is obstructed and an emergency laryngectomy has to be carried out. Serious complications can arise if a toxin (poison) produced by the bacilli enters the bloodstream.

The conventional treatment is with penicillin and diphtheria anti-toxin.

In the unlikely event of a diphtheria epidemic, and if an infant has not been immunized against the disease, homeopathy can be considered, but it should only be used in an emergency, while awaiting medical help. Using the 6c potency, give one dose every 15 minutes until help arrives.

### *Apis mellifica* (honey bee)

This remedy picture describes a red throat with stinging pains on swallowing, which are relieved by drinking cold liquids. Children quickly become very ill, and the backs of their throats become swollen.

### *Lachesis* (bushmaster snake venom)

This remedy picture describes a sore throat with the pain extending into the ear. The exterior of the throat is so sensitive that children loosen any clothing worn around this area.

### *Mercurius cyanatus* (mercury cyanide)

This remedy picture describes a sore throat with particular destruction of the soft palate. This remedy was used exclusively to treat diphtheria before any immunisation programme was started and before penicillin was discovered.

### *Measles*

This highly infectious viral disease is spread by droplet infection from the upper respiratory tract. Breastfed infants are protected from this illness by the antibodies contained in their mothers' milk. The early stages of this illness, which has an incubation period of 10 or 11 days, give symptoms of a sore throat and runny eyes, followed a day later by a very high temperature and the appearance of Koplick's spots, tiny grey-white spots inside the cheeks. These spots allow the positive diagnosis of measles even before the characteristic rash appears, starting on the face and spreading to the trunk. It is red, flat and not itchy. The rash begins to fade after about three or four days, at which time the fever begins to drop. The child remains infectious for five days from the onset of the rash.

The infant is best nursed in a darkened room as the eyes become very sensitive to light (*photophobia*). There is no conventional treatment for measles, apart from establishing the diagnosis and checking to make sure no complications are developing, such as EAR INFECTIONS (*otitis media*; *see above*), chest infections, FEBRILE CONVULSIONS and, relatively rarely, encephalitis (a form of brain infection). There are conventional treatments for these conditions as well as homeopathic remedies where appropriate; see the relevant sections.

The homeopathic treatment for measles varies according to the stage of the illness:

BEFORE ANY SYMPTOMS
- If children have not been immunized against measles and there is a current epidemic, it is possible to give *Morbillinum* (measles virus nosode) in the 30c potency to protect them from catching the disease. One dose of this preparation is given every 12 hours, for three doses.

PRE-RASH STAGE
- *Aconitum napellus* (monk's-hood) or *Belladonna* (deadly nightshade): the indication for either of these remedies is a sudden onset of fever with symptoms of an upper respiratory tract infection. Using the 30c potency, give one dose daily for three days.
- All feverish children should be encouraged to drink plenty of fluids. If they are not thirsty, give *Pulsatilla* (wind flower). Using the 30c potency, give one dose a day for three days.
- If children have red, sore eyes that are running a lot, give *Euphrasia* (eyebright). Using the 6c potency, give one dose every two hours.

RASH STAGE
- *Bryonia* (wild hops): this remedy picture describes a rash that appears suddenly. The children are irritable with a high fever, and they feel better with cold things. Using the 6c

potency, give one dose four times a day for a maximum of twelve doses.
- *Pulsatilla* (wind flower): this remedy is useful for treating coughs after an attack of measles. Using the 30c potency, give one dose daily for three days.
- *Sulphur*: this remedy can be used to help clear the skin of a residual rash. Using the 30c potency, give one dose twice a day for two days.

### Meningitis

This condition is an inflammation of the lining of the brain (meninges) and it occurs in epidemics. It can be either viral (from which a full recovery is usually made) or bacterial, which can be life-threatening. The only way of distinguishing between the two is by a lumbar puncture, during which a sample of the cerebrospinal fluid that bathes the brain and spinal cord is taken from the lower part of the spine and examined. This will show whether or not meningitis is present and whether it is bacterial or viral. In the Western world, two types of bacterial meningitis are common: the one due to meningococcal infection and the one caused by *Haemophilus influenza* b (Hib) infection. There is now a vaccine for the latter (*see box*).

**Bacterial meningitis is very serious, requiring immediate diagnosis and treatment.** The symptoms are: a very high temperature, nausea and vomiting, a dislike of light (photophobia), headache with neck stiffness and increasing drowsiness. In about 50 per cent of cases, there is also a blotchy red rash. The possible complications of bacterial meningitis are brain damage, deafness or even death.

The conventional treatment, which is the first choice, is with antibiotics. Homeopathic treatment can be given after emergency medical help has been summoned. Select the remedy by matching its picture with the physical symptoms as closely as possible. Using the 6c potency, give one dose every 15 minutes.

### Apis mellifica (honey bee)

This remedy picture describes children who push their heads

backwards into their pillows. They are unable to hold their heads upright.

### Belladonna (deadly nightshade)

This remedy picture describes children who pull at their hair and complain of a throbbing, hammering headache that is worse at the sides of their heads (the temples). The headache is made worse from any movement and is made slightly easier by putting a band on to their heads and by bending their heads backwards.

### Gelsemium (yellow jasmine)

This remedy picture describes children with headaches situated at the backs of their heads, associated with dilated pupils. Later they develop a pressure pain on the tops of their heads, which extends into their shoulders. Following on from this, they notice a pain at the sides of their heads (temples), which extends into their ears, noses and finally their chins. Finally they notice soreness of their scalps before becoming drowsy.

### Veratrum viride (white American hellebore)

This remedy picture describes children who develop giddiness with nausea and sudden prostration. These symptoms are made worse when they close their eyes and when they rest their heads. Their heads are forced backwards as they begin to notice pain in the backs of their heads, associated with a dimming of vision.

#### Mumps

This viral condition causes swelling of the parotid glands (located just inside the angles of the jaws) and, sometimes, the ovaries, testes and pancreas. It is spread by droplet infection from the upper respiratory tract. The incubation period is between 14 and 28 days and children remain infectious for as long as the swellings are present. Apart from these symptoms, fever is common, and there is the possibility of "mumps meningitis", which usually clears up with no ill effects. Children can be immunized against mumps (*see box*).

Even though the reproductive organs are affected, sterility is a very rare occurrence.

The treatment, both conventional and homeopathic, is to make children rest and give them plenty of fluids. It is advisable not to give any liquids with a citric taste as this will stimulate the salivary glands, causing extra pain.

The homeopathic nosode is *Parotidinum* (parotid gland infected with mumps). Using the 30c potency, give one dose every 12 hours, for three doses.

The following specific homeopathic remedies can be given to help alleviate the symptoms of mumps. Match the picture of the remedy with the physical symptoms. Using the 6c potency, give one dose daily for seven days.

## Mercurius solubis (black oxide of mercury)

This remedy picture describes parotid glands swollen mainly on the right side, associated with dry lips that may become cracked in the corners. The children's mouths emit a foul odour and their tongues become floppy. They commonly say that they have a metallic taste in their mouths.

## Phytolacca (poke root)

This remedy picture describes salivary glands under the jaw – the submandibular salivary glands – which are swollen: These can be quite hard but tender to the touch, and the pain from them is commonly referred to the ears.

## Rhus toxicodendron (poison ivy)

This remedy picture describes a left-sided parotid gland infection. Children may feel that there is something in their ears (when there isn't).

## Sulphur iodatum (sulphur iodide)

This remedy picture describes a persistently enlarged parotid gland following a bout of the mumps.

## Rheumatic fever

This condition occurs particularly in children who live in damp conditions and represents an allergic reaction induced by a streptococcal sore throat. The initial symptoms include: a sore throat with a fever, tender, swollen joints and a red, blotchy rash. The long-term problems that this illness can cause give this illness its importance. It can cause RHEUMATIC HEART DISEASE and brain damage – in particular, Sydenham's CHOREA.

The conventional treatment is with penicillin and bedrest. To prevent the long-term complications, penicillin will continue to be prescribed for months or even years.

The homeopathic approach includes bedrest together with the following remedies.

### Aconitum napellus (monk's-hood)

The remedy picture describes a very anxious child. This remedy is given in the immediate feverish stage. Using the 6c potency, give one dose every 30 minutes, for a maximum of six doses.

### Bryonia (wild hops)

This remedy picture describes irritable children whose joint pains are made worse from the slightest movement. This makes them antisocial, wishing to be left alone. They desire long drinks, particularly cold ones, although their tongues remain dry. Using the 30c potency, give one dose daily, for a maximum of seven doses.

### Dulcamara (bittersweet)

This remedy picture describes an illness brought on by damp weather. Using the 6c potency, give one dose four times a day, for a maximum of 12 doses.

### Mercurius solubis (black oxide of mercury)

This remedy picture describes children who sweat profusely, and whose sweat smells offensive. They also produce a lot of saliva. Using the 30c potency, give one dose twice a day for a maximum of twelve doses.

### *Pulsatilla* (wind flower)

This remedy picture describes children who feel better in the fresh air and feel worse when exposed to a hot environment and after eating fatty foods. They are very tearful and respond positively and eagerly to being cuddled. Using the 6c potency, give one dose four times a day for three days.

#### *Roseola infantum*

This viral infection produces a fever that lasts four or five days; when it drops, a rash appears that lasts a day or two. There may also be a sore throat and swollen neck glands.

The conventional treatment is to sponge the child's body with tepid water and to give paracetamol, both of which should help to lower the body temperature.

The homeopathic treatment is to use one of the following remedies. Select the picture that most closely matches the physical symptoms. Using the 6c potency, give one dose four times a day, for a maximum of ten doses.

### *Belladonna* (deadly nightshade)

This remedy picture describes children with *Roseola infantum* who become delirious with the fever, having widely dilated pupils and a rapid heart rate.

### *Phytolacca* (poke root)

This remedy picture describes children with *Roseola infantum* who have particularly tender and swollen lymph glands under their jaws, the pain of which is referred into their ears on swallowing. These painful symptoms are relieved when swallowing cold drinks.

### *Pulsatilla* (wind flower)

This describes children with *Roseola infantum* whose general nature is to be very much in need of physical comfort. They prefer fresh air, dislike hot environments and have no thirst.

### Rubella (German measles)

This viral illness has an incubation period of between 14 and 21 days and is spread by oral droplet infection. The symptoms are mild, lasting a few days only. There is a mild fever, swollen glands behind the ears and a fine reddish non-itchy rash that starts on the face and then spreads to the rest of the upper body. The only serious complication is a rare form of encephalitis.

This mild illness is really only significant because of the damage it can cause to unborn babies when pregnant women catch rubella within the first three months of pregnancy. This damage can include deafness, heart disease, mental handicap, cataract and other eye disorders, cerebral palsy and bone abnormalities. All pregnant women are given blood tests to check their immunity against rubella. Ideally this check should be made before conception so that immunization (*see box*) can be offered.

The homeopathic immunization would be to use **Rubella** nosode. Using the 30c potency, give one dose every 12 hours, for three doses.

When children catch rubella, the most that can be done is simply to make them comfortable, as it is such a mild illness.

The following homeopathic remedies will help shorten the duration of the illness. Select the remedy by matching its picture to the physical symptoms. Using the 6c potency, give one dose four times a day for two days.

### Belladonna (deadly nightshade)

This remedy picture describes excitable children who have become distressed with the fever. Their pulse rates are high and their pupils are widely dilated.

### Bryonia (wild hops)

This remedy picture describes irritable children who dislike being touched or picked up.

### Pulsatilla (wind flower)

This remedy picture describes children who prefer being in the fresh air and dislike fatty food and a warm environment. They have no thirst for liquids.

A common problem following a bout of rubella is that children complain of joint pains. The conventional treatment is with paracetamol. The homeopathic treatment is described in the section on OSTEOARTHRITIS.

### Scarlet fever and scarlatina

Scarlet fever, a streptococcal infection, was once a very serious illness. However, over the last 30–40 years, it has become far less dangerous (and far less common), and so some people now call it "scarlatina" to signify its lessened virulence.

The symptoms of scarlet fever include fever, sore throat, flushed face (except around the mouth), a white-coated tongue with red spots (the "strawberry tongue") that later becomes completely bright red, and a widespread red rash. When skin covered by this rash is pressed, the area remains white for some time, and when the rash fades, the skin – particularly of the hands and feet – may peel. The possible rare computations are RHEU-MATIC HEART DISEASE and NEPHRITIS.

The conventional treatment is penicillin or erythromycin.

The homeopathic treatment is with one of the following remedies. Using the 6c potency, give one dose every 30 minutes. If there is no sign of improvement after ten doses, seek medical help.

### Ailanthus glandulosa (Chinese sumach)

This remedy picture describes an irregular-shaped, livid red rash that disappears on pressure.

### Apis mellifica (honey bee)

This remedy picture describes a rosy red skin that is sensitive, sore and hot and breaks into a sweat frequently.

### *Belladonna* (deadly nightshade)

This remedy is the usual homeopathic remedy for this condition. The skin is bright red and quite dry. The child becomes delirious with a rapid heart rate and widely dilated pupils. This remedy can also be given to protect children who have come into contact with others with scarlet fever: using the 30c potency, give one dose daily for one week.

### *Tetanus*

This condition occurs when the spores of the bacterium *Clostridium tetani* get into the bloodstream via a dirty wound. The toxin released by the spores causes the muscles of the body to go into spasm, beginning with those of the throat and resulting in " lockjaw". **This is potentially a life-threatening illness, requiring immediate medical attention.** This means immediate intubation to sustain the airway. The person is nursed in a darkened room, sedated with a muscle relaxant (diazepam) and given antitoxin therapy.

Virtually all babies in the developed world are immunized against tetanus (*see box*); booster injections are recommended every ten years. The homeopathic equivalent is a nosode preparation of *Clostridium* spores. Using the 30c potency, give one dose every 12 hours, for a maximum of three doses.

The following homeopathic remedies can be given to children suspected of developing tetanus. Using the 6c potency, give one dose every five minutes, having first called for medical help.

### *Belladonna* (deadly nightshade)

This remedy picture describes spasms of the limbs. Sufferers sit with their legs crossed and are unable to uncross them.

### *Cicuta virosa* (water hemlock)

This remedy picture describes jerking movements of the arms and fingers. The feet and toes turn inwards and upwards in spasm.

## *Hydrocyanic acid* (prussic acid)

This remedy picture describes spasmodic constriction of the larynx (voicebox), giving a feeling of suffocation. This is rapidly followed by spasms all over the body and collapse.

## *Strychninum* (alkaloid of Nux vomica)

This remedy picture describes spasms and twitching of the whole body, with an inability to breathe properly. The person sweats profusely.

### *Whooping cough (pertussis)*

This highly infectious bacterial illness mainly affects babies and young children, although it can also affect adults. It can be fatal in very young babies if the complication of pneumonia sets in. The incubation period is between one and two weeks, and sufferers remain infectious for as long as they have the characteristic whoop. The illness starts with a mild fever, runny nose and a general feeling of not being well. After three days, this progresses to the spasmodic cough with the characteristic "whoop" when sufferers inhale. While coughing continuously, their faces go red and they usually vomit. The conventional treatment is to give antibiotic therapy for the acute attack.

Routine immunization with the triple vaccine (diphtheria, tetanus and whooping cough) is the conventional method of prevention. The whooping cough (pertussis) vaccine is prepared from attenuated strains of the bacteria that cause whooping cough. There was once much concern about the side-effects of the vaccine, principally brain damage, but these have been much reduced. Therefore, conventional immunization is highly recommended. The homeopathic way of preventing whooping cough – using the nosode *Pertussin* (**whooping cough bacteria**) – has been discontinued.

An attack of whooping cough can be treated homeopathically. Giving children antioxidant therapy (*see* p. 25) and probiotics (*see* p. 27) will help boost their weakened immune systems. Ideally specialist homeopaths should be consulted, who will be able to give the children their constitutional remedies. If this is not possible, one of the following remedies can be used. Select the appropriate one by matching its picture to the physical symptoms. Using the 6c potency, give one dose every four hours for two days, reducing to one dose four times a day until the coughing begins to subside.

### *Belladonna* (deadly nightshade)

This remedy picture describes whooping cough with pain in the stomach before each attack. Coughing up blood (haemoptysis) is common in this remedy picture. The cough is worse at night.

### *Carbo vegetabilis* (vegetable charcoal)

This remedy picture describes whooping cough in which the children's faces have a bluish look.

### *Cina* (worm seed)

This remedy picture describes whooping cough that causes children to produce a lot of tears and gives them such pain in the breast bone (sternum) that they feel as if something has been torn off. They are afraid to speak or move for fear of bringing on another attack of coughing. After each coughing attack, they moan, gasp for air and turn pale.

### *Drosera* (sundew)

This remedy picture describes whooping cough sufferers who feel as if a feather is in their larynxes (voiceboxes); this is made worse when they lie down and particularly after midnight. Because they feel that the cough is coming from their stomachs, they hold their sides. The cough is always followed by retching and vomiting.

### *Ipecacuanha* (ipecac root)

This remedy picture describes whooping cough associated with nose bleeds and bleeding from the mouth. The children retch and stiffen, finally vomiting. They feel better by stepping outside into the fresh air.

### *Mephitis* (skunk)

This remedy picture describes whooping cough with very few coughing attacks during the day but many at night. The attacks are made worse when sufferers talk or drink.

### *Nux vomica* (poison-nut)

This remedy picture describes whooping cough that produces a splitting headache so that sufferers have to hold their heads while they cough.

### *Pulsatilla* (wind flower)

This remedy picture describes whooping cough in which sufferers feel better when sitting upright and worse in hot conditions. The cough is looser in the morning and tends to be dry in the evening and at night.

### *Stramonium* (thorn apple)

This remedy picture describes whooping cough that is made worse when sufferers look at light, a fire or bright objects. The cough causes jerking movements of their lower limbs while they are sitting.

### *Veratrum album* (white hellebore)

This remedy picture describes whooping cough that may have been diagnosed late. The spasmodic cough causes retching which is worse when sufferers drink cold fluids. They commonly lose the use of their voices. The coughing bouts are made worse whenever they move from a cooler room to a warmer one.

After the attack, infants are prone to develop recurrent upper and lower respiratory tract infections. These are treated homeopathically as described on pp. 9–38 and pp. 93–124.

# Sleep problems

NIGHT CRYING has already been discussed in the section on newborn babies. In infants, the same homeopathic remedies can also be used, but other indications may be apparent, and for this reason, other homeopathic remedy pictures will be described. Using the 6c potency, give one dose one hour before the child goes to bed.

### Aconitum napellus (monk's-hood)

This remedy is applicable whenever an infant has been subjected to a frightening experience.

### Chamomilla (camomile)

This remedy picture describes an infant who can only settle down to sleep after being carried around the bedroom.

### Coffea cruda (unroasted coffee)

This remedy picture describes a sleepless infant who has been overstimulated during the day.

### Nux vomica (poison-nut)

This remedy picture describes an infant who persistently wakes up at about 4.00 am.

# Still's disease

This condition is an autoimmune disease that usually begins in children aged between the ages of two and four or at puberty. The symptoms are similar to those of adult RHEUMATOID ARTHRITIS. The disease begins with sudden joint stiffness and swelling, accompanied by a fever, and it usually spontaneously subsides after several years.

The conventional treatment is with nonsteroidal anti-inflammatory drugs, and possibly steroid therapy as well.

The homeopathic approach is to give antioxidant supplements (*see* p. 25) and an appropriate diet (raw organic carrots, vitamin C, vitamin E with selenium), recognizing that this illness is an autoimmune disease. The child's constitutional remedy should be assessed by a specialist homeopath. If this is not possible, the following remedies can be used. Select the appropriate one by matching the physical symptoms with its remedy picture. Using the 6c potency, give one dose twice a day.

### *Aconitum napellus* (monk's-hood)

This remedy picture describes children who suddenly develop this form of arthritis in cold, dry weather. They have a high temperature (104°F/40°C), are thirsty but are not sweaty. They are restless and anxious, and the symptoms are worse during the night.

### *Belladonna* (deadly nightshade)

This remedy picture describes acute rheumatoid arthritis in children whose affected joints are red, hot and sore and burn. The pains come and go suddenly and are made worse from movement or the slightest jar to the body. This remedy picture has two peculiar symptoms: sufferers crave lemon juice, which makes the joint pains better; and the symptoms are made worse when they get their hair wet or have their hair cut.

433

### Bryonia (wild hops)

This remedy picture describes children with red, swollen and stiff joints that give a stitching pain that is made worse from the slightest movement. They are thirsty for large volumes of liquids, yet have a dry coated tongue. They prefer to be left alone.

### Cimicifuga racemosa (black snake root)

This remedy picture describes rheumatoid arthritis, the symptoms of which are mainly in the muscle bulk. It particularly affects sufferers' necks and they cannot turn their heads. The symptoms are made worse from damp, cold conditions and from any mental stress.

### Ledum (marsh tea)

This remedy picture describes children whose arthritis is relieved by cold applications. The pains are worse at night, particularly from the heat of the bedclothes so that sufferers prefer to be uncovered. This last symptom is shared with *Mercurius solubis*, except that the *Ledum* remedy picture does not include sweating.

### Manganum aceticum (manganese acetate)

This remedy picture describes acute rheumatoid arthritis in children, where the outer lining of their bones (periosteum) is sore, particularly that covering the bones of their lower legs. The bones are sensitive to the touch, and the arthritis wanders from joint to joint. Sufferers cannot bear their weight on their heels and so walk tip-toe. They have a fear that "something is going to happen" and feel better physically and emotionally when lying down.

### Mercurius solubis (black oxide of mercury)

This remedy picture describes children with acute rheumatoid arthritis who have thickly coated tongues and produce a profuse amount of offensive sweat, particularly when covered by their bedclothes at night.

## *Pulsatilla* (wind flower)

This remedy picture describes rheumatoid arthritis, the symptom picture of which changes quickly from joint to joint. The symptoms are made worse by complete bedrest and are improved by slow, gentle movement. Heat and wet weather make the joint symptoms worse. The child whom this remedy suits has no thirst.

## *Rhus toxicodendron* (poison ivy)

This describes children whose rheumatoid arthritis is worse on initial movement but is relieved by continued movement until the joints become fatigued and painful again. They are restless, trying to create the conditions that they know will alleviate the pain. Symptoms are improved by heat and made worse from anything cold. Sufferers dislike bathing and washing.

# Teething

This can cause sore gums, irritability and gastrointestinal upsets with a fever. The child's face becomes red (occasionally one cheek is red while the other is of normal colour) and he or she is miserable. The first tooth appears about the age of six months and all the "milk" teeth are through by the age of about three years. Sucking a plastic ring containing frozen fluid helps soothe sore gums. Homeopathic remedies are also helpful. Using the 6c potency, give one dose hourly for a maximum of six doses in any day.

## *Aconitum napellus* (monk's-hood)

This remedy picture describes children with fever and a dry, hot skin, who gnaw their fists and cry incessantly. They are likely to have a FEBRILE CONVULSION if they have already suffered from one. Certainly they will show jerking and twitching movements.

### *Belladonna* (deadly nightshade)

This remedy picture describes children with red faces, dry, hot skin, widely dilated pupils and, like *Aconitum*, jerky, twitchy movements. The fever can make them delirious, in which case they bite and strike out as if they want to escape.

### *Calcarea carbonica* (calcium carbonate)

This remedy suits children who are overweight and fair-haired and sweat profusely from their heads. In this type of child, teething is associated with a cough or diarrhoea.

### *Chamomilla* (camomile)

This remedy is the most commonly used to help teething, and it is particularly useful in treating diarrhoea in young children when it is associated with teething. The picture describes children who are oversensitive to pain and become very irritable as a result. They can only be quietened by being carried around or cuddled. Typically one cheek is hot and red while the other is normal in colour and cold. Temperamentally, these children are frantic, as if they "cannot bear it anymore". Abdominal COLIC is usually present, as is vomiting, and there may be fever.

### *Kreosotum* (beechwood kreosote)

This remedy picture describes diarrhoea occurring in the teething infant. The diarrhoea is extremely offensive in smell and is associated with incessant vomiting. Not unnaturally, the infant is very irritable (as with *Chamomilla*) and feels better by being wrapped up warmly and from being carried around.

## Delayed eruption of teeth

As children develop, their teeth should appear in a definite order. If there is a delay, *Calcarea carbonica* (calcium carbonate) can be taken. Using the 30c potency, give one dose twice a week (but not on consecutive days) as a long-term therapy.

## Temper tantrums

These occur if the immediate needs of the infant are not met, leading to outbursts of emotion that can be vocal and/or physical. They can be very trying for parents who have to find a compromise between defining boundaries and giving unconditional love.

Food allergies are a possible cause of this unsociable behaviour, and the exclusion of junk foods, many of which contain great numbers of additives, is an immediate and important first step. Applied kinesiology can be used to identify other possible food allergies.

The following homeopathic remedies will help. Using the 6c potency, give one dose twice a day for ten days. Should the condition still be causing difficulties, consult a specialist homeopath.

### *Chamomilla* (camomile)

This remedy picture describes impatient, angry children who are impossible to please and can only be settled by being carried around.

### *Cina* (worm seed)

This remedy picture describes temper tantrums in chubby infants whose appetites are variable and who may grind their teeth at night, are generally excitable but irritable and may even suffer from FEBRILE CONVULSIONS. This remedy picture also includes infants infested with THREADWORMS, which may be the trigger for their behaviour.

### *Nux vomica* (poison-nut)

This remedy picture describes easily excitable infants who become much more difficult after a large meal and after drinking a cola drink (which contains caffeine).

## *Tuberculinum* (nosode from tubercular abscess)

This remedy picture describes contradictory infants who become irritable, particularly when woken up. They have a particular fear of dogs and of animals in general. They have episodes of showing a violent temper, wanting to fight and throw anything at anyone without necessarily needing a cause. They are always dissatisfied and are continually looking for something new to do, finding great difficulty in settling down to anything constructive. They may wake up in the middle of the night, screaming with anxiety.

# *Children*

T his section deals with difficulties in children between the
 ages of five and eleven.

## Abdominal migraine

In this condition, children suffer from periodic attacks of abdominal pain associated with nausea and possibly vomiting. They
look pale during an attack and may also have a fever. The attacks
may be precipitated by stress. This form of MIGRAINE may lead
on to the adult form.

The conventional treatment is with tranquillizers, possibly
rectal diazepam.

It is important to reassure affected children that there is
nothing seriously physically wrong with them. This reassurance
can be reinforced by appropriate psychotherapy.

Ideally these children should be taken to a specialist homeopath, who will be able to prescribe a constitutional remedy. If this
is not possible, one of the following homeopathic remedies may
help acute attacks. Using the 6c potency, give one dose every 15
minutes for four doses, reducing to one dose every hour for four
doses.

### *Argentum nitricum* (silver nitrate)

This remedy picture describes nervous children who fear heights
and crowded places and like sweets, for which they have a craving. Pain may radiate from a spot on their stomachs over their
abdomens. The picture describes nausea, retching and vomiting.
The children may also develop colicky pains in their abdomens,
associated with much wind. This pain is mainly sited under the
left ribs.

### *Cina* (worm seed)

This remedy picture describes children who are so stressed that they won't allow themselves to be touched. They seem to be hungry all the time, sometimes just after eating a meal. This remedy picture characteristically describes children who have THREADWORMS.

### *Colocynthis* (bitter cucumber)

This remedy picture describes children who can become easily stressed when irritated. They develop colicky abdominal pains that are only eased when they bend double, thereby putting pressure on their abdomens.

### *Magnesium phosphoricum* (magnesium phosphate)

This remedy picture describes children who develop colicky abdominal pains that are mainly relieved by direct warmth. They are unable to sleep or think clearly about anything other than the pain.

### *Pulsatilla* (wind flower)

This remedy picture describes children who develop stomach ache particularly after they have eaten a meal rich in fatty food. They cry easily and often, and crave physical reassurance and comfort. They prefer fresh air and dislike warm environments.

### *Staphysagria* (stavesacre)

This remedy picture describes children who are impetuous and have violent outbursts of passion. They are very sensitive to what others say about them. They develop abdominal migraine in the form of colicky abdominal pains after they have been angry.

# Asthma

This causes wheezy breathing as well as a persistent cough without any noticeable wheeze. Allergies are a possible cause: clues for the guilty allergen are found by taking a detailed personal history and, possibly, skin testing and applied kinesiology.

The conventional treatment is described on p. 94.

Homeopathic treatment includes miasm assessment (see p. 000) as well as symptomatic assessment, which will be obtained by consulting a specialist homeopath. The following homeopathic remedies should be considered after using the miasmic remedies where appropriate. Using the 6c potency, give one dose four times a day for one week, reducing to one dose twice daily for a further week.

### *Chamomilla* (camomile)

This remedy picture describes children who have asthma attacks after a fit of anger. Their breathing sounds as if the trachea (windpipe) has been tied up with string. They breathe easier when they hold their heads back and by breathing cool air and drinking cold water. They are irritable, hard to please and generally miserable and feel comforted by being carried around. Characteristically they have one flushed cheek while the other is normal in colour.

### *Ipecacuanha* (ipecac root)

This remedy picture describes children who, when having an asthma attack at night, have to sit up in order to breathe. They prefer to gasp for air at an open window and feel worse in a warm environment. While coughing, they often gag and vomit.

### *Natrum sulphuricum* (sodium sulphate)

This remedy picture describes breathing that is worse in damp weather and from damp housing conditions. The children feel worse lying on their left sides and, while lying down at night, are commonly seen to spring up in bed clutching their chests, saying that there is a pain in their lower left chest. The worst time for breathing is between 4.00 and 5.00 am.

### *Sambucus nigra* (elder)

In this remedy picture, children's general behaviour during asthma attacks includes suddenly springing out of bed. An attack usually starts at 3.00 am, quite suddenly and in a typical way: the children gasp for breath, begin to turn blue and seem to be dying; they then fall back to sleep, having stopped gasping and regained their normal colour, only to wake up again with another attack. This cycle is repeated over and over. These suffocative attacks may well not occur when the children are awake, but as soon as they fall asleep, the suffocative attacks restart. The skin of these children is dry and hot when they are asleep, but when they are awake, they sweat profusely.

## Constipation

Constipation in children is defined as delay or difficulty in defecation that causes them to become distressed. (It is not necessarily a description of the hardness of the stool, although the stool is often hard.) This constipation can cause soiling and ENCOPRESIS. If constipation in childhood is not treated correctly, it can lead on to megacolon (a grossly enlarged colon), impacted rectum and colon, and an increased incidence of ENTEROCOLITIS and possible perforation of the colon. Therefore it is important to treat childhood constipation seriously.

If there is any psychological reason for the constipation – such as school phobia or family stress – this must be adequately explored as an adjunct to practical treatment. The natural laxatives described on pp. 159 should be considered initially. The broad guidelines about diet and probiotic therapy, also found on those pages, apply to children, too.

There are several homeopathic remedies that can be used

alongside these laxatives. Using the 6c potency, give one dose four times a day until the constipation improves. At this stage, the dose can be slowly reduced. All these remedies can be given in liquid form to babies and very young children; one dose equals one drop.

### *Collinsonia canadensis* (stone-root)

This remedy picture describes children who may complain of a sensation of sharp sticks pressing into the rectum, which makes defecation difficult. This causes a build-up of faeces in the colon.

### *Parafene* (purified paraffin)

This remedy picture describes an obstinate constipation. The children have a frequent desire to defecate but with no result. They notice a pain in their lower abdomen, extending into their genital area, coccyx and rectum.

### *Psorinum* (scabies vesicle)

This remedy picture describes children whose constipation makes them cold so that they prefer to be wrapped up warmly. They probably have a sickly appearance.

The remedies contained in the main section on constipation (*see* p. 158) are also useful in childhood constipation.

## Growth problems

The heights and weights of children are usually assessed regularly throughout their development. The measurements are plotted on a "centile chart", one that gives the average measurements for height and weight for each age of a child. If children begin to "fall away" from their point on the graph, it is important to find out why. For this reason, a conventional medical work-up is essential.

Homeopathy can give an added boost to the general well-being of children through a constitutional remedy obtained from a specialist homeopath. If this is impossible, the following homeopathic remedies can be used. Using the 30c potency, give one dose weekly.

### *Baryta carbonicum* (barium carbonate)

This remedy picture describes children whose growth, both mental and physical, becomes retarded. These children tend to have repeated attacks of TONSILLITIS, which wears them down.

### *Calcarea carbonica* (calcium carbonate)

This remedy picture describes fat, sweaty children who may have large heads. Their scalps sweat a lot. Their milk teeth erupted later than normal, and they probably started walking later than normal as well.

### *Calcarea phosphorica* (calcium phosphate)

This remedy picture describes children who are delicate and either tall and thin or simply scrawny. Their skin is a dirty colour. They easily become anaemic following an illness.

### *Medorhinum* (gonorrhoea bacteria)

This remedy picture describes children who slowly lose weight because of a gradual loss of appetite. This appetite is stimulated when they are at the seaside.

### *Phosphoricum acidum* (phosphoric acid)

This remedy picture describes children who grow rapidly but become stressed physically and mentally from life in general and particularly following an illness.

### Phosphorus

This remedy picture describes children who grow rapidly and tend to stoop, but whose weight begins to lag behind. This remedy suits children who have a particular fear of thunderstorms.

### Silicea (pure flint)

This remedy picture describes children who are not gaining weight satisfactorily due to imperfect assimilation of their food during digestion. These children tend to have large heads, and they sweat profusely, particularly their feet. Generally they lack energy.

### Thyroidinum (extract from sheep's or cow's thyroid gland)

This remedy picture describes quick weight loss in children who develop a craving for huge quantities of sugar.

# Lack of confidence

At this stage of life, children begin to make friends, and peer group pressures start to emerge. Usually children are able to cope with these, but sometimes it can be a hard struggle. Gentle reassurance may be all that is necessary, but occasionally psychotherapy is needed.

Homeopathy is helpful in giving children a mental boost. Constitutional homeopathic remedies are the best way of doing this, and a consultation with a specialist homeopath is required. If this is not possible, the following homeopathic remedies can be used. Select one by matching its remedy picture with the physical symptoms. Using the 30c potency, give one dose twice a week, but not on consecutive days.

### *Anacardium* (marking nut)

This remedy picture describes ill-natured children who swear and curse a lot. They are particularly fearful of examinations as they find that they easily forget whole sections of work previously learned. They can give the impression of being absent-minded.

### *Argentum nitricum* (silver nitrate)

This remedy picture describes children who, for reasons they can't fathom, find going to school a terrifying experience. This difficulty is often associated with diarrhoea. These children seek comfort in sweets, and they also have a fear of heights and crowded places.

### *Causticum* (Hahnemann's mixture of quicklime [calcium oxide] with potassium bisulphate)

This remedy picture describes children who find that the least thing makes them cry. They feel sad and are burdened by the suffering of others. Thinking about their problems only makes their difficulties worse. WARTS are a common feature, particularly on the tips of the fingers.

### *Lycopodium* (club moss)

This remedy picture describes children who have an anticipatory anxiety, and yet, when the feared task has been completed, it is done successfully. They tend to write the wrong syllables of a word because they write in such a hurry, and they have difficulty in reading what they have written. They dislike being left alone, and prefer warm food and particularly sweet foods.

### *Pulsatilla* (wind flower)

This remedy picture describes children who cry easily and often. They are not particularly emotionally demonstrative, yet repeatedly want to be comforted physically. They dislike warm environments and prefer the fresh air. This remedy particularly suits blond-haired, blue-eyed children.

# Sleeping difficulties

This problem is usually the result of emotional difficulties, including school phobia. These need to be properly explored in order to understand the basis of the underlying difficulty. Reassurance and tolerance are the keynotes of treatment.

Simple methods of helping children to recover their sleeping patterns include:

- redefining bedtimes
- reducing the hours of television viewing
- making a reduction in the intake of caffeine (in, for example, cola drinks, chocolate, tea and coffee)
- avoiding late meals
- having a warm milky drink before going to bed
- taking a warm bath just before getting into bed

Conventional sleeping drugs are not recommended.

The following homeopathic remedies can be used as well as the above general advice. Using the child's constitutional remedy is the best way of helping him or her overcome this difficulty. This will be obtained by consulting a specialist homeopath.

If this is not possible, give one of the following homeopathic remedies, matching its picture with the physical symptoms. (Some of these remedies are also applicable to children who sleep walk.) Using the 6c potency, give one dose an hour before the child goes to bed.

### *Aconitum napellus* (monk's-hood)

This remedy picture describes sleeping difficulties in a child who has been subjected to a severe shock.

### *Argentum nitricum* (silver nitrate)

This remedy picture describes nervous children who find sleep difficult because they are worried about anything and everything. They crave sweets and dislike the heat. They have a particular fear of heights.

### *Calcarea carbonica* (calcium carbonate)

This remedy picture describes obstinate children who become anxious, particularly towards evening, and are easily frightened and commonly cry out in the night. The child that this remedy will suit sweats easily from the head, has a tendency to be overweight and is constipated.

### *Cina* (worm seed)

This remedy picture describes children who have THREAD-WORMS, which makes them irritable and quick-tempered. They are restless and have difficulty in falling asleep.

### *Cocculus* (Indian cockle)

This remedy picture describes children who can easily become overexcited, finding sleep difficult, and therefore become over-tired, starting a vicious circle.

### *Coffea cruda* (unroasted coffee)

This remedy picture describes bright children with overactive personalities and physical actions. They are happy to be awake at night, while other people in their house try to sleep in vain.

### *Gelsemium* (yellow jasmine)

This remedy picture describes children who become delirious on falling asleep, which makes them wake up screaming as though they are frightened of falling.

### *Ignatia* (St Ignatius' bean)

This remedy picture describes children who find difficulty with sleep following a shock, grief or disappointment over a broken friendship.

### *Kali bromatum* (potassium bromide)

This remedy picture describes children who are prone to sleep-walking. On other occasions, they wake up with night terrors and are generally very restless and fidgety.

### *Nux vomica* (poison-nut)

This remedy picture describes children who, in the middle of the night, become wide awake. If they are able to return to sleep, they do so deeply and are difficult to rouse in the morning. In general, they tend to be very critical of others and have high expectations of themselves.

### *Silicea* (pure flint)

This remedy picture describes children who show a tendency towards sleepwalking. The head of the child that this remedy will suit is large compared with their trunk. Their feet sweat easily and probably smell.

## Stammering

This speech impediment causes children much embarrassment, particularly when their peers mimic them. It is as if these children are thinking too quickly to formulate the proper word so that it comes out as a stammer. The precise cause for this difficulty is uncertain.

The conventional treatment is speech therapy.

The homeopathic approach is to use constitutional remedies, particularly when the child demonstrates underlying insecurities or nervousness. This will be obtained by consulting a specialist homeopath.

If this is not possible, the following homeopathic remedies may be tried. Match the remedy picture with the physical symptoms. Using the 6c potency, give one dose twice a day for up to one month.

### *Agaricus muscarius* (toadstool)

This remedy picture describes children who have generalized trembling and twitching that particularly affect their tongues. As a result of this, they stammer. This remedy also applies to children who have developed their walking and talking skills at a late stage.

### *Belladonna* (deadly nightshade)

This remedy picture describes excitable children who rush around generally, speak rapidly and often stammer as a result.

### *Bovista* (puff ball)

This remedy picture describes children who stammer. It also describes ECZEMA and a problem of easy bleeding.

### *Digitalis* (foxglove)

This remedy picture describes children who are worried about the future and find themselves stammering when talking to strangers.

### *Hyoscyamus* (henbane)

This remedy picture describes children who stammer only when they are talking very loudly.

### *Lycopodium* (club moss)

This remedy picture describes children who stammer on the last word of a sentence.

### *Mercurius solubis* (black oxide of mercury)

This remedy picture describes children who are nervous and talk in a hurried fashion. They have muscular tremors, particularly of their tongues, and as a result, they stammer. They produce a lot of saliva.

### *Nux vomica* (poison-nut)

This remedy picture describes children who stammer when they become angry. They are overly critical of others and can easily be irritated.

### *Stramonium* (thorn apple)

This remedy picture describes children who go completely over the top with violent muscular movements and vocal actions, which include a tendency to stammer.

# Threadworms

These tiny, shiny-white worms, about 2 cm (3/4 in) long, live in the rectum causing anal irritation and occasionally abdominal COLIC. When children scratch the anus and then suck their fingers, they reinfect themselves, creating a vicious circle.

The conventional treatment is to use anti-worm medications, as well as giving children explicit advice on the importance of handwashing after going to the toilet.

There are several homeopathic remedies that can be used to eradicate threadworms. Choose one by matching the physical symptoms to the remedy picture. Using the 6c potency, give one dose three times a day for at least two weeks. As with the conventional treatment, give specific advice about personal hygiene.

### *Caladium seguinum* (American arum)

This remedy picture describes itchiness in the genital area following infestation with threadworms.

### *Calcarea carbonicum* (calcium carbonate)

This remedy picture describes children who have a crawling sensation in their rectums, causing anal itchiness. The head of the child whom this remedy suits is large compared with their trunk; scalp perspiration is pronounced. He or she also has an obstinate personality.

### Cina (worm seed)

This remedy picture describes children with an itchy anus, whose stools contain threadworms. They also get colicky pains around their tummy button, which is eased by pressure. This remedy picture also describes an itchy nose that the children tend to pick at.

### Ferrum metallicum (iron)

This remedy picture describes threadworms in the stools of children who tend to have diarrhoea in the summer. The children are sensitive emotionally and excitable (which is aggravated by the least contradiction) and think that they are always in the right.

### Ratanhia (krameria-mapato)

This remedy picture describes children who feel as if their rectums are full of broken glass, and after they have passed a stool, they have a painful ache for hours afterwards. There is faecal oozing from the anus, which contains threadworms.

### Sabadilla (cevadilla seed)

This remedy picture describes children who have a crawling, itchy sensation in their anal area, which alternates with itchiness in their ears or noses. Threadworms are the cause of the anal symptoms. The child whom this remedy suits will also have violent sneezing attacks.

### Santoninum (santonin)

This remedy has a specific homeopathic action on the bladder (causing irritation), on threadworm infestations and on muscles (causing twitchy activity). It should be considered as the main alternative should the other remedies not work.

### *Teucrium marum* (cat thyme)

This remedy picture describes children who have an itchy anal area that keeps them awake at night. Their stools are found to contain threadworms.

### *Urtica urens* (stinging nettle)

This remedy picture describes children who have intense itching in their anuses due to the presence of threadworms. This remedy suits the child whose skin is very sensitive and who is allergic to many things.

# Tonsillitis

In children, tonsillitis is only a problem if it keeps recurring. Sometimes GLANDULAR FEVER presents as acute tonsillitis, and in these cases, the spleen will be enlarged. From all points of view, a precise diagnosis is important, and throat swabs – to culture the bacteria causing the acute tonsillitis, usually a streptococcus – and a blood test to rule out a diagnosis of glandular fever must be carried out.

The conventional approach is to treat each acute attack of tonsillitis with penicillin and to consider the surgical removal of the tonsils (tonsillectomy).

Because the tonsils are part of the immune system, some parents look to homeopathy to provide a different form of treatment for acute tonsillitis (*see* SORE THROATS AND TONSILLITIS). For recurrent attacks of tonsillitis, the opinion of a specialist homeopath is necessary. He or she will approach the problem from a miasmic angle (*see* p. 95), as well as giving dietary advice.

# *Adolescents*

This section covers young people between the ages of 11 and 18, after which their illnesses are classed as adult.

## Acne vulgaris

This condition of septic spots mainly on the face and back occurs at puberty and usually subsides as the person gets older, although occasionally it persists into later life. The spots can leave disfiguring scars. The primary causes of acne are a hormonal imbalance and mental stress, especially at examination times and, in young women, just before a period. It is important to lead a balanced life with sufficient amounts of rest and exercise and a good nutritious diet. Multi-vitamin and multi-mineral supplements are also helpful.

Should a septic spot arise, personal hygiene is important, particularly when a spot is squeezed (a practice to be discouraged). The conventional treatment is to use long-term antibiotic therapy, antiseptic soaps and creams, or preparations based on vitamin A. For women, there is a particular oral contraceptive pill that has a beneficial effect on acne as well as providing contraception.

As an alternative, there are a number of homeopathic remedies that can be used with success. It is best to consult a specialist homeopath who will be able to advise the correct remedy for the individual as well as prescribing their own constitutional remedy. If this is not possible, the following remedies may be used. Select one by matching the remedy pictures with the physical symptoms. Using the 6c potency, give one dose twice a day.

### *Antimonium tartaricum* (antimonium tartrate)

This remedy picture describes a pustular eruption on the skin that leaves a blush-red mark. The person is extremely drowsy and has an irresistible inclination to sleep. The skin problem is made worse by warmth, damp weather, sour foods and milk.

### *Berberis aquifolium* (mountain grape)

This remedy picture describes pimply, rough skin. The pimples extend from the face to the neck and may go into the scalp. Sufferers feel as though a band is firmly in position just above their ears, and they tend to suffer from headaches that make them vomit.

### *Calcarea sulphurica* (calcium sulphate)

This remedy picture describes a skin that has many pimples under the skin, which do not produce pus. These tend to bleed when scratched, and the resulting wounds are slow to heal, forming septic spots on which yellow crusts form.

### *Hepar sulphuris* (Hahnemann's calcium sulphide)

This remedy picture describes serious pustular eruptions on the face and back that look like boils. The skin is unhealthy and the slightest cut or scratch becomes infected. The person feels better with the head wrapped up warmly.

### *Kali arsenicum* (Fowler's solution)

This remedy picture describes acne that is worse during MEN-STRUATION.

### *Kali bichromium* (potassium bichromate)

This remedy picture describes an eruption on the face formed of small, solid, slightly raised areas, which have a tendency to ulcerate. The ulcers, which have a characteristic appearance of punched-out edges, tend to penetrate deeply into the skin.

### *Kali bromatum* (potassium bromide)

This remedy picture describes an eruption of pus-filled blisters that are prominent on the chest, shoulders and face. Each eruption is itchy. Sufferers are drowsy and yet find sleep difficult as they have horrible dreams. They may grind their teeth during sleep and are fidgety during the day.

### *Ledum* (marsh tea)

This remedy picture describes acne on the forehead that give sticking pains. The person may also develop itching on their feet and ankles that is made worse by scratching and by warmth.

### *Lycopodium* (club moss)

This remedy picture describes acne associated with urinary or digestive disorders.

### *Pulsatilla* (wind flower)

This remedy picture describes acne that is made worse by eating fatty foods and by warm environments. The person prefers the fresh air.

### *Silicea* (pure flint)

This remedy picture describes skin that is delicate, pale and waxy in appearance. The acne spots become pustular, remain in this form for a long time and cause long-lasting scars. The person sweats easily, particularly from the feet (which smell).

### *Sulphur*

This remedy picture describes spotty-faced individuals who dislike washing their faces (or hair). Warmth tends to make the condition worse, as those whom this remedy will suit tend to sweat easily and don't feel the cold even when everyone else does.

Should the acne form permanent scars, the following remedy is helpful. It is also useful in helping to resolve ABDOMINAL ADHESIONS. Using the 6c potency, give one dose twice a day for several weeks.

*Thiosinaminum* (chemical derived from oil from mustard seed)

This remedy acts by resolving scar tissue both externally (skin) and internally (adhesions caused through abdominal surgery).

The following two remedies are useful for treating scars that are not as superficial as those that can be treated by *Thiosinaminum*:

*Graphites* (black lead)

This remedy is indicated when the scar begins to weep a honey-coloured exudate.

*Silicea* (pure flint)

This remedy is indicated in scars that suddenly become itchy or inflamed.

# Examination nerves

At this critical period of adolescents' lives, examinations take on increasing importance. They have feelings of "butterflies in the stomach", and they worry that, when they sit down to do their exams, their minds will go blank and they will forget everything they have learned.

Conventional treatment with tranquillizers is unhelpful because of the sedating side-effect. There are stress management courses available to help students cope with exam nerves.

Homeopathic remedies are available which do not have any sedating side-effect. Select one by matching the symptoms with the remedy picture. Using the 30c potency, give one dose the evening before the examination and another one in the morning. Then, using the 6c potency, give a final dose immediately before the examination.

### *Anacardium* (marking nut)

This remedy picture describes adolescents who find it difficult to settle down to the necessary revision work prior to the exam. Already they are finding it difficult to recall work previously learned.

### *Argentum nitricum* (silver nitrate)

This remedy picture describes adolescents who, already nervous about the approaching examination, develop diarrhoea.

### *Gelsemium* (yellow jasmine)

This remedy picture describes adolescents who have studied hard and conscientiously but, at the examination, become paralysed with fear (like "stage fright"). Their legs and arms just won't function properly.

### *Lycopodium* (club moss)

This remedy picture describes already anxious adolescents who compensate for their anxieties by showing off and bragging about their knowledge to their peers. They compensate for their fear of the forthcoming examination by eating sweets.

### *Pulsatilla* (wind flower)

This remedy picture describes adolescents who develop headaches whenever they study for long periods. These headaches are relieved by going out into fresh air and by cold applications.

### *Silicea* (pure flint)

This remedy picture describes adolescents who develop headaches from studying for long periods. These headaches are relieved by warm applications and by wrapping up the head or wearing a hat. The adolescent that this remedy particularly suits has sweaty, smelly feet.

# Masturbation

Here we are not giving moral guidelines but homeopathic remedies that are available for certain difficulties. This normal sexual activity only becomes a problem when performed in antisocial situations.

The conventional treatment is with psychotherapy.

The homeopathic approach is to not only use psychotherapy but also to consult a specialist homeopath who will be able to assess the person generally as well as their specific problems. If this is not possible, the following homeopathic remedies can be used. Select one by matching its picture with the physical symptoms. Using the 30c potency, give one dose twice a week but not on consecutive days.

### *Bufo* (poison of the toad)

This remedy picture describes male adolescents who have a tendency to fondle their genitalia and become sexually aroused and masturbate.

### *Caladium seguinum* (American arum)

This remedy picture describes a female adolescent who has a discharge from her vagina which is itchy, and as a result of this itchiness, she scratches her vulval area and masturbates.

### *Calcarea carbonica* (calcium carbonate)

This remedy picture describes adolescents who are fat and tend to sweat easily from their scalps, and who have a problem with masturbation.

### *Origanum* (sweet marjoram)

This remedy picture describes an adolescent who has excessively aroused sexual impulses and masturbates frequently and openly.

### *Platina* (platinum)

This remedy picture describes children who masturbate before they reach the age of puberty.

### *Staphysagria* (stavesacre)

This remedy picture describes an adolescent who is angry and full of resentment and whose sexual activity is increased, including overt masturbation.

### *Zincum metallicum* (zinc)

This remedy picture describes a female adolescent whose sexual desire increases during menstruation as does her need to masturbate.

# Menstrual difficulties

*Painful ovulation (Mittelschmerz syndrome)*
About 14 days following the onset of menstrual bleeding, ovulation occurs, when the ovary sheds an egg (ovum). At this point in their menstrual cycles, some young women develop colicky pains in the lower abdomen, which are not associated with any other symptoms or physical signs.

The conventional treatment is explanation, reassurance and simple painkillers.

In the homeopathic approach, explanations and reassurance are also given, together with a homeopathic remedy if necessary. Select one by matching its remedy picture with the physical symptoms. Before it can be taken, the young woman must keep track of her menstrual cycle for several cycles. Then, using the 6c potency, one dose of the remedy should be taken the day before ovulation occurs (usually on or about day 13 after the onset of the last period) and one dose on the day of ovulation (day 14).

### *Cimicifuga racemosa* (black snake root)

This remedy has a specific action on the ovaries. Its picture describes a neuralgic pain in the lower abdomen in the region of one of the ovaries. It also describes shooting colicky pains radiating from hip to hip, as well as facial blemishes in young women.

### *Colocynthis* (bitter cucumber)

This remedy picture describes a boring pain in the region of one of the ovaries, which forces the woman to bend double; this pressure on her abdomen eases the pain slightly. The woman is generally irritable, particularly when being questioned.

### *Lycopodium* (club moss)

This remedy picture describes right-sided abdominal pain in the region of the ovary. This pain becomes worse during the late afternoon and early evening (between 4.00 and 8.00 pm.) The woman that this remedy suits likes sugar, warm drinks and food, and is generally apprehensive, with a particular fear of loneliness.

### *Naja tripudians* (cobra venom)

This remedy picture describes a young woman with pains in her left lower abdomen in the region of her ovary. These pains can extend into the groin but more usually radiate upwards to the heart.

### *Palladium* (palladium metal)

This remedy picture describes low right-sided abdominal pain in the region of the ovary. This leads to a cutting pain in the uterus and to generalized pains in the entire pelvic area. These pains are relieved when the woman rubs the painful region.

### *Painful periods (dysmenorrhoea)*
The early periods are generally painless and remain so until the ovaries begin to release their eggs. At this point, the onset of

461

blood flow is accompanied by cramping pains, medically called *dysmenorrhoea*.

The conventional treatment is with painkillers mainly of the nonsteroidal anti-inflammatory type.

The homeopathic approach is to advise the woman to take evening primrose oil: at least 2 grams a day, in divided doses. Consultation with a specialist homeopath is also recommended; he or she will be able to devise the appropriate constitutional remedy for the young woman. However, if this is not possible, the following homeopathic remedies can be given. Choose one by matching its picture with the physical symptoms. Using the 6c potency, give one dose four times a day just before the period is due.

### *Cactus grandiflorus* (night-blooming cereus)

This remedy picture describes a young woman who cries with the pain at the onset of bleeding, which feels as though a vice is gripping her womb (uterus).

### *Calcarea phosphorica* (calcium phosphate)

This remedy picture describes a young woman who initially has an irregular menstrual cycle and experiences pain when the cycle settles down to a regular rhythm.

### *Chamomilla* (camomile)

This remedy picture describes a young woman who develops dysmenorrhoea whenever she gets angry.

### *Graphites* (black lead)

This remedy picture describes a young woman who develops dysmenorrhoea together with a throbbing headache and possible eczema on her nipples.

### *Pulsatilla* (wind flower)

This remedy picture describes dysmenorrhoea in a young woman who weeps easily and often. She probably has blonde hair and blue eyes, dislikes fatty foods and the heat and prefers the fresh air. She has no thirst.

## Sulphur

This remedy picture describes dysmenorrhoea in a young woman who also feels a burning, itchy sensation in her vagina and general vulval area. These symptoms are worse when she sits down, so that she can hardly keep still. She also has a bearing-down sensation whenever she stands up.

## Viburnum opulus (cramp bark)

This remedy picture describes severe cramp-like pains in the uterus that radiate down the young woman's thighs and through to her back.

## Xanthoxylum (prickly ash)

This remedy picture describes a young woman who develops a violent, agonizing, grinding dysmenorrhoea that is not relieved by moving to any position. The pains radiate down her thighs or over her whole body, including her heart.

### Pre-menstrual syndrome (PMS)

The distressing symptoms of this syndrome – depression, irritability, tension, fatigue, bloating, breast tenderness, headache, backache and lower abdominal pain – can interfere with study and examinations.

The conventional treatment is the prescribing of progesterone-based hormonal drugs.

The homeopathic approach is initially with supplements of evening primrose oil (at least 2 grams each day in divided doses) and daily multi-mineral and multi-vitamin tablets, particularly the vitamins B, C (at least 2 grams a day) and E. Consultation with a specialist homeopath is the ideal; he or she will be able to match the qualities of the person as a whole with her physical difficulty.

If this is not possible, the following homeopathic remedies can be considered. Match the presenting symptoms with the remedy picture. Using the 200c potency, give one dose every 12 hours for three doses in the middle of the menstrual cycle (approximately 14 days after the onset of bleeding). This is to coincide with ovulation.

## *Lachesis* (bushmaster snake venom)

This remedy picture describes a young woman who becomes quite violent pre-menstrually, hitting out at people with her arms, feet and any objects lying around. This violence can become serious when knives are used and cause actual physical harm.

## *Natrum muriaticum* (sodium chloride)

This remedy picture describes a young woman who does not express her emotions but bottles them up, silently seething. She is able to bear a grudge should anyone cross her path. Physical comfort in the form of a hug is not appreciated; she feels that she can manage on her own. Anecdotally, this remedy can be summarized by the statement: "She is nice to know but difficult to live with." The added feature of this remedy picture, and of the person that this remedy will suit, is a liking for salt.

## *Pulsatilla* (wind flower)

This remedy picture describes a young woman who cries easily but more so pre-menstrually. She enjoys physical comfort and fresh air and dislikes fatty foods.

## *Sepia* (inky juice of cuttlefish)

This remedy picture describes a young woman who becomes indifferent to her best friends and loved ones, retreating into her own private space. She becomes tearful and resists all attempts to comfort her physically (by giving her hugs). Premenstrually, she develops a craving for vinegar and possibly chocolate as well.

# PART III

# *Special Disorders of Adults*

# Men

This section includes difficulties of the younger and older man. The male urogenital tract consists of the penis, two testicles in the scrotum and the prostate gland that surrounds the urethra at the base of the bladder.

## HIV (human immunodeficiency virus) infection

This viral infection is acquired by transmission of blood or other body fluids either by contaminated intravenous needles, administration of contaminated blood products or unprotected sexual activity (i.e. not using a condom). It can be caught by both men and women (and passed on to babies at birth by infected mothers), but the vast majority of those who have contracted this infection are male.

The virus lives in the T4 lymphocytes – some of the white blood cells that make up the body's immune system – and these are progressively destroyed as the virus multiplies. After an average of ten years, this leads to the development of AIDS (acquired immune deficiency syndrome). The mean survival time from the onset of AIDS is about three years.

Basic treatment, both conventional and homeopathic, is to provide psychological and social support, and to encourage those infected to eat a nutritious diet, including probiotic therapy (*see* p. 27), raw organic carrots, and vitamin and mineral supplements according to the antioxidant therapy described on p. 25. A reasonable amount of exercise is also beneficial.

The conventional drug regime has recently been revised and consists of anti-retroviral drugs given in combination. Homeopathic treatment is complicated, requiring consultation with a specialist homeopath.

# Impotence

This describes the inability of a man's penis to develop an erection when he wants sexual activity. This can be caused by a neurological problem or DIABETES MELLITUS or other hormonal disorder, because of the taking of certain drugs or because of ALCOHOLISM. Treatment of impotence with these causes involves treatment of the primary disorder. However, most cases of impotence are due to psychological difficulties, and in these, psychotherapy together with homeopathic remedies will be helpful.

The homeopathic treatment should be obtained by consulting a specialist homeopath who will be able to make an overall assessment of the person. If this is not possible, select one of the following homeopathic remedies, matching its remedy picture with the physical symptoms. Using the 6c potency, give one dose twice a day.

### Baryta carbonicum (barium carbonate)

This remedy picture describes a man who is generally sexually inactive (and can even fall asleep while having sexual intercourse!). He can occasionally find himself impotent.

### Conium (poison hemlock)

This remedy picture describes a man whose sexual desire is definitely present but who is sexually nervous and has a feeble erection.

### Lycopodium (club moss)

This remedy picture describes a man who is generally nervous and feels particularly distressed when left on his own. He likes sweet foods and prefers it warmed. He becomes somewhat depressed between 4.00 and 8.00 pm. He either suffers from premature ejaculation or is unable to maintain an erection.

### Nux vomica (poison-nut)

This remedy picture describes an overactive man who finds himself impotent as a result of too much alcohol and caffeine. He also smokes far too many cigarettes.

### Sulphur

This remedy picture describes a man with a very laid-back attitude to life. He enjoys drinking beer and eating fatty foods, and enjoys sweets and a good joke. He complains of a stitching pain in his penis and an itching discomfort on his scrotum when he goes to bed. His penis remains relaxed and impotent when he wants an erection.

# Penis problems

The penis consists of a shaft through which runs a central canal called the urethra. It is through this channel that urine flows when the man wishes to urinate. When the penis is erect for sexual activity, sperm flows through the urethra as an ejaculation. The covering of the tip of the penis (the *glans penis*) is the foreskin, which should be fully retractable. Some men have had their foreskins surgically removed (CIRCUMCISION).

Any part of the penis can become infected. Infection of the urethra is known as URETHRITIS. The glans penis can become infected with a number of things, including bacteria, trichomonas (a protozoan pathogen), yeast and one type of virus (herpes). These infections are collectively known as BALANITIS.

# Chlamydial infection

This is the commonest sexually transmitted bacterial infection in the United Kingdom. In men it causes URETHRITIS, presenting as a urethral discharge with painful urination (dysuria) two to three weeks following sexual exposure.

As with all other sexually transmitted diseases, the conventional treatment is the first choice. This usually involves a week's course of the antibiotic tetracycline, but a recent advance is to give a single oral dose of azithromycin; this is more effective since, with tetracycline, patients are less likely to finish taking the drug. It is important to treat the sexual partner as well.

Homeopathic options are very much second choice. Remedies that are appropriate are discussed under URETHRITIS (see p. 213).

# Genital warts

Genital warts are caused by the human papilloma virus (HPV), which is transmitted by direct skin contact. These warts appear either singly or as a massed collection anywhere on the external genitalia or in the urethra or rectum.

In the conventional treatment – the first choice – liquid nitrogen is applied to the wart, which when frozen is removed. Homeopathic treatment involves the use of constitutional remedies for which the man must see a specialist homeopath. If this is not possible, select the appropriate remedy from the section on WARTS (see p. 291).

# Gonorrhoea

This bacterial infection causes urethritis with or without painful urination (dysuria) after an incubation period of three to five days. It is always sexually acquired. In untreated cases, it can lead to prostatitis.

The conventional treatment is with penicillin. Because of its importance as a sexually transmitted disease, conventional treatment is recommended to eradicate the infection, as well as following up and treating the man's sexual contacts. Homeopathic treatment is very much the second choice. Use the remedies for URETHRITIS (see p. 213) and PROSTATITIS (see p. 477).

# Herpes infection

The *Herpes simplex* virus that causes genital herpes is the same one that causes cold sores on the mouth, and it can affect both men and women. It is possible to have a primary vaginal or penile herpes infection without any sexual contact, but the usual cause is through sexual contact. There are two types of the *Herpes simplex* virus – HSV-1 and HSV-2 – the former being the commonest in sexually transmitted diseases. There is a new blood test that can distinguish between the two and is useful in monitoring the prevalence of this illness. The risk of contracting a herpes infection is increased if the person has multiple sexual partners.

In men, the physical symptoms range from a mild BALANITIS to blister formation on the glans penis followed by ulceration and subsequent crust formation. Occasionally more severe and generalized infections such as MENINGITIS can occur as a result of the herpes virus, and there can also be retention of urine, a dangerous condition that can lead to kidney damage. Once infected, the virus remains in the body and the person can suffer recurrent attacks of herpes, although the symptoms won't last as long as they did in the initial attack. The trigger factors for recurrences include stress, exposure to ultraviolet light and sexual activity.

The conventional treatment is the first choice, and involves the taking of anti-viral tablets. Homeopathic treatment, which is very much the second choice, consists of the remedies given for the treatment of SHINGLES, which is caused by the closely related *Herpes zoster* virus.

# Non-specific urethritis (NSU)

This form of urethritis is sexually transmitted but no definite microbe is known to cause it. The incubation period between sexual contact and the appearance of symptoms may be as long as three months. In men, the symptoms are not very severe: a mild urethral discharge and mild discomfort when passing urine.

In women, no symptoms at all may appear, but they should be tested and treated if their male partners develop NSU.

The conventional treatment is with tetracycline.

The homeopathic treatment, which is very much the second choice of therapy, comprises the remedies given for URETHRITIS.

# Priapism

In rare circumstances, the penis remains painfully erect even though the man has lost all his sexual drive. If such an erection remains untreated for four hours or more, permanent damage can take place to the shaft of the penis.

This condition demands immediate conventional medical attention. This will result in a surgical procedure to help restore the normal blood circulation in the penis.

While awaiting conventional medical treatment, the following homeopathic remedies can be given. Select the appropriate remedy, matching its remedy picture with the profile of the man. Using the 6c potency, give one dose every ten minutes.

### *Cannabis sativa* (hemp)

This remedy picture describes a man who can get an erection without having any amorous thoughts. His sexual desire is increased, his foreskin is often swollen and he easily develops priapism. His mind is in a daze.

### *Cantharis* (Spanish fly)

This remedy picture describes a rapid, violent state of sexual activity that is not subdued by sexual intercourse. The man often pulls at his penis, commonly has blood in what he ejaculates, often has pain in his urethra following sexual intercourse and easily develops priapism.

### *Graphites* (black lead)

This remedy picture describes a man who dislikes sexual intercourse even though his sexual desire is increased. As a result of excessive masturbation, he tends to suffer from IMPOTENCE when he attempts sexual intercourse. When he finally does have it, he suffers from premature ejaculation and develops cramps in his calf muscles. He also suffers from priapism.

### *Pulsatilla* (wind flower)

This remedy picture describes a man who commonly develops pains down his left side to his left testicle. He usually has a gentle, mild nature and weeps easily, dislikes hot environments and fatty foods and prefers fresh air. He can develop priapism.

# Syphilis

Most cases of syphilis affecting men are transmitted through homosexual contact. The incubation period is two to four weeks, after which a painless genital ulcer – a chancre – appears, which heals over a period of three to eight weeks. This stage is known as primary syphilis. Because of this seemingly spontaneous recovery, the person is often tempted not to seek treatment. However, six to eight weeks later, the chancre is followed by a skin rash, enlarged lymph glands and mouth ulcers. This is known as secondary syphilis. All the mouth ulcers are infectious. After a "latent" period of 10 to 40 years, tertiary syphilis appears. The symptoms of this stage are seen in the nervous and cardiovascular systems, and spots filled with pus, known as *gummata*, appear on the skin and in the bones. Among other terrible effects, tertiary syphilis can lead to brain damage and general paralysis.

All stages of syphilis should be treated conventionally with intramuscular penicillin.

The only indication for homeopathic remedy treatment is when treating a known descendant of an infected person for an unrelated problem. This person's family history makes syphilis a significant factor, in which case the use of the nosode *Syphilinum* is important as a prelude to any subsequent treatment. This homeopathic therapy should only be used under the guidance of a specialist homeopath.

# Thrush

The tip of the penis – the glans penis – can become infected with a yeast-like fungal organism called *Candida albicans*. This infection is much more common in an uncircumcised man, whose foreskin provides the warm, moist environment in which the *Candida* thrives. The symptoms are itchiness, redness and a milky discharge.

The infection can occur spontaneously or may be sexually acquired. If it has been acquired sexually, the woman needs treatment for her vaginal thrush as well as the man. To prevent this infection from occurring spontaneously, it is important for the man to be scrupulous about his personal hygiene: the foreskin has to be retracted daily so that the glans penis can be adequately washed and dried.

The conventional treatment is to prescribe an anti-fungal cream.

The homeopathic approach is to advise the man to reduce his intake of refined sugar and his consumption of alcohol and to start probiotic therapy (*see* p. 27). A cream containing zinc and caster oil should be applied to the glans penis twice a day for three to five days. If there is no improvement, the following homeopathic remedy can be used. Using the 6c potency, give one dose three times a day for three days.

### *Mercurius solubis* (black oxide of mercury)

This remedy picture describes a glans penis with itchy red spots and a discharge of pus and mucus.

For recurrent attacks of penile thrush occurring spontaneously, it is possible to use a homeopathic preparation of **Candida albicans**. Using the 6c potency, give one dose twice a day for one month.

## Trichomonas infection

This sexually transmitted infection usually causes no symptoms in the man but sometimes there is redness and itchiness of the glans penis associated with a discharge of pus and mucus. The woman needs treatment as well (*see below*).

The conventional treatment is with drugs, mainly metronidazole or one from the tetracycline group.

Although it must remain the second choice, the homeopathic treatment available for this condition involves the use of the following remedy:

### *Mercurius solubis* (black oxide of mercury)

This remedy picture describes an itchy glans penis with red spots, associated with a discharge of pus and mucus. Using the 6c potency, give one dose three times a day for three days.

## *Prostate problems*

## Enlarged prostate

The prostate is a gland wrapped around the urethra at the neck of the bladder in men. From the age of 45 onwards, it begins to enlarge as the level of testosterone begins to fall and the influence of oestrogen begins to exert its effect. This enlargement results in a reduced urine flow and an increased frequency of urination; this is particularly noticeable at night (when it is called *nocturia*). The obstruction at the neck of the bladder leads to stagnation of urine in the bladder itself, providing an ideal environment for the growth of bacteria.

The diagnosis of an enlarged prostate is made by a rectal examination by a medical practitioner. Further tests will probably be made to check on kidney function, as well as ultrasound investigation to check on the entire urinary tract. To exclude cancer of the prostate, a sample of tissue (a biopsy) may be taken from the prostate, and a blood test may be carried out to identify the SPA-specific prostate antigen.

Conventional treatment will be the primary choice after these tests. If they show that there is no cancer, an operation may be recommended to reduce the size of the prostate gland. This can be done through the urethra route or by abdominal surgery to remove the entire prostate gland. A very new form of treatment is to subject the prostate gland (via the urethra) to high temperatures (60°C/140°F), which shrinks the gland. In addition, alpha blocker drugs have been shown to be effective.

There are homeopathic remedies that have an effect on the symptoms of an enlarged prostate. Using the 6c potency, give one dose four times a day for three weeks, and then reduce to twice a day as a long-term strategy. Fluid intake must also be maintained at a reasonable level to avoid dehydration and urine stagnation. About 250 ml (9 fl. oz) of cranberry juice should be drunk four times a day.

### *Ferrum picricum* (iron picrate)

This remedy picture describes a man who frequently urinates at night and also has a feeling of fullness and pressure in the rectum. There is a sensation of pain along the whole length of the urethra, and a smarting sensation at the neck of the bladder. Retention of urine within the bladder is common.

### *Populace tremuloides* (American aspen)

This remedy picture shows a man who has to strain considerably to urinate and whose urine is painful and scalding. He is aware of a pain behind the pubic bone (pubis) as he finishes urinating. Medical examination reveals an enlarged prostate gland.

### *Sabal serrulata* (saw palmetto)

This remedy picture describes a man with a constant desire to urinate, particularly at night, when there can also be incontinence. He shows a hesitancy in starting to urinate and has a weak urine stream that cannot be stopped without terminal dribbling. He has a lack of sexual power, and if ejaculation occurs, it is painful. There is a feeling of coldness about the genital organs, including the prostate. The picture also describes CYSTITIS in a man with an enlarged prostate.

## Prostate cancer

If tests show that there is prostate cancer, the conventional treatment is either radiotherapy or surgical castration (this will remove any testosterone from the body, which can cause the cancer to grow). However, it has been shown that, in older men, they are more likely to die from a pre-existing problem such as heart disease than from the cancer of their prostate. Therefore no treatment for the cancer is given unless they develop severe bone pains, indicating that the cancer has spread into their bones. In this case, the conventional treatment involves injections of an oestrogen-based drug given as subcutaneous injection therapy.

Homeopathic treatment is only available through a specialist homeopath. The basic treatment is with *Iscador* (mistletoe) given as injections or tablets.

## Prostatitis

This is an infection of the prostate gland, usually due to an infection in another part of the urinary tract. It causes pain at the base of the penis, and fever may be present.

The conventional treatment is with antibiotics and prostatic massage and occasionally surgery to help drain the infection.

The following homeopathic remedies can be used either as a

complementary form of treatment or on their own. Using the 6c potency, give one dose twice a day.

### *Chimaphila umbellata* (pipsisewa)

This remedy picture describes a smarting pain in the urethra, from the neck of the bladder to the tip of the penis. Urine flow is scanty, and it feels as if there is a ball in the perineum, the area between the base of the penis and the anus. The man is unable to urinate without standing with his feet wide apart and his body leaning forward.

### *Pulsatilla* (wind flower)

This remedy picture describes a man who has an increased desire to urinate but only passes urine in drops, the stream being interrupted. There is also pain and urgency when urinating. All of these symptoms are worse when he is lying on his back. The man whom this remedy will particularly suit dislikes the heat and fatty foods, feeling better in the fresh air.

### *Sabal serrulata* (saw palmetto)

This remedy picture describes a man who has a constant desire to urinate at night (nocturia), and there may be urinary incontinence, particularly at night.

### *Thuja occidentalis* (arbor vitae)

This remedy picture describes pain and a burning sensation near the neck of the bladder. There is a frequent and urgent desire to urinate, but the urine stream cannot be controlled, being split and weak. Symptoms are suggestive of an ENLARGED PROSTATE. There may be an associated infection of the foreskin and the glans penis.

# Swellings in the scrotum

It is important that an accurate diagnosis of these swellings is made so that cancer of the testicles can be excluded. Young men should regularly examine their testicles for lumps – gentle squeezing of the testicles should be painful. Cancer of the testicles presents itself as a painless lump on one of the testicles in young men aged between 20 and 35. The conventional treatment is surgical removal of the affected testicle, combined with radiotherapy and chemotherapy. Provided that this cancer is diagnosed at an early stage, the outlook is excellent.

## Epididymal cysts

The epididymis is a coiled tube that lies behind the testicle, and if it is normal, it feels like a cord with no noticeable lumps or tenderness. A painless lump felt in the testis is usually an epididymal cyst.

The conventional treatment of an epididymal cyst is surgical drainage.

The following homeopathic remedies can be tried initially to see whether this will reduce the cyst. Select the remedy by matching its picture with the physical symptoms. If this doesn't work, surgical drainage becomes necessary.

### *Apis mellifica* (honey bee)

This remedy picture describes cysts within the scrotum. This man is restless and can easily get jealous. Using the 6c potency, give one dose twice a day for one month.

### *Graphites* (black lead)

This remedy picture describes cystic swellings within the scrotum. The man does not show much enthusiasm for sexual intercourse. Using the 6c potency, give one dose twice a day for one month.

# Epididymitis

When the epididymis becomes tender to the touch, the cause is an infection, usually due to a urinary infection with the symptoms of frequency and urgency of urination.

The conventional treatment is to use antibiotic therapy.

Homeopathic treatment can be tried for 24 hours to see if there is any improvement. See the section on CYSTITIS (p. 216) for appropriate homeopathic remedies for urinary infections. Specific remedies for treating epididymitis are described below. Select one by matching its picture with the physical symptoms. Using the 6c potency, give one dose four times a day for one week. If there is no improvement after 24 hours, seek conventional medical treatment.

### *Belladonna* (deadly nightshade)

This remedy picture describes a hot tender testicle that is probably developing a reddish colour. The man finds the slightest movement incredibly painful.

### *Hamamelis virginica* (witch hazel)

This remedy picture describes such severe pain in the testicle that the man feels as if he has been kicked by a horse.

### *Pulsatilla* (wind flower)

This remedy picture describes pain in the testicle that becomes swollen and hot. The pain radiates upwards into the abdomen.

# Hydrocoele

In this condition, excess fluid forms within the scrotum around the testicle, giving a painless swelling that progressively enlarges as more fluid accumulates. This is a benign condition and is treated conventionally by drawing off the fluid at intervals or, more permanently, by a surgical procedure.

The following homeopathic remedies can be given to reduce the accumulation of fluid. Using the 6c potency, give one dose twice a day for two weeks every month.

### Digitalis (foxglove)

This remedy picture describes a hydrocoele on the left side of the scrotum. The man is unhappy and worried about his future. His pulse rate is either slow or irregular.

### Helleborus (Christmas rose)

This remedy picture describes a man who can develop a hydrocoele on either side. The person that this remedy suits has generalized muscular weakness and is not mentally "switched on".

### Rhododendron (snow rose)

This remedy picture describes a man with a hydrocoele that begins to ache before a thunderstorm. The hydrocoele in this picture is more commonly found on the left side.

### Rhus toxicodendron (poison ivy)

This remedy picture describes a man who develops a hydrocoele because he has been over-exerting himself when lifting something.

### Sambucus nigra (elder)

This remedy picture describes a man who develops a hydrocoele through a physical injury to his testicles.

### Silicea (pure flint)

This remedy picture describes a hydrocoele in a man who has itchy, moist spots on his scrotum. He also suffers from severe exhaustion following sexual intercourse, taking up to ten days to recover.

# Women

S ome of the conditions mentioned in this section apply to both younger and older women. This section discusses problems of the breasts and the female genitals. Disorders of pregnancy are dealt with in the next section.

The female genitals consist of an outer vulval area into which the urethra (the end of the urinary tract) emerges. The clitoris, the centre of sexual stimulation in women, is located underneath the urethra and extends into the vagina. The tube-like vagina goes upwards, backwards and slightly to the left, ending at the cervix, the neck of the uterus (womb).

The two ovaries are sited in the lower abdomen and secrete the hormone oestrogen, which has a protective effect on the heart and circulatory system, keeps the woman's skin and hair healthy and is responsible for the lubrication of the vagina, particularly during sexual intercourse. It is from the ovaries that the ova (eggs) are shed at approximately monthly intervals. These find their way down one of the Fallopian tubes (right and left) and end up in the uterus. If an ovum is fertilized by a sperm that has been ejaculated into the vagina, the woman becomes pregnant. If there is no fertilization, the woman ultimately menstruates.

## Breast problems

### Breast cysts

Women should regularly examine their breasts for lumps. If one is found, immediate medical advice should be obtained. The critical question is whether this lump represents a cancer. Physical examination can reveal whether the lump is solid or cystic. If it is a cyst, the medical practitioner can drain it by a needle aspiration. The fluid will be sent away for cytological examination in order to exclude a cancer.

Some women have recurrent benign cysts in their breasts. There is no conventional treatment to stop these breast cysts from coming back.

The homeopath is able to offer constitutional remedies that will help an individual woman. This will mean a consultation with a specialist homeopath. If this consultation is not possible, the following homeopathic remedies can be used. Select one by matching its picture with the physical symptoms. Using the 6c potency, give one dose twice a day.

### Conium (poison hemlock)

This remedy picture describes recurrent breast cysts that cause discomfort just before a menstrual period. This causes the woman to press her breast firmly with her hand in order to obtain relief.

### Graphites (black lead)

This remedy picture describes breasts with cysts. Both nipples are cracked with a surrounding area of eczema.

### Phytolacca (poke root)

This remedy picture describes breasts with cysts, with the breasts sensitive to the touch and having a purple coloration.

## Breast size

The breasts of a non-pregnant/non-breastfeeding woman consist mainly of fat, and as fat distribution is primarily genetically determined, losing or gaining weight will not necessarily change the shape of a woman's breasts very much.

Plastic surgery can be carried out to enlarge the breasts with silicon implants. However, the use of silicon is not recommended by this author, because of its side-effects. Plastic surgery can be beneficial for those women who have large breasts in comparison with the rest of their body and who, as a result, develop neck and shoulder ache. In this case, of course, the object is to reduce the size of the breasts.

A consultant homeopath will be able to devise a constitutional remedy to help a woman with this difficulty. If it is impossible to arrange this consultation, there are several homeopathic remedies that may influence the size of the breasts; these can be tried for one month to see if they have any effect. Select the remedy according to its picture and match this with the physical symptoms. Using the 6c potency, give one dose twice a day.

### *Calcarea carbonica* (calcium carbonate)

This remedy picture describes an obese woman with heavy breasts. She is likely to be obstinate, sweats easily around her head and tends to be constipated.

### *Carbo animalis* (animal charcoal)

This remedy picture describes a woman's breasts that have darting pains within them, particularly on the right side. This right breast can also become hardened. The pains within the breast can give the woman breathing difficulties. Either breast can develop painful lumps.

### *Conium* (poison hemlock)

This remedy picture describes two different types of breasts. One type are enlarged and become painful before and during a menstrual period. This pain is made worse from any movement, but the woman finds it helpful to press her breasts firmly with her hands. The other type are lax and shrunken, and the woman may have lost her sexual desire. Her nipples become hardened and may crack.

### *Iodum* (iodine)

This remedy picture describes breasts that slowly diminish in size. They always feel hot and probably have red (non-malignant) lumps under the skin.

### *Natrum muriaticum* (sodium chloride)

This remedy picture describes a woman's breasts that shrink in size but swell again if she retains fluid. In any case, her nipples ache generally.

### *Sabal serrulata* (saw palmetto)

This remedy picture describes two types of breasts. One type are sore and tender, symptoms that are made worse from the cold. The other type are small and undeveloped. Both types have a similar characteristic in that one breast is larger than the other. Another feature that is common to both types is that the woman has a furious sexual passion.

# Disorders of the cervix

## Cervical cancer

It is very important to diagnose problems of the cervix so that cervical cancer can be excluded. This is done by having a regular cervical smear examination. This is a simple test during which cells are scraped off the surface of the cervix with a wooden spatula. This test and a vaginal examination are carried out either by a trained nurse or by a medical practitioner.

Sometimes this test will reveal cervical dysplasia – abnormal cervical cells – which are examined and assigned a specific "stage" according to the risk of malignant change. Cervical dysplasia produces no symptoms. The treatment for this condition is strictly conventional. The suspect area of the cervix is either removed surgically or treated by laser therapy.

In the UK, cervical testing first occurs one year after a woman becomes sexually active, and then the test is repeated every three to five years until she is well into the menopause. The test should be carried out more frequently when there is cervical dysplasia, when there is a history of GENITAL WARTS in either partner or when the woman has had multiple sexual partners.

# Cervical erosion

This condition, in which glandular tissue appears on the outside of the cervix, causes the woman to have a watery vaginal discharge with, possibly, bleeding between periods or after sexual intercourse.

The conventional and preferred method of therapy is with cauterization, a painless procedure in which the glandular tissue on the surface of the cervix is burned away.

While waiting for this, the following homeopathic remedies can be used to lessen the symptoms. Select the remedy by matching its picture with the physical symptoms. Using the 6c potency, give one dose twice a day.

### *Alumina* (aluminium)

This remedy picture describes a profuse burning vaginal discharge that makes the woman want to scratch her vulva. The symptoms are worse during the daytime, and are eased when she washes her vulva with cold water. She has a strong need for an embrace.

### *Calcarea carbonica* (calcium carbonate)

This remedy picture describes a thick, milky discharge that increases in volume whenever the woman urinates. This discharge causes itching and burning in the vulva.

### *Cinchona officinalis (China)* (Peruvian bark)

This remedy picture describes a bloody discharge that sometimes appears to take the place of a normal period. The woman may notice heaviness in her lower abdomen and in her pelvis.

### *Nitric acidum* (nitric acid)

This remedy picture describes a brown watery discharge that

leaves a stain surrounded by a black margin on the woman's underwear. The discharge may contain strings of mucus.

### Phosphorus

This remedy picture describes a profuse vaginal discharge that contains blood, particularly after sexual intercourse. The woman may find her sexual appetite is increased.

## Endometriosis

This condition occurs when patches of the lining of the uterus – the endometrium – appear on the Fallopian tubes and the ovaries and/or in the abdominal cavity. These patches are known as "chocolate cysts" and respond to the normal hormonal cycle of the woman – that is, they bleed and are shed, just as the lining of the uterus does during a period. This causes pain, and can result in infertility due to the patches obstructing the Fallopian tubes and adhering to the ovaries.

The conventional treatment is with a hormonal drug or the oral contraceptive and, in more severe cases, surgery to remove the cysts or, if the woman does not want children or is nearing the menopause, surgery to remove the uterus.

Homeopathic treatment requires consultation with a specialist homeopath, who will prescribe the woman's constitutional remedy as well as treating specific symptoms. If this is not possible, the remedies found in the section on PAINFUL PERIODS (see p. 461) can be used.

## Hormone imbalance

Any upset in the delicate balance between the brain and ovaries can give a woman symptoms such as fluid retention, breast tenderness and a variable mood pattern. Many of these symptoms are linked with the menstrual cycle and have been discussed in the section on PREMENSTRUAL SYNDROME (*see* p. 463). Many of the remedies found there will help, but if none does, the following remedy should be considered:

### *Folliculinum* (preparation from ovarian follicle)

This remedy picture describes a woman who has fluid retention, breast tenderness and a variable mood pattern. Fourteen days after the period has finished, and using the 200c potency, give one dose every 12 hours, for a maximum of three doses.

# *Menopause problems*

The "menopause" is the term commonly used to describe the time when a woman's ovaries begin to decline, usually at the age of about 55, and the monthly periods stop. (Medically, the term "menopause" is used for the precise moment that periods end; the time leading up to this is known as the "climacteric".) Should any bleeding occur after this, it should be fully investigated as it may indicate cancer.

The menopause is a natural event, and many women adjust to it with no difficulty. However, as the level of oestrogen in the body falls, a number of secondary symptoms may become apparent. Conventional treatment is with hormone replacement therapy (HRT), which will resolve virtually all the problems of the menopause. But HRT does have side-effects, notably pulmonary embolism (a clot of blood that has moved from the venous system into the lungs), which, although rare, can be fatal. For this reason, many women look for safe alternative forms of therapy. Below, various symptoms of the menopause are dealt with, including the appropriate homeopathic remedies.

## Osteoporosis

This condition occurs when calcium is leached out of the bones; although the bones remain the same shape, they are substantially weakened and so are much more likely to fracture, particularly the hip. While osteoporosis occurs in astronauts who stay weight-less in space for long periods (weight-bearing exercise is good at preventing it), it is primarily a problem of women entering the menopause and of people who take steroids for a long time. Ageing is a significant feature of osteoporosis in both sexes, but the condition is more common in women: women over the age of 80 will have lost between 25 and 50 per cent of their bone density.

Osteoporosis is most frequently found in the following types of women:

- those who have a family history of osteoporosis.
- those who have had an early menopause (before the age of 45), including those who have had their ovaries removed during a full hysterectomy.
- those who are particularly thin.
- those who have missed many periods for reasons other than pregnancy (this is particularly true of women athletes).

Certain other factors increase the risks in men and women:

- having to take steroids for a long time.
- heavy cigarette smoking.
- excessive drinking of alcohol
- a previously fractured bone or a serious fall.

The conventional treatment is hormone replacement therapy (HRT) and physical exercise. It is advisable for women to exercise to the point of breathlessness for at least 30 minutes a day, but the exercise must be weight-bearing – e.g. brisk walking, aerobic exercises, cycling – to have an effect on the bones. Therefore, swimming (in all other respects an excellent form of exercise) is not helpful in preventing osteoporosis.

An adequate diet is also important in minimizing the calcium loss from bones. This loss can be increased by diets particularly high in protein from animal sources because animal protein contains excess phosphorus. Therefore, it is advisable that a good proportion of the protein in the diet should come from vegetable sources, notably pulses, tofu, soya and nuts. Refined sugar also increases calcium loss from the body (although the natural sugars in fruit are fine), as do caffeine-containing and carbonated drinks. Foods rich in calcium include whitebait (860 mg per 100 g), Cheddar cheese (400 mg per 50 g), tinned sardines (350 mg per 70 g) and milk (350 mg per 285 ml). Calcium supplements of 1,500 mg per day are also recommended as a long-term approach to prevent osteoporosis.

Magnesium controls the uptake of calcium by the body, and a daily intake of 300–450 mg of this mineral should be the aim. Magnesium is best obtained from unprocessed whole food: millet (370 mg per 230 g), lima beans (125 mg per 170g), Brazil nuts (80 mg per 10 nuts), plain low-fat yoghurt (40 mg per 285 ml), dark green-leafed vegetables (20 mg per 100 g). The trace mineral boron, also necessary for the metabolism of calcium, is found in vegetables but a supplement of 1–3 mg daily guarantees the daily quantity necessary.

Vitamin D is closely involved in the absorption of calcium by the body. This nutrient is naturally obtained through exposure to sunlight. However, sunlight is now known to promote skin cancer, so as an alternative, a supplement can be taken, either in cod liver oil or in a multi-vitamin. Aim for a daily intake of 200–400 iu.

Homeopathic treatment is directed exclusively towards women nearing the age of menopause and post-menopausal women, and involves homeopathic hormone replacement with *Wild Yam* cream. Rich in progesterone, this has been shown to increase bone density.

Women who are beginning to show signs of the menopause but who are still menstruating can be given the hormones that their ageing ovaries are beginning to fail to supply. These naturally occurring hormones would be inappropriate to give in any other than the homeopathic form because of their potentially serious side-effects. However, the homeopathic way of preparation results in products that are so diluted that there are no molecules of the original substances left, yet they still have a therapeutic effect.

The following homeopathic remedies can be given instead of the *Wild Yam* cream.

- *Oestrogen*: 12c potency to be given once a day for three weeks, starting as soon as menstruation has started.
- *Progesterone*: 6c potency to be given twice a day for one week, following the three-week cycle of oestrogen.

The following homeopathic remedy is given on its own to women who are still menstruating as well as to those whose periods have stopped.

- *Oestradiol* (naturally occurring hormone): Using the 12c potency, give once a day for one month to post-menstruating women and thereafter once a week. For women who are menstruating, give one dose a week.

The choice between these two methods of treatment depends on the person's individual choice – one treatment may suit one woman better than another. Using the *Wild Yam* cream on its own seems to suit those women who have minor depression or breast tenderness, possibly before their menstrual cycle, or a past medical history of depression.

## Stiff and painful joints

Maintenance of an ideal body weight is important as this will help take the load off the joints. Supplementing the diet with evening primrose oil (at least 1,000 mg per day) will be beneficial.

Conventional treatment will also include nonsteroidal anti-inflammatory drug therapy.

Homeopathic remedies that will be helpful in treating these symptoms will be found in the appropriate section on OSTEOAR-THRITIS (*see* p. 321).

## Vaginal dryness

The woman may notice dryness of her vagina, which can make it more vulnerable to infection and can make sexual intercourse painful.

A topical homeopathic treatment is to use *Calendula* (marigold) ointment daily as required spreading it directly in the vagina. For sexual lubrication, use a bland, water-based jelly (*not* petroleum jelly).

The following homeopathic remedies can also be helpful. Select one by matching its picture with the physical symptoms. Using the 6c potency, give one dose twice a day.

### Ferrum phosphoricum (iron phosphate)

This remedy picture describes a pale woman who is excitable and whose vagina is dry and feels hot. If sexual intercourse takes place, it is painful, causing the woman to have VAGINISMUS (*see below*).

### Graphites (black lead)

This remedy picture describes a woman with a marked aversion to sexual intercourse. Her vagina is dry and she commonly has eczema on her vulva. She is overweight and her nipples are cracked with eczema, which may ooze a honey-coloured exudate.

### Lycopodium (club moss)

This remedy picture describes a woman whose vagina is dry during and following intercourse. She commonly has a burning vaginal discharge that is worse during a full moon.

### Natrum muriaticum (sodium chloride)

This remedy picture describes a woman who develops a burning, smarting sensation in her vagina during sexual intercourse, caused by vaginal dryness, and, as a result, has an aversion towards sex. The general characteristics of the women whom this remedy will particularly suit are that they like salt, are shy and are capable of bearing a grudge.

# Hot flushes

With the decrease in the production of oestrogen by the ovaries, hot flushes become prominent, causing reddening of the face, neck and upper trunk and a sensation of heat and sweating.

The following homeopathic remedies may be used to help control these flushes. Select one by matching its picture with the physical symptoms.

### *Amyl nitrosum* (amyl nitrate)

This remedy picture describes rapidly dilating capillaries (the smallest blood vessels), giving flushes of the face with heat and sweat. Using the 6c potency, give one dose every ten minutes as required.

### *Lachesis* (bushmaster snake venom)

This remedy picture describes a woman who suddenly develops hot flushes, together with headaches and fainting spells. She feels especially worse if her clothes are tight around her neck or waist. This remedy particularly suits the woman who chats a lot. She can become violent on occasions (*see* PREMENSTRUAL SYNDROME). Using the 6c potency, give one dose every hour as required.

### *Sanguinaria* (blood root)

This remedy picture describes a woman with disturbances in the blood vessels, giving her red cheeks and a sensation of blood rushing to her head. At the same time, she feels hot and as if her whole body is throbbing. She commonly has a painful vaginal discharge and a particular soreness under her right nipple. Using the 6c potency, give one dose every four hours as required.

### *Sepia* (inky juice of cuttlefish)

This remedy picture describes a woman who develops sudden

flushes of heat and sweating with a feeling of weakness and exhaustion. She finds that her vagina becomes painfully sensitive after sexual intercourse. She prefers sitting with her legs crossed as she feels as if her womb (uterus) will fall out from between her legs. Using the 6c potency, give one dose every hour as required.

### Sulphur

This remedy picture describes a woman who suddenly develops redness in her face and sweats on her face, scalp, back and thighs. She has a definite point of view and enjoys a joke and a drink, and her house has a lived-in feeling. Using the 6c potency, give one dose twice a day.

# Menstrual difficulties

## Heavy periods (menorrhagia)

A woman can bleed so excessively at each menstrual period that she can become anaemic. She will need to see her medical practitioner for blood tests to find out the level of her anaemia, and she will also need to be examined vaginally so that the uterus can be assessed for any abnormality (e.g a FIBROID) that could be the cause of the menorrhagia.

The conventional treatment depends on the severity of the periods and the age of the sufferer. Hormones may be prescribed, which will reduce the amount of bleeding. The other options are surgical: either removal of the lining of the uterus (the endometrium) or of the uterus itself (hysterectomy).

The homeopathic treatment that should be given following surgery consists of the following two remedies:

### Arnica (leopard's bane)

This remedy will reduce bruising. Using the 6c potency, give one dose before surgery and two further doses following it, the first as soon as possible and the second six hours later.

### Hypericum (St John's wort)

This remedy will help any skin incision to heal quicker and will also help reduce the pain from the incision. Using the 6c potency, give one dose with each dose of *Arnica*.

The following homeopathic remedies all have menorrhagia in their pictures, and they can be tried instead of surgery. Select one by matching its picture with the physical symptoms. After the onset of bleeding from a menstrual period, and using the 6c potency, give one dose twice a day for two weeks; repeat for three cycles. After this time, it is possible to assess the effect of this form of therapy. If it has been successful, this dosage schedule can be continued.

### Belladonna (deadly nightshade)

This remedy picture describes menorrhagia where the blood is bright red, as well as flowing profusely and quickly. The woman is aware of the heat of the blood. She also feels as if her uterus is going to protrude through her vulva.

### Calcarea carbonica (calcium carbonate)

This remedy picture describes a woman with menorrhagia whose breasts become swollen and tender before her menstrual cycle begins. Menstruation may make her feel dizzy. She probably has a problem with her weight and sweats easily, particularly from her feet and scalp.

### Cinchona officinalis (China) (Peruvian bark)

This remedy picture describes menorrhagia that produces large, dark clots of blood. Menstruation is associated with much pain and swelling of the abdomen, and the woman feels faint. She also notices a bloody vaginal discharge at the time of ovulation.

### Crocus sativa (saffron)

This remedy picture describes a woman with menorrhagia where the blood flows so quickly that it could be classified as a uterine haemorrhage. The blood is very dark in colour and slimy and contains long strings of blood. The woman notices a jerking pain in her left breast, as if it is being drawn towards her back by means of a thread. She may also notice a sensation in her right breast as though something is alive in it.

### Ipecacuanha (ipecac root)

This remedy picture describes a woman with menorrhagia who bleeds bright red blood, whose blood flow is profuse (like *Belladonna*) but who feels nauseated.

### Platina (platinum)

This remedy picture describes a woman who is arrogant and proud. She has menorrhagia associated with blood clots and painful uterine spasms. Her vagina and her vulva are very sensitive to the touch even when she is not menstruating, so that sexual intercourse becomes very difficult.

### Sabina (savine)

This remedy picture describes a woman with menorrhagia whose sexual desire increases during menstruation. The blood flow, which contains clots of blood, is made worse from the slightest movement yet can be improved by walking. The woman notices pain from her lower back radiating to her pubic bone or a pain that shoots up her vagina. She may also find her vulva very itchy at all times.

### Sanguinaria (blood root)

This remedy picture describes a woman with menorrhagia who is just becoming menopausal and may be having hot flushes already. Her breasts are sore under the nipples, particularly the right one.

Further homeopathic remedies for menstrual difficulties can be found under PAINFUL PERIODS (p. 461), PAINFUL OVULATION (p. 460) and PREMENSTRUAL SYNDROME (p. 463).

# Ovarian cysts

These can cause pain and must be accurately diagnosed to exclude cancer. This is done by a vaginal examination and, if indicated, a computerized scan with a follow-up biopsy. If cancer is found, surgery to remove the ovary may be recommended.

Homeopathic treatment is second choice and begins (having excluded cancer) with constitutional prescribing from a specialist homeopath. If this is not possible, the following remedies can be tried, matching the remedy picture with the physical symptoms. Using the 6c potency, give one dose twice a day.

### *Apis mellifica* (honey bee)

This remedy picture describes lower abdominal tenderness (from ovarian cysts) and swelling of the lips of the vulva (the labia). The woman also suffers from PAINFUL PERIODS (dysmenorrhea).

### *Cimicifuga* (black snake root)

This remedy picture describes pain in the lower abdomen from the ovaries, which shoots upwards and downwards into the woman's thighs.

### *Colocynthis* (bitter cucumber)

This remedy picture describes pains in the lower abdomen from the ovaries, which are eased from firm pressure obtained when the woman bends double.

### *Iodum* (iodine)

This remedy picture describes pains in the lower abdomen from the ovaries, which the woman describes as if a wedge is being driven between her ovary and her womb (uterus).

### *Lachesis* (bushmaster snake venom)

This remedy picture describes a tender left ovary that is swollen from multiple cysts. The pain from this ovary is worse in the morning, tending to wake the woman, but wears off during the course of the day.

## Pelvic inflammatory disease (PID)

This is a bacterial infection of the genital tract. It is most common in younger women and is sexually transmitted. It causes pain and can lead to infertility.

The conventional treatment is with appropriate antibiotic therapy.

The homeopathic approach is to use the woman's constitutional remedy, particularly when she suffers from recurrent attacks. For this, she is advised to see a specialist homeopath. Bedrest is also important for an acute attack, as is avoidance of sexual intercourse until the pain has subsided.

The following homeopathic remedies can be used to treat the acute attack. Select the remedy by matching the picture to the physical symptoms. Using the 6c potency, give one dose every two hours. If there is no sign of any improvement, consult your medical practitioner.

### *Aconitum napellus* (monk's-hood)

This remedy picture describes a sudden onset of symptoms with a possible fever. The woman is very anxious, even fearful of dying, and the symptoms are made worse by anything cold.

### *Apis mellifica* (honey bee)

This remedy picture describes pains in the pelvic region that have a stinging quality. The woman is not very thirsty, and her pains are made worse from heat of any form.

## *Belladonna* (deadly nightshade)

This remedy picture describes a sudden onset of lower abdominal pain that is associated with a fever, making the woman's face go red and her pupils dilate widely. She finds that the pains are made worse from the slightest jarring of her body.

## *Colocynthis* (bitter cucumber)

This remedy picture describes pelvic pain that is relieved by firm pressure, particularly when the woman bends double.

## *Mercurius corrosivus* (corrosive sublimate of mercury)

This remedy picture describes pelvic pains as well as the characteristic feature of this remedy, which is profuse, foul-smelling sweat.

# Sexually transmitted diseases

These have been covered in the section on adult MEN, and the same remedies and advice apply for women except for the following conditions.

## Chlamydia

The importance of chlamydial infection is very significant in women because it has serious consequences if it remains undiagnosed: 30 per cent of women inadequately treated for this infection go on to develop PELVIC INFLAMMATORY DISEASE (PID), and of these, one-fifth become infertile and one-tenth suffer an ECTOPIC PREGNANCY.

The symptoms of this infection vary from a vaginal discharge and URETHRITIS to no specific symptoms at all. For this reason, a woman who has had multiple sexual partners is recommended to attend a clinic that will screen for this infection. The treatment for this infection is as described on p. 469.

# Thrush

In women, this infection, caused by the yeast-like fungus *Candida albicans*, produces an itchy vaginal discharge that consists of a thick white-yellow material. As with all sexually acquired diseases, the male partner must be treated as well as the woman.

The conventional treatment is an anti-fungal ointment and a pessary that is placed in the vagina.

The homeopathic approach is to follow the dietary advice given on p. 474. The following homeopathic remedies can also be given. Select one by matching its picture with the physical symptoms. Using the 6c potency, give one dose three times a day.

### *Alumina* (aluminium)

This remedy picture describes a woman whose vaginal discharge is profuse and burning and runs down her legs and is therefore worse during the day. Before her menstrual period, it is made better by washing her vulva with cold water. She develops an itching and tickling sensation in her vulva and, at the same time, has an overwhelming need for an embrace.

### *Calcarea carbonica* (calcium carbonate)

This remedy picture describes a woman whose vaginal discharge is thick and gushing and is either yellow or milky in colour. The discharge causes itching and burning, sensations that are made worse when the woman urinates.

### *Hydrastis* (golden seal)

This remedy picture describes a woman who has an itchy, profuse vaginal discharge that is worse after she menstruates.

### *Kreosotum* (beechwood kreosote)

This remedy picture describes a vaginal discharge that is either yellow or green and stains the woman's underwear considerably. It causes a corrosive feeling in the vagina and makes the vulva swell. The woman develops a violent itching between her thighs.

### *Pulsatilla* (wind flower)

This remedy picture describes a vaginal discharge that comes on when the woman gets her feet wet, when she is mentally run down or if she becomes anaemic. The discharge is watery and is worse just before and immediately after her menstrual period.

### *Sepia* (inky juice of cuttlefish)

This remedy picture describes a vaginal discharge that is yellow-ish and causes the woman's vulva to itch and produces a sharp, stinging pain in her uterus. Walking makes her symptoms worse, and her abdomen becomes distended during the day.

### *Sulphur*

This remedy picture describes a woman whose vaginal discharge is worse a week before her menstrual period. It can be either white or yellow, but always causes cramping in her abdomen or a pinching sensation around her tummy button.

## Trichomonas infection

This infection produces a greenish or yellowish vaginal discharge in women. It is diagnosed by taking a swab of the discharge, culturing it and then examining this microscopically. The conventional treatment is with a course of an antibiotic, tetracycline or metronidazole.

The following homeopathic remedies can be used instead. Select one by matching its picture with the physical symptoms. Using the 6c potency, give one dose three times a day.

### *Bovista* (puff ball)

This remedy picture describes a woman with a yellow-green

vaginal discharge that causes a stinging, smarting sensation and is worse whenever she walks about. The discharge stains her underwear green.

### Carbo vegetabilis (vegetable charcoal)

This remedy picture describes a burning, green vaginal discharge that particularly occurs before the woman's menstrual period.

### Mercurius corrosivus (corrosive sublimate of mercury)

This remedy picture describes a yellow-green vaginal discharge, the smell of which makes the woman feel sick. The discharge may contain solid matter, and the woman alternates between feeling cold and sweating.

### Nitric acidum (nitric acid)

This remedy picture describes a vaginal discharge that is brown or flesh-coloured. It stains the woman's underwear yellow or leaves spots with black borders. This discharge is stringy and is more profuse following a menstrual period.

# Uterine problems

## Fibroids

These are growths within the muscle of the uterus, which are almost always non-malignant. They can cause infertility and HEAVY PERIODS (menorrhagia).

The conventional treatment is surgery. When the woman wants to become pregnant, this can involve the simple removal of the fibroid. The alternative is removal of the uterus by a hysterectomy.

The ideal homeopathic treatment is to prescribe the woman's constitutional remedy, which necessitates a consultation with a specialist homeopath. The following homeopathic remedies may be tried for a short time. Using the 6c potency, give one dose three times a day for six weeks. If there is no sign of improvement, conventional treatment should be pursued.

### Aurum muriaticum (sodium chloroaurate)

This remedy picture describes a uterus that becomes bony hard and fills up the whole of the woman's pelvis. The cervix commonly ulcerates, and the vagina develops spasmodic contractions.

### Calcarea iodata (iodide of lime)

This remedy has a specific action on the uterus and is specially useful in the treatment of small fibroids. This remedy picture also describes cramps.

### Fraxinus americana (white ash)

This remedy has a specific action on uterine muscle. It describes a woman with fibroids that give her a bearing-down sensation that may be located in the groin. She may also have PAINFUL PERIODS (dysmenorrhoea) and a watery vaginal discharge.

## Prolapsed uterus and vagina

The muscles and ligaments that keep the uterus in place become slack with age, and especially so if the woman has given birth. To prevent this from occurring, exercises should be performed that will strengthen the pelvic floor muscles. This is done by squeezing the cheeks of the buttocks together frequently during the course of the day. When the prolapse does occur, the cervix protrudes to varying degrees through the vagina.

The conventional treatment is to hold the uterus in position by inserting a plastic pessary ring into the top of the vagina. Alternatively, a hysterectomy or vaginal repair may be performed.

Homeopathic remedies can be used in the early stages to help prevent further deterioration, with the woman having been encouraged to do pelvic floor muscle exercises. Select the remedy by matching its picture with the physical symptoms. Using the 6c potency, give one dose twice a day for one month. If there is no improvement, conventional methods must be used.

### *Aloe* (socotrine aloes)

This remedy picture describes a uterus that feels heavy, a symptom that is worse when the woman stands up or walks about; for this reason, she tries to stay still by sitting down. There is also a bearing-down sensation in the rectum, which is worse during the woman's menstrual period.

### *Argentum metallicum* (silver)

This remedy picture describes a bearing-down pain due to a prolapsed uterus. The woman has a sore feeling throughout her abdomen, which is made worse by any jarring movement.

### *Argentum nitricum* (silver nitrate)

This remedy picture describes a prolapsed uterus with an ulcerated cervix. It also includes a nervous woman who desires sweets and is particularly nervous of heights and crowds.

### *Aurum metallicum* (gold)

This remedy picture describes a woman who is seriously depressed. Her uterus feels enlarged and prolapses.

### *Belladonna* (deadly nightshade)

This remedy picture describes a woman who feels that her genitals will fall out of her vagina. The reality is that her uterus often does prolapse. She is easily excited.

### Calcarea carbonica (calcium carbonate)

This remedy picture describes a woman with a prolapsed uterus. She tends to be overweight and easily sweats from the head. She is an obstinate woman who tends to be constipated.

### Lilium tigrinum (tiger lily)

This remedy picture describes a woman with a prolapsed uterus, who has an irresistible urge to replace it physically herself. Her vulva itches, and she has a frequent desire to urinate and defecate; she has a generalized pain in her lower abdomen. She is excitable and irritable.

### Pulsatilla (wind flower)

This remedy picture describes a woman in the early stages of developing a prolapsed uterus. She has a bearing-down sensation in her genital area, associated with backache. These symptoms are made worse whenever she lies down, has a menstrual period or enters a warm environment (she feels better in the fresh air). She has a tendency to weep a lot.

### Sepia (inky juice of cuttlefish)

This remedy picture describes a woman who feels as if her uterus will fall out of her vagina. For this reason, she prefers to sit with her legs crossed. Her pelvic floor muscles are relaxed, and prolapse of the uterus is common. This woman definitely prefers her own space.

# Vaginal disorders

## Bartholin's abscess

The two pea-sized Bartholin's glands are situated at the entrance of the vagina, and ducts from them secrete fluid to lubricate the vagina during sexual intercourse. Either of these glands can become infected, causing pain and, possibly, fever.

The conventional treatment is with antibiotics, with follow-up surgery (if necessary) to widen the opening of the duct, convert the duct into an open pouch or remove the gland entirely.

Homeopathic treatment, which is only to be used in a complementary way with the conventional treatment, will hasten the woman's recovery. Using the 6c potency, give one dose three times a day for three days.

### *Belladonna* (deadly nightshade)

This remedy picture describes the early stages of the infection where there is heat, tenderness and swelling at the vaginal entrance.

### *Hepar sulphuris* (Hahnemann's calcium sulphide)

This remedy picture describes an infection that is beginning to create pus. The discharge smells very offensive, like old cheese.

## Vaginismus

This occurs in a woman who, because of spasm of the muscles at the entrance to the vagina, finds penile penetration during sexual intercourse impossible.

Treatment, both conventional and homeopathic, is supportive towards the woman, helping her to understand her underlying anxieties. Psychotherapy may be relevant. The pain of the spasm may be associated with chronic vaginitis (infection of the vagina), THRUSH or VAGINAL DRYNESS, in which case, the underlying cause must be treated.

Conventional drug therapy is with tranquillizers, and with a series of graded dilators, which the woman learns to use until she is comfortable with the largest one – the size of the average penis.

The following homeopathic remedies can be used. Select the

one whose picture matches the physical symptoms most precisely. Using a 6c potency, give one dose daily.

### Cactus grandiflorus (night-blooming cereus)

This remedy picture describes a vagina that goes into spasm whenever sexual intercourse is attempted and therefore it cannot take place. The picture also describes PAINFUL PERIODS (dysmenorrhoea) and constricting pains in the uterus and in the ovarian region (the two lower quadrants of the abdomen).

### Plumbum metallicum (lead)

This remedy picture describes a woman with vaginismus who may also have an underdeveloped uterus and hardened breasts. Her breasts give her stitching pains, and she probably suffers from HEAVY PERIODS (menorrhagia), with a sensation of a string pulling her uterus towards her back.

# Vulval warts

These genital warts are caused by the human papilloma virus (HPV) and are found on the lips of the vulva (the labia) and in the entrance to the vagina. They are sexually acquired.

The conventional treatment is by freezing them off with liquid nitrogen.

The homeopathic treatment for treating genital warts has already been discussed in the section on MEN (*see* p. 470).

---

Genital warts in women have been linked with cases of CERVICAL CANCER (*see above*). Therefore, a woman who has had genital warts, or whose partner has had these warts, should have annual cervical smear tests.

---

# Pregnancy, Delivery and After

This section explains how homeopathic therapies can complement conventional obstetric treatments during pregnancy and for the first few weeks following delivery.

Before conception, the woman should stop smoking; this has been shown to reduce placental blood flow to the baby. She should also eat a diet rich in folic acid – obtained from green-leafed vegetables and nuts – as this has been shown to reduce neural tube abnormalities in the baby, notably spina bifida. Conventional treatment is to advise that the woman takes a folic acid supplement as soon as she decides to become pregnant. Once she is pregnant, it will be too late to take folic acid supplements, as the beneficial effect of protecting against neural tube defects has been lost. Eating a folic acid-rich diet should ensure an adequate intake of this important B vitamin without needing a supplement. It is, however, possible to obtain a homeopathic preparation of folic acid: using the 6c potency, take one dose twice a day as soon as the decision has been made to conceive.

She should also check, by means of a blood test, that she has had RUBELLA (German measles). If she hasn't, she can arrange to be immunized before becoming pregnant.

When the woman has become pregnant, she should go to see her medical practitioner and arrange for a midwife, so that she can have the necessary blood tests and physical checks.

Pregnancy lasts for about 40 weeks. The expected date of delivery – the EDD – is calculated from the first day of the woman's last menstrual period.


## Common problems in the first trimester

The first trimester covers the pregnancy up to the 14th week.

# Anaemia

When a woman becomes pregnant, her blood naturally becomes diluted so that her blood count is lower than when she isn't pregnant. There are, however, two more serious types of anaemia found in pregnancy.

**Megaloblastic anaemia** is due to folic acid or vitamin $B_{12}$ deficiency. Folic acid deficiency is caused by a lack of this nutrient in the diet (*see above*, where this is discussed in connection with neural tube development). Far more worrying is vitamin $B_{12}$ deficiency, which is due to a primary problem of the gastrointestinal tract and requires detailed investigation. The only treatment is conventional, by appropriate injection therapy.

**Iron-deficiency anaemia** is a common occurrence during pregnancy. There are two reasons for giving conventional iron supplements (which can cause CONSTIPATION as a side-effect) at this time:

- if it is a multiple pregnancy (i.e. twins, triplets or more).
- if there is a past history of iron-deficiency anaemia.

For women who make an informed decision not to take these conventional tablets, the following homeopathic remedies are available. Select one matching its picture with the physical symptoms. Using the 6c potency, give one dose twice a day.

### *Ferrum metallicum* (iron)

This remedy picture describes a woman who is restless and has an aversion to eating eggs.

### *Ferrum phosphoricum* (iron phosphate)

This remedy picture describes a woman who feels weak, flushes easily and yet looks pale.

# Ectopic pregnancy

This occurs when the fertilized egg becomes implanted in a place other than the uterus, usually one of the Fallopian tubes. This causes severe pain as well as collapse if the pregnancy breaks through the tube, leading to haemorrhage. This is life-threatening and requires immediate hospitalization for surgery.

The only homeopathic remedy to be considered is:

### *Aconitum napellus* (monk's-hood)

This remedy picture describes a sudden illness causing extreme anxiety with a fear of dying. Using the 30c potency, give one dose every 15 minutes while waiting for the ambulance.

# Fatigue

This is a common symptom in the early stages of pregnancy. Provided that the blood tests are normal, showing that the woman is not anaemic, a constitutional remedy – obtained after consultation with a specialist homeopath – will help alleviate this symptom. If this is not possible, the following homeopathic remedies can be tried. Using the 30c potency, give one dose daily for five days, and then repeat the dose monthly throughout the pregnancy.

### *Argentum nitricum* (silver nitrate)

This remedy picture describes a woman who has a marked anticipatory anxiety. She is particularly fearful of heights and crowded places. She dislikes hot environments and desires refined sugar.

### *Arsenicum album* (arsenic trioxide)

This remedy picture describes an excessively neat and tidy woman who is also house-proud. She is very restless and sensitive to the cold weather. Any symptoms that she may have are magnified out of all proportion. She enjoys sips of warm water, and feels worse late at night.

## *Natrum muriaticum* (sodium chloride)

This remedy picture describes a woman who has greasy skin and characteristically has a crack in the middle of her lower lip. Outwardly she gives the impression of being sociable, but this conceals an inner shyness and a lack of confidence. She easily becomes distressed if she is left out of things and can bear a grudge. Paradoxically, any attempt to console her will make her feel worse. Typically she is "nice to know but difficult to live with". She may suffer severe throbbing headaches. She has a desire for salty foods and feels worse in extremes of temperature (either hot or cold).

## *Nux vomica* (poison-nut)

This remedy picture describes an ambitious woman who, because she is a perfectionist, finds that, on becoming pregnant, she cannot cope with the stresses and strains on her life. She feels better in wet weather, provided that the rain is not associated with a cold wind. She has a desire for stimulants such as alcohol, coffee and, probably, cigarettes.

## *Phosphorus*

This remedy picture describes a woman who is very sensitive and is able to give and receive emotional support easily. She likes company and has an active social life. She has artistic qualities and may have a tint of red in her hair. She tends to tire easily, but responds to short naps. She has a particular fear of thunderstorms.

## *Pulsatilla* (wind flower)

This remedy picture describes a woman who tends to cry easily and often. She positively dislikes hot places, much preferring the fresh air. She dislikes any arguments, seeking harmony at all times. She is not particularly thirsty nor is she particularly emotionally demonstrative, much preferring to be supported emotionally and physically by someone else. She dislikes fatty foods, and is at her worst in the late afternoon.

### Sepia (inky juice of cuttlefish)

This remedy picture describes a woman who feels completely overburdened and that no one else is pulling their weight. She retreats into her own private space, away from all her loved ones. She feels tired all the time, which sleep doesn't help but dancing or physical exercise does. Her taste is for vinegary foods.

### Sulphur

This remedy picture describes a woman who has a ruddy complexion and is not particularly fussy about her personal appearance. She is always happy to have people visiting her and doesn't care about the tidiness of her surroundings. She enjoys a joke, alcohol and, particularly, beer and fatty food, but finds that cow's milk disagrees with her. She has a definite point of view.

# Heartburn

The primary symptom is a burning pain behind the breastbone (sternum) whenever the woman belches.

The conventional treatment is with an antacid.

The following homeopathic remedies can be used. Select one by matching its picture with the physical symptoms. Using the 6c potency, give one dose as often as required.

### Asafoetida (gum of the stinkasand)

This remedy picture describes a woman with considerable flatulence and regurgitation of stomach contents. She tends to behave irrationally.

### *Capsicum annuum* (cayenne pepper)

This remedy picture describes an obese woman who characteristically has a burning sensation on the tip of her tongue. She is thirsty but drinking causes shivering.

### *Carbo vegetabilis* (vegetable charcoal)

This remedy picture describes a woman who passes a great deal of wind, both upwards and downwards. She feels worn out and is improved when air is fanned over her face.

# Miscarriage

This is defined as the loss of the foetus before the 28th week of pregnancy. At least 10–30 per cent of all pregnancies end in miscarriage, usually before the tenth week. The symptoms are bleeding from the vagina, cramping and pain. Miscarriages are classified as either threatened, inevitable or missed, and are distinguished by a vaginal examination and by the symptoms. In a threatened miscarriage, the foetus remains alive despite bleeding from the vagina; vaginal examination reveals that the neck of the womb is closed and the pregnancy will very likely go successfully to term. In an inevitable miscarriage, cramping uterine pains are felt as the foetus (which has died) is expelled from the uterus; examination reveals that the neck of the cervix is open. In a missed miscarriage, the foetus has died but has not been expelled; it will have to be removed surgically.

A threatened miscarriage is treated, both conventionally and homeopathically, with bedrest.

The following homeopathic remedies can also be used. Select one by matching its picture with the physical symptoms.

### *Aconitum napellus* (monk's-hood)

This remedy picture describes severe anxiety and a particular fear of dying. Using the 30c potency, this remedy should be given immediately and repeated every 15 minutes, for a maximum of six doses.

### *Arnica* (leopard's bane)

This remedy should be used whenever there has been any injury preceding the threatened miscarriage. Using the 30c potency, give one dose immediately and repeat twice at four-hour intervals.

### *Belladonna* (deadly nightshade)

This remedy picture describes a woman undergoing a threatened miscarriage who has a red, flushed face. Her pulse rate is high and her pupils are dilated. Using the 30c potency, give one dose immediately and repeat three times at six-hour intervals.

### *Ipecacuanha* (ipecac root)

This remedy is indicated when the woman feels nauseated and may even vomit. Using the 30c potency, give one dose immediately and repeat at hourly intervals, for a maximum of three doses.

### *Secale cornutum* (ergot)

This remedy picture describes blood loss that is profuse and blackish, leaving the woman feeling weak, exhausted and fearful of dying. Clearly the woman in this situation must be assessed by a medical practitioner. When using this remedy, it is important to have regular vaginal checks because, although the bleeding subsides, the cervix might have opened, in which case the miscarriage has become inevitable and the woman possibly requires hospital admission. Using the 30c potency, give one dose immediately and repeat with caution daily, for a maximum of three doses.

### Repeated miscarriage

This needs a detailed gynaecological investigation to check that there are no genetic, hormonal or uterine abnormalities. If there aren't, the best advice is to see a specialist homeopath. If this is not possible, the following homeopathic remedies can be used.

Select one by matching its picture with the physical symptoms. Using the 6c potency, give one dose twice a day.

### *Caulophyllum* (blue cohosh)

This remedy picture describes a woman who has recurrent miscarriages. She may feel needle-like pains in her cervix (neck of the womb). She may also have severe drawing-like pains in the small joints of her fingers and toes.

### *Sepia* (inky juice of cuttlefish)

This remedy has a special affinity for the uterus and helps the foetus stay within it. The remedy is selected primarily from the general features of the woman. She prefers her own space when depressed, goes off those people closest to her and likes vinegar and fresh, sunny, windy weather. She prefers warmth as she is sensitive to the cold. Paradoxically she feels better by eating or drinking small amounts.

## Morning sickness

Nausea and vomiting is very common in early pregnancy, usually starting before the sixth week and discontinuing at about the 12th week, although it can continue throughout the pregnancy. It generally occurs early in the morning, on waking, although it can happen at any time of the day. Sufferers may find that it is relieved if they eat and drink little and often.

Conventional treatment has little to offer most sufferers of morning sickness, as any drugs that might be given could harm the baby.

However, the following homeopathic remedies can be used safely to help reduce this symptom. Select one by matching its picture with the physical symptoms. Using the 6c potency, give one dose three times a day.

### *Arsenicum album* (arsenic trioxide)

This remedy picture describes a woman whose sickness is also probably associated with diarrhoea. The woman is chilly, thirsty, anxious and exceptionally neat and tidy. She is also house-proud.

### *Ipecacuanha* (ipecac root)

This remedy picture describes a woman who feels nauseated all the time. Even vomiting doesn't bring any relief.

### *Natrum muriaticum* (sodium chloride)

This remedy picture describes a woman with morning sickness who has a craving for salt. She has greasy skin and a characteristic crack in the centre of her lower lip. She is shy, but overcomes this by producing an artificial sense of gaiety. She is very sensitive to loud noises and can bear a grudge should anyone cross her path.

### *Nux vomica* (poison-nut)

This remedy picture describes a woman with morning sickness whose abdomen feels bloated and is particularly tender to firm pressure. She belches and this gives her a bitter taste in her mouth. The woman is ambitious and enjoys alcohol and coffee (and possibly finds it difficult to stop smoking or eating chocolates).

### *Phosphorus*

This remedy picture describes a woman whose nausea and vomiting is worse towards evening. It may be brought on by salty foods and by cold food or liquids, which are vomited as they warm up in her stomach. This remedy describes a woman who is fearful of thunder, has a wide circle of friends and tires easily but recovers quickly after a short nap.

### *Pulsatilla* (wind flower)

This remedy picture describes a woman who becomes nauseated when eating or smelling fatty food. She feels better in the fresh air and worse in hot environments. She weeps easily and responds well to a reassuring cuddle.

### Sepia (inky juice of the cuttlefish)

This is the classic remedy for morning sickness as the remedy picture describes a woman who feels sick at the sight, smell or even the thought of food. However, this symptom is improved when she has a small amount to eat or drink. She needs her own space and can easily become depressed.

# Common problems in the second trimester (14 weeks to 28 weeks)

This section covers difficulties that a pregnant woman may discover from the 14th to the 28th week.

## Urogenital tract disorders

### Vaginal discharge

It is important to make an accurate diagnosis of any vaginal discharge – by taking swabs of the discharge, culturing these and examining them microscopically – in order to establish the precise cause, which can then be dealt with.

While waiting for the results, the following homeopathic remedies can be used. Select the remedy by matching its picture with the physical symptoms. Using the 6c potency, give one dose four times a day.

### Hydrastis (golden seal)

This remedy picture describes a thick, ropey, yellow discharge that causes a marked irritation of the vagina and the surrounding vulva.

### *Kreosotum* (beechwood kreosote)

This remedy picture describes a discharge that is particularly smelly and stains the woman's underwear a dark colour.

### *Nitricum acidum* (nitric acid)

This remedy picture describes a vaginal discharge that causes a pricking sensation in the woman's vagina, which may also be ulcerated.

### *Pulsatilla* (wind flower)

This remedy picture describes a vaginal discharge that is bland in colour and non-irritant. The profile of the woman is helpful when selecting this remedy: she is gentle, dislikes the heat and prefers fresh air, and dislikes fatty foods.

### *Sepia* (inky juice of cuttlefish)

This remedy picture describes a vaginal discharge that is jelly-like. The woman may feel that her vagina is PROLAPSED. She can become moody, retiring into her own private space. Things can get on top of her, and she can emotionally switch off those people closest to her.

### Recurrent thrush

This is a frequently recurring infection with the yeast-like fungus *Candida albicans*. When this occurs despite the woman (and her sexual partner) having adequate conventional treatment, it is important for the woman to reduce her intake of refined sugar as this creates a favourable environment in which *Candida* thrives.

The following homeopathic remedy may be given, as well as those listed for vaginal discharge (*see above*). Select one by matching its picture with the physical symptoms.

### *Helonias* (unicorn root)

This remedy picture describes a woman who has a copious vaginal discharge causing marked irritation and itchiness of the whole of her vulva, which becomes swollen and tender. The woman herself becomes miserable and can only cope by keeping herself busy. Using the 6c potency, give one dose twice a day for up to two weeks.

If the swabs show that the discharge is due to *Candida* that hasn't responded to conventional treatment, give a homeopathic preparation of *Candida albicans*, using a potency of 6c and giving one dose twice a day for two weeks.

### *Cystitis*

It is important to have a medical practitioner do a urine test to find out if there is any bacterial cause for the symptoms of needing to urinate frequently and urgently and pain on passing urine (dysuria). If there is a bacterial basis for the infection, conventional antibiotic therapy must be considered as the first choice.

Drinking barley water helps alleviate the symptoms, and if the woman has recurrent infections, the regular drinking of cranberry juice is important.

The following homeopathic remedies can be given while waiting for the result of the urine test. Select the remedy by matching its picture with the physical symptoms. Using the 6c potency, give one dose twice a day for up to five days.

### *Cantharis* (Spanish fly)

This remedy picture describes violent irritation in the bladder causing frequent urination and pain on passing urine.

### *Sarsaparilla* (similax)

This remedy picture describes pain occurring towards the end of urination.

## *Staphysagria* (stavesacre)

This remedy picture describes pain along the urethra, the tube leading from the bladder, which is eased when the woman passes urine.

### Incontinence

A pregnant woman can become incontinent of urine whenever she coughs, sneezes or lifts anything. This annoying symptom can be helped by the following homeopathic remedies. Select one by matching its picture with the physical symptoms. Using the 6c potency, give one dose twice a day for one week, reducing the frequency to once a day.

## *Causticum* (Hahnemann's mixture of quicklime [calcium oxide] with potassium bisulphate)

This remedy picture describes a woman who, finding it difficult to start passing urine, may go into acute retention of urine. She more commonly suffers from stress incontinence of urine.

## *Natrum muriaticum* (sodium chloride)

This remedy picture describes a woman who suffers from stress incontinence of urine but also finds it difficult to pass urine in the presence of other people. She has greasy skin and probably has a crack in the middle of her lower lip. The general profile of this woman, which will help in the selection of this remedy, is that she is basically shy but is able to put on a front to give the impression of sociability. She has a craving for salty foods.

## *Pulsatilla* (wind flower)

This remedy picture describes a woman who suffers from stress incontinence of urine whenever she laughs or passes wind. The general profile of the woman, which will help in the selection of this remedy, is that she is mild and gentle and has a tendency to weep. She dislikes arguments, the heat and fatty foods.

# Abdominal symptoms

### Abdominal colic

This pain can arise from constipation (*see below*) or from diarrhoea. It is important for an accurate diagnosis to be made so that a more serious condition such as APPENDICITIS is not overlooked. The following homeopathic remedies can be used while waiting for medical assessment. Using the 6c potency, give one dose every 30 minutes.

### Colocynthis (bitter cucumber)

This remedy picture describes colicky pain that forces the woman to bend double; this firm pressure relieves the pain. She tends to be irritable and angry.

### Magnesium phosphoricum (magnesium phosphate)

This remedy picture describes colicky pains that are relieved by warmth rather than by pressure.

### Constipation

It is important for pregnant women to follow the dietary advice on p. 158, which encourages the eating of a high-fibre diet, so that they don't become constipated. If they do, natural laxatives include molasses, linseed and dried apricots.

The following homeopathic remedies can also be used. Select one by matching its picture with the physical symptoms. Using the 6c potency, give one dose daily.

### Alumina metallicum (aluminium)

This remedy picture describes a woman who has lost all expulsive power to defecate despite having the urge to do so. An unusual symptom that she may have is that potatoes disagree with her.

## Nux vomica (poison-nut)

This remedy picture describes a woman who has a frequent desire to defecate but is left feeling as if her rectum is never properly emptied. The general profile of the woman, which will help in the selection of this remedy, is that she is ambitious and has a strong desire for alcohol, coffee and cigarettes. She is sensitive to cold weather and feels more comfortable in wet weather, provided that the wind chill factor is not significant.

## Silicea (pure flint)

This remedy picture describes a stool that appears only to retreat back into the anus – the so-called " bashful stool". The general profile of the woman will help in the selection also of this remedy. She shows a lack of confidence and a general lack of "go", just letting life drift by. However, when particularly irritated, she can lose her temper.

### Cravings

Some pregnant women at this stage have a craving for certain types of food. While this is not a specific problem in itself, the woman and her family might find it one.

Each of the following homeopathic remedies has an indication for a particular source of a craving. Using the 30c potency, give one dose every time the woman has an irresistible desire for her particular craving.

- **Beer and brandy**: *Nux vomica* (poison-nut)
- **Caffeine**: *Angusturavera* (bark of *Galipea cusparia*)
- **Chocolate**: *Nux vomica* (poison-nut)
- **Cigarettes**: *Nux vomica* (poison-nut)
- **Eggs**: *Calcarea carbonica* (calcium carbonate)
- **Fat**: *Nitric acidum* (nitric acid)
- **Ice cream**: *Phosphorus*
- **Oysters**: *Lachesis* (bushmaster snake venom)
- **Raw food**: *Sulphur*
- **Refined sugar**: *Sulphur*

- **Salt**: *Natrum muriaticum* (sodium chloride) or *Phosphorus*. The general profile of the woman will help distinguish these two remedies. The *Phosphorus* woman has a particular fear of thunderstorms. The *Natrum muriaticum* woman has greasy skin and possibly a crack in the middle of her lower lip, and she can bear a grudge against people who have crossed her.
- **Smoked food**: *Causticum* (Hahnemann's mixture of quicklime [calcium oxide] with potassium bisulphate)
- **"Strange" food**: *Lyssin* (saliva from rabid dog). The woman may also do strange things.
- **Sweet food**: *Argentum nitricum* (silver nitrate) or *Cinchona officinalis (China)* (Peruvian bark) or *Lycopodium* (club moss). The remedy picture for *Argentum nitricum* describes anxiety and a fear of heights and of crowds. The remedy picture for *Cinchona officinalis (China)* describes a woman who feels exhausted from loss of body fluids, possibly sweat, or a woman who is recovering from a recurrent illness. *Lycopodium* suits a woman who has an anticipatory anxiety that, in reality, is baseless.
- **Vinegar**: *Sepia* (inky juice of cuttlefish)
- **Whisky**: *Sulphur*
- **Wine**: *Phosphorus* or *Sulphur*. The distinguishing features of the woman will help select the specific remedy. The *Phosphorus* woman has a particular fear of thunderstorms. The *Sulphur* woman has a ruddy complexion and isn't concerned with her appearance.

*Haemorrhoids (piles)*

This condition is common in all pregnant women as their babies grow in their abdomens, causing pressure to build up in the veins around their anuses.

The conventional treatment is with soothing creams that may contain steroids.

The homeopathic treatment is to ensure that the woman is not constipated and therefore straining to defecate (*see* p. 158 for advice). The following homeopathic preparations can also be taken. Select the appropriate remedy by matching its picture with the physical symptoms. Using the 6c potency, give one dose three times a day.

### *Aesculus hippocastanum* (horse chestnut)

This remedy picture describes haemorrhoids that produce sharp shooting pains that radiate up the woman's back.

### *Nux vomica* (poison-nut)

This remedy picture describes a woman with haemorrhoids who never feels that her rectum has properly emptied whenever she defecates. Her haemorrhoids may or may not bleed. The general profile of the woman is helpful when selecting this remedy. She is ambitious and finds faults in other people. She feels better when overindulging in alcohol, caffeine and cigarettes, and after a short sleep, provided she is allowed to finish it. She also feels better in damp, wet weather.

### *Paeonia* (peony)

This remedy picture describes very itchy haemorrhoids, causing a burning feeling after the woman has defecated. This remedy can also be given as an ointment, to be used as often as necessary.

### *Sulphur*

This remedy picture describes haemorrhoids that bleed and produce a burning and itchy feeling in the anus. The woman also has painless diarrhoea in the morning, which often forces her to rush out of bed. The general profile of the woman will also help in the selection of this remedy. She tends to have a ruddy complexion and is not particularly concerned about her appearance. She sweats easily. She enjoys alcohol and sweets, but milk may disagree with her. She enjoys a joke and has a definite point of view.

## Circulatory problems

*Cramps*
Cramps can be painful and cause much distress. They may be

associated with VARICOSE VEINS, in which case, the woman is advised to wear support stockings. For other causes, the following homeopathic remedies can be used. Using the 6c potency, give one dose immediately. If the cramps occur regularly, give one dose twice a day as a preventive measure.

### Arnica (leopard's bane)

This remedy picture describes a woman who develops cramps and whose legs always feel tired.

### Coffea cruda (unroasted coffee)

This remedy picture describes a woman who easily develops cramps. She is overactive and finds it difficult to get to sleep, tossing around, unable to relax.

### Cuprum metallicum (copper)

This remedy picture describes a woman who develops cramps that come in repeated spasms. This remedy can be combined with *Chamomilla* (camomile) and given at monthly intervals by injection. This preparation is useful where *Cuprum metallicum* is not working on its own.

### Nux vomica (poison-nut)

This remedy picture describes a woman who develops cramps in her calf muscles and also in the soles of her feet. Her arms tend to "go to sleep". The general profile of the woman describes someone who is ambitious and a perfectionist and indulges in alcohol, coffee and cigarettes.

### Fainting

It is important to distinguish fainting from an epileptic fit (*see* EPILEPSY). The immediate treatment for a pregnant woman who has just had a simple faint is to make sure her head is kept below her heart, ideally with her head between her knees.

Provided it is a simple faint, the following homeopathic remedies can be used to help prevent this from recurring. Select one by matching its picture with the physical symptom. Using the 6c potency, give one dose twice a day.

## Aconitum napellus (monk's-hood)

This remedy picture describes a woman who has fainted and wakes up feeling anxious and fearful of dying.

## Belladonna (deadly nightshade)

This remedy picture describes a woman who faints whenever she gets hot, either from a warm environment or from a fever.

## Cinchona officinalis (China) (Peruvian bark)

This remedy picture describes a woman who sweats heavily and, as a result of losing this body fluid, becomes exhausted and faints.

## Ignatia (St Ignatius' bean)

This remedy picture describes a woman who faints easily from any form of unhappiness, especially grief.

### Palpitations
This form of heart irregularity must be accurately diagnosed as conventional treatment might be more appropriate.

If the irregularity is not serious, the following homeopathic remedies may be used. Select one by matching its picture with the physical symptoms. Using the 6c potency, give one dose twice a day.

## Aconitum napellus (monk's-hood)

This remedy picture describes a woman who develops palpitations from an emotional shock or because of great apprehension.

### Arsenicum album (arsenic trioxide)

This remedy picture describes a woman who develops palpitations towards midnight and whenever she lies on her right side. Their recurrence is reduced by her keeping herself warm. The general profile of the woman for whom this remedy will suit is someone who is excessively neat and tidy and shows a marked sensitivity to cold environments.

### Lycopodium (club moss)

This remedy picture describes a woman who develops palpitations between 4.00 and 8.00 pm and when she lies on her left side. The woman whom this remedy will particularly suit has an anticipatory anxiety, is fearful of being left on her own and feels better by being uncovered in order to cool down.

### Natrum muriaticum (sodium chloride)

This remedy picture describes a woman who has palpitations that cause her bed to throb. Emotional support and physical comfort make her feel worse.

### Pulsatilla (wind flower)

This remedy picture describes a woman who develops palpitations from eating rich, fatty foods and also from hot environments. She gets better when she receives emotional and physical support.

### Phlebitis

This condition occurs when part of the wall of a VARICOSE VEIN (*see below*) becomes inflamed. Both conventional and homeopathic forms of treatment include the advice to wear support stockings. Homeopathic treatment also comprises the remedies given below to treat varicose veins. Using the 6c potency, give one dose three times a day for two weeks, reducing to one dose twice a day.

### Pre-eclampsia and essential hypertension

Conventional treatment is the first choice in the management of these two serious problems. Meditation, yoga and sauna sessions are helpful ways of relaxing.

Homeopathy is only to be used as a complementary form of therapy, working alongside conventional treatment, and it can only be obtained through consultation with a specialist homeopath.

### Varicose veins

These appear in some women as their pregnancies proceed, with the pressure in their abdomens increasing as their babies gain weight. Such women are advised to wear support stockings, and the following homeopathic remedies may also help. Using the 6c potency, give one dose twice a day.

### Arsenicum album (arsenic trioxide)

This remedy picture describes a woman who develops varicose veins. Her general profile will help select this remedy. She is very sensitive to the cold, house-proud and thirsty for sips rather than gulps of fluid.

### Carbo vegetabilis (vegetable charcoal)

This remedy picture describes a woman whose varicose veins have ulcerated.

### Fluoricum acidum (hydrofluoric acid)

This remedy picture describes a woman who develops varicose veins and has a sensation as if hot water is coming out of all the pores of her leg.

### Hamamelis virginica (witch hazel)

This remedy picture describes a woman who has developed varicose veins and whose leg muscles feel tired. She also has a cold sensation running down the backs of her legs and neuralgic pains going down the inside of both legs.

### *Pulsatilla* (wind flower)

This remedy picture describes a woman who develops painful varicose veins. She notices a cold sweat on her legs and her feet also produce a foul-smelling sweat. Her legs become numb whenever she stands for long periods. The general profile of the woman is that she is mild and gentle, disliking any conflict. She dislikes fatty foods and a hot environment, feeling comfortable in the fresh air.

### *Sepia* (inky juice of cuttlefish)

This remedy picture describes a woman with varicose veins who has the sensation that a mouse is running up and down her legs. The general profile of the woman will help select this remedy. She can easily become moody, seeking her own private space. She goes off the people closest to her and shuns any physical comfort.

## Skin changes

When a woman becomes pregnant, she will notice certain skin changes. The following homeopathic remedies will help resolve some of these difficulties. Using the 6c potency, give one dose daily.

### *Arsenicum album* (arsenic trioxide)

This remedy picture describes a woman whose scalp is so sensitive that she finds it difficult to comb or brush her hair.

### *Lachesis* (bushmaster snake venom)

This remedy picture describes a woman whose skin has purple blotches on it, which are more prominent when she wakes up in the morning.

### Nux vomica (poison-nut)

This remedy picture describes a woman whose skin problem is worsened by drinking alcohol and coffee.

### Sepia (inky juice of cuttlefish)

This remedy picture describes a freckly rash shaped like a butterfly, which appears over the woman's nose and spreads on to her cheeks.

### Sulphur

This remedy picture describes a woman who has dry skin that is made worse whenever she washes herself. She tends to blush easily. The general profile of the woman will help in the selection of this remedy. She is a jolly person who enjoys a joke and has a definite point of view, and is not particularly concerned about her appearance.

## Common problems in the third trimester (from 28 weeks to delivery)

## Backache

Some women find this a problem at this point in their pregnancies. The following homeopathic remedies can be used to help. Select one by matching its symptoms with the physical symptoms. Using the 30c potency, one dose should be sufficient to ease the backache. If it isn't, use the 6c potency and give one dose twice a day for up to one week.

### Kali carbonicum (potassium carbonate)

This remedy picture describes a woman who develops a pain in the small of her back, which radiates into both hips. Her symptoms tend to change with the weather, being worse when it is cold, particularly if there are cold winds.

### Natrum muriaticum (sodium chloride)

This remedy picture describes a woman who has pain in the small of her back, which is relieved by firm pressure.

### Rhus toxicodendron (poison ivy)

This remedy picture describes a woman whose backache is worse whenever she begins to move, improving on subsequent movement only to return when she becomes tired. She tends to be restless because she knows that moving will help ease her pain.

## Braxton–Hicks' contractions

These contractions are not labour pains but can cause the woman to become physically distressed. There is no conventional therapy.

The following homeopathic remedy helps alleviate these symptoms. Using the 6c potency, give one dose daily.

### Cimicifuga racemosa (black snake root)

This remedy picture describes shooting pains across the woman's abdomen.

## Emotional difficulties

The conventional treatment is either by tranquillizers, psychotherapy or antidepressant drugs.

Such difficulties are best treated homeopathically by consultation with a specialist homeopath who will be able to assess the woman as a whole. If this is not possible, the following homeopathic remedies may be used. Select one by matching its picture with the physical symptoms. Using the 30c potency, give one dose daily for one week, reducing to one dose of the 30c potency twice a week thereafter.

### *Aconitum napellus* (monk's-hood)

This remedy picture describes a woman who has a major unresolved anxiety that continues to escalate as the delivery date gets nearer. She also is afraid that she is going to die.

### *Argentum nitricum* (silver nitrate)

This remedy picture describes a woman with generalized anxiety causing her to urinate frequently. She has a desire for sweets and a fear of heights and crowds, and she dislikes hot environments.

### *Arsenicum album* (arsenic trioxide)

This remedy picture describes a woman who is exceptionally neat and tidy and has marked anxiety and restlessness. There is a deterioration of these symptoms towards midnight. She is physically cold, and enjoys sips of fluid.

### *Gelsemium* (yellow jasmine)

This remedy picture describes a woman who has a marked anticipatory anxiety, giving her butterflies in her stomach – it is as if she is going to take an examination. She prefers to be left on her own, and causes much concern because of her lack of thirst.

## Malpresentation

If the baby's head is not in the correct position within the pelvic cavity by the 36th week (when it should have "engaged" – that is, descended into the pelvis) and its bottom is the presenting feature, the woman's obstetrician may consider it necessary to turn the baby around.

When this has been done, the following homeopathic remedy can be given to help maintain the corrected position. Using the 6c potency, give one dose twice a day.

### *Pulsatilla* (wind flower)

If the baby is in a totally unstable position, using this remedy will help tone up the uterine muscles to encourage the baby's head to find the right position. Using the 6c potency, give one dose twice a day.

## Preparation for labour

At the 37th week, a pregnant woman should take the following homeopathic remedy. It makes for an easier labour by strengthening uterine muscular activity during labour and by softening the cervix (neck of the womb), which allows the baby to descend quicker. It will reduce the necessity for an episiotomy, for a forceps delivery and for a Caesarean section. Using the 30c potency, give one dose twice a week until labour starts.

### *Caulophyllum* (blue cohosh)

This remedy picture describes extreme rigidity of the cervix and weak uterine muscular activity during labour. The remedy itself is able to revive labour pains if they start to diminish. It also acts on the joints of the fingers and toes, which may be stiff and painful. This remedy classically describes the homeopathic principle of "like cures like".

## *Problems during labour and delivery*

Every woman should be encouraged to have a supply of the following homeopathic remedies immediately to hand so that she can take them when she goes into labour and into hospital. All these remedies should be in the 30c potency.

### *Arnica* (leopard's bane)

This remedy will help reduce bruising to the vulva and also reduce uterine bleeding.

### *Hypericum* (St John's wort)

This will help the healing of any vulval tissue damage, including a surgical cut from an episiotomy or from a Caesarean section.
    Single doses of these two remedies can be taken together as soon as labour begins. The *Hypericum* can be repeated twice a day if there have been any skin lacerations or cuts.

### *Staphysagria* (stavesacre)

This remedy, which can only be obtained from a specialist homeopath, is to be given as a 10m potency (a dilution of 1 in 1000) on the fourth or fifth day following delivery. It will help reduce any damage to the urethra if the woman was catheterized during labour. It will also help prevent any post-delivery "blues", particularly if labour did not follow the woman's prepared birth plan.

## Hypotonic uterine activity

Sometimes, when a woman is in established labour, her contractions disappear for no obvious reason. The conventional treatment is to give her the drug syntometrine by drip. The following homeopathic remedies can be given to encourage the labour pains to become re-established.

*Caulophyllum* (blue cohosh) is the first choice of the remedies and should be given as a single dose in the 30c potency. If, after 30 minutes, nothing has happened, single doses of the following remedies can be given, using the 30c potency: *Natrum muriaticum* (sodium chloride) and then *Pulsatilla* (wind flower).

# Backache during labour

This distressing symptom can be helped by massaging the woman's back. The following homeopathic remedy will also help:

### *Natrum muriaticum* (sodium chloride)

This remedy is particularly helpful in those cases where the baby is moving down the birth canal bottom first. Using the 30c potency, give a single dose. If, after one hour, there has been no improvement, the dose can be repeated.

# Pain relief during labour

This is usually managed with conventional pain-relieving drugs and "gas and air".

The following homeopathic remedy can be used with conventional drugs or on its own if the woman decides to use only gas and air.

### *Belladonna* (deadly nightshade)

This remedy picture describes a woman who is red-faced and moaning, and whose thoughts and behaviour may have become irrational. Her labour pains come and go frequently. Using the 30c potency, give one dose immediately, and repeat every 30–60 minutes as required.

# Afterpains

These gripping pains in the uterus can follow delivery.

The conventional treatment is with paracetamol or nonsteroidal anti-inflammatory drugs.

Homeopathic treatment involves the use of one of the following remedies. Select it by matching its picture with the physical symptoms. Using the 6c potency, give one dose every two hours as required.

### *Caulophyllum* (blue cohosh)

This is the first choice of remedies. It is particularly useful where there has been a prolonged labour.

### *Sabina* (savine)

This remedy picture describes intense afterpains that feel worse for the least movement and better when the windows of the room are wide open, allowing cool, fresh air to enter.

### *Secale* (ergot)

This remedy picture describes a woman with afterpains that are worse when she is covered with the bedclothes and are relieved when she is lying on her back, exposed.

## Emergencies

In these two extremely serious conditions, homeopathic remedies should be only given *after* calling an obstetrician for urgent help.

*Retained placenta*

### *Sabina* (savine)

This remedy can be given as a single 30c potency dose to help the normal expulsion of the placenta (afterbirth) following delivery. This would then make manual extraction of the placenta unnecessary.

*Post-partum haemorrhage*
When the amount of blood lost following delivery exceeds 300

millilitres, or when vaginal bleeding continues following the delivery of the placenta, the woman is said to be suffering post-partum haemorrhage. This is an emergency, requiring immediate medical help. The following homeopathic remedy can be given after this help has been summoned.

### Secale (ergot)

This remedy should be given as a single dose of the 30c potency. Its remedy picture describes stopping uterine blood loss. The woman feels unhappy by being covered with bedclothes because of the warmth, and so she pushes them away, preferring to lie exposed, particularly on her back.

# Breastfeeding difficulties

### Sore nipples

The conventional and homeopathic treatment is to use nipple shields and to apply creams to soften the nipples. The homeo-pathic cream is *Calendula* (marigold), applied as often as neces-sary.

The following homeopathic remedies can also be taken orally. Using the 30c potency, give two doses at hourly intervals, redu-cing to the 6c potency and giving one dose daily.

### Chamomilla (camomile)

This remedy picture describes nipples that are inflamed, making them so tender that the woman prevents her baby from suckling from them. In this situation, the mother becomes increasingly irritable.

### Nitric acidum (nitric acid)

This remedy picture describes nipples that are very cracked so that, when the baby suckles from them, the mother feels a severe pricking sensation as if splinters are piercing her nipples.

*Excessive milk production*
The following homeopathic remedies can be given to those mothers who produce too much breast milk.

### *Calcarea carbonica* (calcium carbonate)

This remedy picture describes a woman who tends to be obese and shows marked perspiration on her face and scalp. Her breasts are swollen, and although there is a free flow of milk, her baby cries and refuses to suckle. As a result, the mother commonly has tears silently trickling down her face. Using the 30c potency, give one dose only.

### *Lac caninum* (dog's milk)

This is a powerful remedy and may cause the milk to dry up completely. For this reason, only a single dose of the 6c potency should be given.

*Loss of breast milk*
The woman should be encouraged to drink plenty of fluid and reduce the amount of exercise she does. The following homeopathic remedies can be used. Select one by matching its picture to the physical symptoms. Using the 6c potency, give one dose twice a day, for a maximum of 12 doses.

### *Agnus castus* (chaste tree)

This is the first choice of treatment. In this remedy picture, the mother is particularly sad.

### *Lac defloratum* (skimmed milk)

This remedy picture describes a generalized loss of milk, with the woman's breasts decreasing in size. She may also be experiencing throbbing headaches, which are associated with a profuse flow of urine.

## *Pulsatilla* (wind flower)

This remedy picture describes a woman who is tearful and feels worse in a hot, stuffy room. She prefers the fresh air and her bedroom window open.

### *Mastitis*

This is caused by a blockage in a milk duct. It is treated conventionally with antibiotics. General advice is for the woman to wear a well-fitting maternity bra at all times and to offer the affected breast initially to the baby when breastfeeding. The following remedies can be used. Select one by matching its picture with the physical symptoms. Using the 6c potency, give one dose twice a day, for a maximum of 12 doses.

## *Belladonna* (deadly nightshade)

This remedy picture describes a woman who has engorgement of her breasts with an over-production of breastmilk. Her breasts are inflamed and tender, and the woman herself is flushed and may become feverish.

## *Bryonia* (wild hops)

This remedy picture describes breast pain that is made worse by the slightest movement and is eased by rest. This remedy follows on well from *Belladonna* in helping to resolve any residual mastitis.

## *Hepar sulphuris* (Hahnemann's calcium sulphide)

This remedy picture describes a breast that has a single area of mastitis. The woman is unduly irritable and thirsty, craving sour fluids, especially vinegar. She also tends to sweat profusely, and the sweat has a particularly offensive smell.

### *Phytolacca* (poke root)

This remedy picture describes a breast that is hard and lumpy. The woman has tender glands in the armpit closest to the affected breast. Pressure on the nipple causes pain to be referred over the woman's entire body.

### *Silicea* (pure flint)

This remedy picture describes a breast that has developed mastitis, and where the nipple has also become cracked. The woman feels totally exhausted. This remedy follows on well from *Hepar sulphuris* in resolving any residual mastitis.

# Problems of the Elderly

This section describes homeopathic remedies that can be helpful in treating certain conditions that are particularly common among people over the age of 65.

## Alzheimer's disease and other forms of dementia

There are a number of forms of dementia, some of which occur because of brain cell degeneration due to ATHEROSCLEROSIS of the blood vessels to the brain. It comes on slowly, with the person simply just becoming forgetful.

In Alzheimer's disease, there is such a loss of brain cells that the unfortunate sufferers become totally disoriented in time and space – that is, they don't know where they are or what the time of day is. They are unable to recognize close members of their family. They dress inappropriately, wander around, putting themselves in possible danger, and they may become incontinent of urine and faeces. Because of all of these symptoms and because they tend to wander, they need specialized nursing and residential care. Although this is uncommon, the disease can affect people below the age of 65.

These conditions are diagnosed and distinguished by a specialized brain scan. The conventional drug therapy is with sedation and antidepressants as required.

The early stages can be treated by giving the brain exercises to do such as crossword and jigsaw puzzles and by encouraging sufferers to read a daily newspaper. It is helpful for the time, date and day to be prominently displayed. A balanced diet containing enough protein, non-refined carbohydrates and fats is also important. Multi-mineral and multi-vitamin tablets should be taken every day. A daily capsule of ginkgo should also be included in this regime as it has been shown to improve brain function.

The following homeopathic remedies will also be helpful. Select one by matching its picture with the physical symptoms. Using the 6c potency, give one dose daily.

### *Anacardium* (marking nut)

This remedy picture describes people with impaired memory, where chunks of recent memory just disappear. They can also develop hallucinations as if their minds are possessed by another. They feel anxious when walking, believing that they are being followed. They have a lack of confidence that makes them anxious and sad. They can occasionally become physically violent and verbally abusive, using foul language.

### *Baryta carbonicum* (barium carbonate)

This remedy picture describes people whose memories have deteriorated. They have lost confidence in themselves, feeling shy of meeting strangers. They become very upset over the least thing.

### *Belladonna* (deadly nightshade)

This remedy picture describes people with deteriorating memories, who lives in a world of their own. They tend to laugh, dance, sing and whistle. They have a peculiar symptom: they commonly sit and break pens. They have a desire to escape or hide themselves. They are excitable and weep easily and are quarrelsome.

### *Lycopodium* (club moss)

This remedy picture describes people who become confused over daily affairs, are sad and are afraid to be on their own. Men are afraid of their own shadows. They are suspicious, find faults in everything and generally find everyone distasteful.

### *Nux moschata* (nutmeg)

This remedy picture describes people who have confused minds with impaired memory. They are very changeable, alternating between crying and laughing. They feel as if they are in a dream, and sometimes think that their bodies have two sets of hands.

### *Phosphorus*

This remedy picture describes people whose brains feel tired, and who have a cold feeling at the back of their heads. Their memories are grossly impaired.

# Bladder difficulties causing urine incontinence

With ageing, the muscular sphincter control of the rectum and, particularly, the bladder can become unreliable, causing incontinence.

In both men and women, urinary infection must be excluded initially as the cause of urine incontinence. The typical symptoms of CYSTITIS (frequency and urgency) are not always present in the older person.

In men, the usual cause of urine incontinence, finally leading to retention of urine, is an ENLARGED PROSTATE.

Paralysis of the bladder muscles occurs in older women more often than in men. This makes satisfactory emptying of the bladder impossible. The volume of urine is profuse but only emerges drip by drip, leading to incontinence. The conventional treatment in this case is to use incontinence appliances. However, there are homeopathic remedies that can work in a complementary way in this situation. Select one by matching its picture with the physical symptoms. Using the 6c potency, give one dose twice a day.

### *Baryta carbonicum* (barium carbonate)

This remedy picture describes older people who are beginning to show symptoms of DEMENTIA. They have an urgent desire to urinate as their bladders, which are shrinking in size, are unable to retain much urine. Incontinence of urine is a common occurrence.

### *Causticum* (Hahnemann's mixture of quicklime [calcium oxide] mixed with potassium bisulphate)

This remedy picture describes incontinence of urine when the bladder becomes overstretched when the person forgets to urinate regularly. It also becomes temporarily paralysed, leading to overflow incontinence or acute retention of urine. The picture also describes stress incontinence where the person is incontinent of urine whenever he or she laughs, coughs or sneezes.

### *Plumbum metallicum* (lead)

This remedy picture describes people who produce a lot of urine but can only pass it in very small quantities. They often find that they are incontinent of urine.

## Constipation

With decreasing physical activity, the bowels of older people can become sluggish. It is important to maintain a diet that contains a high level of fibre (roughage). **When elderly people become so constipated that there is no or little regular bowel action, it is important for a medical assessment to be carried out to exclude cancer of the bowel.** Once this possibility has been eliminated, dietary advice is essential to encourage the bowel to develop a regular and convenient pattern of defecation. If the rectum becomes impacted with faeces and the capacity of the bladder is reduced because of this build-up of faeces, the person may become incontinent of urine (*see* BLADDER DIFFICULTIES *above*) as well as having overflow faecal incontinence. Massage with essential oils (aromatherapy) has been shown to help relieve constipation.

The conventional treatment for constipation is to use laxatives, suppositories or enemas.

Homeopathic remedies and natural laxatives are given in the general section on CONSTIPATION (p. 158).

# Depression

This is a problem of older people that is often misdiagnosed (for dementia; *see above*) or simply unrecognized. At this stage of life, people have to cope with so many changes – including the deaths of close friends – that the brave face that they may put on will hide depression.

Conventionally this can be treated with antidepressant tablets.

Homeopathic treatment for depression is discussed in the section on p. 369.

# Giddiness

This dizziness can lead to accidental falls resulting in minor injuries and more serious ones involving fractured bones. The commonest sites for fractures are the neck of the femur (thigh bone), commonly called a "broken hip", and the forearm (known as a "Colles fracture").

Homeopathic remedies applicable for fractures are given in the appropriate section on p. 314.

The underlying cause of the giddiness must be properly evaluated by a medical practitioner. The possibilities include ANAEMIA, ATHEROSCLEROSIS, HIGH BLOOD PRESSURE and OSTEOARTHRITIS of the neck (cervical) bones. The conventional treatment is determined by the diagnosis revealed by this examination.

There are several homeopathic remedies that can work in a complementary way with whatever conventional therapy is suggested. Select one by matching its picture with the physical symptoms. Using the 6c potency, give one dose twice a day. If, after two weeks of this treatment, there is no improvement, it is advisable to consult a specialist homeopath.

### Belladonna (deadly nightshade)

This remedy picture describes giddiness when the person stoops and then rises up.

### Bryonia (wild hops)

This remedy picture describes dizzy turns or fainting whenever elderly people stand up. It is as if all the objects in the room are whirling around them. The symptom can also occur when they are in bed, when it feels as though they are sinking deeper into it; this bedtime symptom is improved by the cold. They actually feel the giddiness at the backs of their heads, and it can leave them with a bursting headache.

### Nux vomica (poison-nut)

This remedy picture describes giddiness during which sufferers notice objects turning in circles around them, resulting in a temporary loss of consciousness. This happens particularly when they have not been eating properly. They can also feel dizzy and faint in crowded places or where there are many bright lights.

### Phosphorus

This remedy picture describes people who feel dizzy on waking up but become better when they have defecated.

### Pulsatilla (wind flower)

This remedy picture describes people who have dizzy turns but feel better in the fresh, open air.

# Skin problems

With increasing age, the skin loses its elasticity and becomes fragile, dry and itchy. The homeopathic and conventional advice is to use a moisturizing cream (such as aqueous cream) on a regular basis. Supplements of evening primrose oil and vitamin C – at least 1 gram daily of each – will also help to maintain the health of the skin.

The following homeopathic remedies can be used specifically to improve elderly skin. Select one by matching its picture with the physical symptoms. Using the 6c potency, give one dose daily.

### *Kali arsenicum* (Fowler's solution)

This remedy picture describes a dry, wilted skin that has a tendency to scale. It itches, and this itchiness is made worse whenever the person undresses.

### *Oleander* (rose laurel)

This remedy picture describes dry, itchy skin that is also made worse by the friction caused by undressing. The person may find temporary relief from scratching, but this causes the skin to bleed.

# Readjustment difficulties

With ageing and retirement from employment, many problems emerge, both physical and mental. For a married couple, retirement makes both partners readjust their daily lives – a well-worn rut suddenly has to be changed. This can lead to resentment on both sides. Careful pre-retirement counselling can help avoid this, and the following homeopathic remedy can also be beneficial.

### *Staphysagria* (stavesacre)

This remedy picture describes people who rage and fume silently, until their pent-up emotions and suppressed feelings finally erupt. They are unable to work or concentrate and are apathetic during the day and sleepless at night. The keynote of this remedy is indignation. Use the 30c potency as a single dose whenever tensions begin to rise on either side.

# Stroke

When ATHEROSCLEROSIS blocks some of the vital capillaries carrying blood (and oxygen) to the brain, that part of the brain becomes starved of oxygen and therefore dies. This leads to a loss of function in the part of the body that was once activated by the affected part of the brain. This is commonly called a "stroke", and one in three attacks are fatal. However, some strokes – known as transient ischaemic attacks (TIAs) – cause only temporary damage, and the person begins to recover within one or two days. However, these TIAs should be seen as warnings of a more serious stroke.

The conventional treatment for TIAs is rest and evaluation of possible causes, such as stress, HIGH BLOOD PRESSURE, obesity and cigarette smoking. It is vital for any sufferer of a stroke or TIA to readjust their life styles appropriately to eliminate these risk factors. In addition, a daily dose of aspirin has been shown to reduce significantly the likelihood of a major stroke.

The immediate homeopathic treatment for TIAs follows the same strategy. In addition, if the person is very anxious and fearful of dying, *Aconitum napellus* (monk's-hood) is indicated. Using the 6c potency, give one dose every 15 minutes, for a maximum of ten doses until medical help arrives.

If the stroke is permanent, immediate nursing care is required, then an evaluation of possible causes and physiotherapy to encourage rehabilitation.

The immediate homeopathic treatment is the same as for the

TIA except that a follow-up consultation with a specialist homeopath is necessary to obtain a constitutional remedy that will aid recovery. If this is not possible, the following specific remedies can be given. Using the 6c potency, give one dose twice a day for one month, reducing to one dose a day for up to three months.

### *Causticum* (Hahnemann's mixture of quicklime [calcium oxide] with potassium bisulphate)

This remedy picture describes two types of paralysis. One is a local paralysis of a single muscle group (such as is found in BELL'S PALSY, where one side of the face becomes paralysed). The other is a more generalized paralysis; this follows a restless night due to tearing pains in the joints, causing the person to feel a progressive weakness in their muscles and finally paralysis.

### *Cocculus* (Indian cockle)

This remedy picture describes people who become paralysed down one half of their body during sleep. Previously they may have suffered from motion sickness.

### *Conium* (poison hemlock)

This remedy picture describes progressive paralysis of one side of the body, starting from the feet and spreading upwards.

### *Gelsemium* (yellow jasmine)

This remedy picture describes generalized weakness in a person who has a sluggish circulation and suffers from attacks of GIDDINESS, trembling legs and ultimately paralysis.

### *Nux vomica* (poison-nut)

This remedy picture describes a person who suffers a stroke after overexertion or becoming soaked through. This picture also describes a stroke that comes on after a heavy meal or over-indulgence with alcohol.

If there is no improvement in the person who has suffeerd the stroke after three weeks, the following can be given:

### *Arnica* (leopard's bane)

This remedy picture describes general weakness with an inability to think clearly. Using the 6c potency, give one dose three times a day for one month.

Following on from the *Arnica*, the following homeopathic remedies can be used. Select one by matching its picture with the physical symptoms. Using the 6c potency, give one dose twice a day.

### *Opium* (dried latex of poppy)

This remedy picture describes a painless paralysis that leaves sufferers feeling that their limbs are severed and belong to someone else.

### *Plumbum metallicum* (lead)

This remedy picture describes a person who has suffered a stroke and is left with pain in the limb that has become paralysed.

### *Rhus toxicodendron* (poison ivy)

This remedy picture describes individuals who have suffered strokes that are usually right-sided. They have been left with the sensation that the affected part of their bodies has gone to sleep. The stroke in this picture usually occurs in cold, damp weather, after a bout of physical exertion or an attack of influenza.

# Further Reading

Berkow, R. *et al.*, *The Merck Manual of General Medicine.*

Boericke, W., *Materia Medica with Repertory*, Boericke & Tafel, Philadelphia, 1927.

Boyd, H., *Introduction to Homoeopathic Medicine*, Beaconsfield, 1981.

Cooper, P. J., *Bulimia Nervosa and Binge-Eating*, Robinson Publishing, 1993.

Corrigan, D., *Ancient Medicine*, Amberwood Publishing, 1993 (ginkgo).

Gemmell, D., *Everyday Homoeopathy*, Beaconsfield, 1987.

Graham, J., *Multiple Sclerosis*, Thorsons Publishers, 1981.

Kent, J. T., *Repertory of the Homoeopathic Materia Medica*, Homoeopathic Book Services, 1986.

Lessell, C. B., *The Dental Prescriber*, British Homoeopathic Association.

Lockie, A. H., *The Family Guide to Homeopathy*, Elm Tree Books, London, 1989.

Phatak, S. R., *A Concise Repertory of Homoeopathic Medicines*, New Delhi, 1963.

Phatak, S. R., *Phatak's Materia Medica of Homoeopathic Medicines*, Foxlee-Vaughan Publishers, 1988.

Scott, G. and Barton, S., *Sexually Transmitted Diseases*, A/M Publishing, 1996.

Tyler, M. L., *Pointers to the Common Remedies*, British Homoeopathic Association.

Webb, P. J., *Homoeopathy for Midwives and for Pregnant Women*, British Homoeopathic Association, 1992.

# Useful contacts

## Homeopathic Associations

The following organizations will be able to provide information on homeopthy. Most if not all of them will also be able to refer you to a properly qualified homeopathic physician in your area.

### United Kingdom

**The British Homoeopathic Association**
27a Devonshire Street
London W1N 1RJ

Tel: (1071) 935 2163

**The Society of Homoeopaths**
2 Artizan Road
Northampton
NN1 4HU

Tel: (01604) 214000
Fax: (01604) 22622

**The Faculty of Homoeopathy**
The Royal London Homoeopathic
Hospital
Great Ormond Street
London WC1N 3HR

Tel: (0171) 837 3091 Ext.7285

**The Homoeopathic Trust**
2 Powis Place
London WC1N 3HT

Tel: (0171) 837 9469
fax: (0171) 278 7900

**Northern Ireland Homoeopathic Society**
1 Cranmore Park
Belfast
BT10 6JF

### Australia

**Australian Homeopathic Association Inc.**
PO Box 806
Spit Junction
NSW 2088
Australia

**Society of Classical Homeopathy**
2nd Floor, Paxton House
90 Pitt Street
Sydney 2000
Australia

### Canada

**SPHQ (Syndicat Professionel des Homéopathes du Québec)**
1600 De Lorimier
Local 295
Montréal, Qc.
Canada H2K 3W5

Tel: (514) 525 2037
Fax: (514) 525 1299

Vancouver Centre for
Homeopathy
2246 Spruce Street
Vancouver, BC
Canada V6H 2P3

### Ireland

Homeopathic Association
92 Connolly Street
Nenagh
Co. Tipperary
Republic of Ireland

### New Zealand

The NZ Homoeopathic Society
Inc.
PO Box 67-095
Mt. Eden
Auckland
New Zealand

### South Africa

Technikon Witwatersrand
Box 17011
Doornfontein
Johannesburg 2028
South Africa

Tel: (011) 406 2911
Fax: (011) 402 0475

### United States

The National Center for
Homeopathy
801 North Fairfax Street, Suite 306
Alexandria VA 22314, USA

Tel: (703) 548 7790
Email: nchinfo@igc.apc.org

American Institute of
Homeopathy
925 East 17th Avenue
Denver, CO 80218, USA

Tel: (303) 321 4105

# Homeopathic Pharmacies in Britain

The following pharmacies aim to give a 24-hour delivery service from the
time that an order has been placed.

Ainsworths Homoeopathic
Pharmacy
36 New Cavendish Street
London W1M 7LH

Tel: (0171) 935 5330
Fax: (0171) 486 4313

Freeman's
20 Main Street
Busby
Glasgow G76 8DU

Tel: (0141) 644 1165
Fax: (0141) 644 5735

Galen Homoeopathics
Lewell-Mill
West Stafford
Dorchester DT2 8AN

Tel: (01305) 265 759 (orders only) or
263 996
Fax: (01305) 250 792

Goulds Homoeopathic Pharmacy
14 Crowndale Road
London NW1 1TT

Tel: (0171) 388 4752 or 387 1888

**Helios Homoeopathic Pharmacy**
97 Camden Road
Tunbridge Wells
Kent TN1 2QR

Tel: (01892) 536393 or 537254
Fax: (01892) 546850

**Nelson's Pharmacies**
73 Duke Street
Grosvenor Square
London W1M 6BY

Tel: (0171) 629 3118

**Weleda (UK) Ltd**
Heanor Road
Ilkeston
Derbyshire DE7 8DR

Freephone: (0800) 626 107
Freefax: (0800) 132 069

The following company is not a pharmacy, but sells antioxidant therapy as well as individual vitamin supplements:

**Lamberts Healthcare Ltd**
1 Lamberts Road
Tunbridge Wells
Kent TN2 3EQ

Tel: (01892) 552 121
Fax: (01892) 515 863

# Internet

A great deal of information is available on the World Wide Web, although sites and their contents change all the time. At the time of writing, the following sites provide useful lists of resources and are good jumping-off points for further connections.

**Homeopathy Home Page**
http://www.dungeon.com/~cam/homeo.html
Homeopathic associations, pharmacies, hospitals, colleges, training courses and much more in many countries around the world. An invaluable source of detailed information.

**Homeopathy Internet Resources List**
http://www.antenna.nl/homeoweb/index.html
Homeopathic resources, conferences, journals and so on.

**National Center for Homeopathy (USA)**
http://www.healthy.net/pan/pa/homeopathic/natcenhom/index.html
The principal homeopathic association in the United States.

Also worth checking is the newsgroup misc.health.alternatives. There is a homeopathy mailing list: information from homeopathy-request@lyghtforce.com.

# Index

# INDEX